Youth Mental Health

A Paradigm for Prevention and Early Intervention

Strüngmann Forum Reports

Julia R. Lupp, series editor

The Ernst Strüngmann Forum is made possible through the generous support of the Ernst Strüngmann Foundation, inaugurated by Dr. Andreas and Dr. Thomas Strüngmann.

This Forum was supported by the
Deutsche Forschungsgemeinschaft

Youth Mental Health

A Paradigm for Prevention and Early Intervention

Edited by

Peter J. Uhlhaas and Stephen J. Wood

The MIT Press

Cambridge, Massachusetts
London, England

Series Editor: J. R. Lupp
Editorial Assistance: A. Ducey-Gessner, M. Turner, C. Stephen
Photographs: N. Miguletz
Lektorat: BerlinScienceWorks

The book was set in TimesNewRoman and Arial.
Printed and bound in the United States of America.

Library of Congress Cataloging-in-Publication Data

Names: Uhlhaas, Peter J., editor. | Wood, Stephen J., editor.
Title: Youth mental health : a paradigm for prevention and early intervention / edited by Peter J. Uhlhaas and Stephen J. Wood.
Other titles: Strüngmann forum reports.
Description: Cambridge, Massachusetts : The MIT Press, [2020] | Series: Strüngmann forum reports | Includes bibliographical references and index.
Identifiers: LCCN 2019034693 | ISBN 9780262043977 (hardcover)
Subjects: MESH: Mental Disorders--therapy | Mental Disorders--diagnosis | Adolescent Health | Congress
Classification: LCC RJ503 | NLM WS 463 | DDC 616.8900835--dc23
LC record available at https://lccn.loc.gov/2019034693

10 9 8 7 6 5 4 3 2 1

Contents

Preface

Science is a highly specialized enterprise—one that enables areas of enquiry to be minutely pursued, establishes working paradigms and normative standards, and supports rigor in experimental research. Yet all too often, "problems" encountered in research fall outside the scope of a single discipline, thus requiring external input to expand conceptualization, increase understanding, and envisage future trajectories for research to pursue.

The Ernst Strüngmann Forum was established in 2006 to address these types of topics. Founded on the tenets of scientific independence and the inquisitive nature of the human mind, it provides a platform for experts to discuss "problems" that require input from multiple areas of expertise. The resulting transdisciplinary discourse (or Forum) is best imagined as an intellectual retreat: Disciplinary idiosyncrasies are put aside and existing perspectives questioned. Consensus is not the goal. Instead, gaps in knowledge are exposed, questions are formulated, and ways are collectively sought to move research forward. The results from the entire process are disseminated to the scientific community to promote further consideration and implementation.

Impetus for this topic came from Peter Uhlhaas and Stephen Wood, who formulated the original proposal. Joining them on the on the program advisory committee were Andrew Chanen, Matcheri Keshavan, and Andreas Meyer-Lindenberg. From July 29 to August 3, 2018, participants gathered in Frankfurt for this 28th Forum to explore the nature of emergent psychopathology underlying causal factors and mechanisms and to develop a framework for prevention and early intervention in youth mental health.

This volume synthesizes the resulting discourse and is comprised of two types of contributions. Background papers, written before the Forum, address key aspects of the overall theme. These chapters have been peer reviewed and subsequently revised. In addition, Chapters 3, 6, 9, and 13 provide an overview of the working groups and expose diverging opinions as well as areas where future attention is needed.

An endeavor of this kind creates its own unique group dynamics and puts demands on everyone who participates. Each invitee played an active role and for their efforts, I am grateful to all. A special word of thanks goes to the program advisory committee, to the authors and reviewers of the background papers, as well as to the moderators of the individual working groups (Alyson Yung, Stephen Wood, Matcheri Keshavan, and Andrew Chanen). Importantly, the rapporteurs of the working groups (Jai Shah, Urvakhsh Meherwan Mehta, Christopher Davey, and John Torous) deserve special recognition, for to draft a report during the Forum and finalize it in the months thereafter is no simple matter. Finally, I extend my appreciation to Peter Uhlhaas and Stephen Wood, whose commitment was essential to this 28th Ernst Strüngmann Forum.

The Ernst Strüngmann Forum is reliant on institutional stability. The generous support of the Ernst Strüngmann Foundation, established by Dr. Andreas and Dr. Thomas Strüngmann in honor of their father, enables the Ernst Strüngmann Forum to pursue its work in the service of science. In addition, the following valuable partnerships are gratefully acknowledged: the Scientific Advisory Board, which ensures the scientific independence of the Forum; the Deutsche Forschungsgemeinschaft, for its supplemental financial support; and the Frankfurt Institute for Advanced Studies, which shares its intellectual setting with the Forum.

Long-held views are never easy to put aside. Yet, when the limits to our knowledge begin to appear and the resulting gaps are identified, the act of formulating strategies to move past this point becomes a most invigorating activity. On behalf of everyone involved, I hope this volume will spur further action to address the myriad issues being faced in youth mental health.

Julia R. Lupp, Director
Ernst Strüngmann Forum
Frankfurt Institute for Advanced Studies (FIAS)
Ruth-Moufang-Str. 1, 60438 Frankfurt am Main, Germany
https://esforum.de/

List of Contributors

Allen, Nicholas B. Department of Psychology, University of Oregon, Eugene, OR 97403-1227, U.S.A.

Alvarez-Jimenez, Mario Orygen and Centre for Youth Mental Health, The University of Melbourne, Parkville VIC 3052, Australia

Amminger, G. Paul Orygen and Centre for Youth Mental Health, The University of Melbourne, Parkville VIC 3052, Australia

Avenevoli, Shelli National Institute of Mental Health, Bethesda, MD 20892, U.S.A.

Behrendt, Hannah F. Child Neuropsychology Section, Department of Child and Adolescent Psychiatry, RWTH, 52056 Aachen, Germany; JARA-Brain Institute II, Molecular Neuroscience and Neuroimaging, Research Center Jülich, 52428 Jülich, Germany

Bella-Awusah, Tolulope Department of Psychiatry, College of Medicine, University of Ibadan, Ibadan, Nigeria

Berger, Maximus Orygen and Centre for Youth Mental Health, The University of Melbourne, Parkville VIC 3052, Australia

Bitanihirwe, Byron K. Y. Centre for Global Health, Trinity College, D02 K104 Dublin, Ireland

Blasco, Drew College of Global Public Health, New York University, New York, NY 10012, U.S.A.

Cahill, John D. Department of Psychiatry, Yale University, New Haven, CT 06519, U.S.A.; Program for Specialized Treatment Early in Psychosis (STEP), New Haven, CT 06519, U.S.A.

Carpenter, Joanne S. Clinical Research Unit, Brain and Mind Research Institute, University of Sydney, Camperdown NSW 2050, Australia

Chanen, Andrew M. Orygen and Centre for Youth Mental Health, The University of Melbourne, Parkville VIC 3052, Australia

Chen, Eric Y. H. Department of Psychiatry, University of Hong Kong, Hong Kong SAR, China

Colombo, Shane D. Columbia University, New York, NY 10027, U.S.A.

Correll, Christoph U. Charité–Universitätsmedizin Berlin, Klinik für Psychiatrie, Psychosomatik und Psychotherapie des Kindes- und Jugendalters, 13353 Berlin, Germany; Departments of Psychiatry and Molecular Medicine, Donald and Barbara Zucker School of Medicine at Hofstra/Northwell, Hempstead, NY 11549, U.S.A.

Davey, Christopher G. Orygen and Centre for Youth Mental Health, The University of Melbourne, Parkville VIC 3052, Australia

Do, Kim Q. Centre for Psychiatric Neuroscience, Department of Psychiatry, Lausanne University Hospital, 1008 Prilly-Lausanne, Switzerland

Fair, Damien A. School of Medicine, Oregon Health and Science University, Portland, OR 97239-3098, U.S.A.

Fisher, Helen L. Social, Genetic and Developmental Psychiatry Centre, Institute of Psychiatry, Psychology and Neuroscience, King's College London, London SE5 8AF, U.K.

Frangou, Sophia Department of Psychiatry, Icahn School of Medicine at Mount Sinai, New York 10029, U.S.A

Gleeson, John School of Behavioural and Health Sciences, Faculty of Health Sciences, Australian Catholic University, Melbourne Campus, Fitzroy VIC 3065, Australia

Heinssen, Robert K. NIMH Division of Services and Intervention Research, National Institute of Mental Health, Bethesda MD, 20892, U.S.A.

Hickie, Ian B. Brain and Mind Centre, University of Sydney, Camperdown NSW 2050, Australia

Iorfino, Frank Brain and Mind Centre, University of Sydney, Camperdown NSW 2050, Australia

Keshavan, Matcheri S. Department of Psychiatry, Beth Israel Deaconess Medical Center and Harvard Medical School, Boston, MA 02115, U.S.A.

Konrad, Kerstin Child Neuropsychology Section, Department of Child and Adolescent Psychiatry, RWTH, 52056 Aachen, Germany; JARA-Brain Institute II, Molecular Neuroscience and Neuroimaging, Research Center Jülich, 52428 Jülich, Germany

Le, PhuongThao D. Johns Hopkins Bloomberg School of Public Health, Baltimore, MD 21205, U.S.A.

Lee, Francis Department of Psychiatry, Weill Cornell Medical College, Cornell University, New York, NY 10065, U.S.A.

Leve, Leslie D. Oregon Social Learning Center, Eugene, OR 97401, U.S.A.

Lieff, Sarah A. New York University, New York, NY 10003, U.S.A.

Liu, Cindy H. Pediatric Newborn Medicine and Psychiatry, Brigham and Women's Hospital, Boston, MA 02446, U.S.A.

Luna, Beatriz Department of Psychiatry, University of Pittsburgh, Pittsburgh, PA 15213, U.S.A.

McGorry, Patrick D. Orygen and Centre for Youth Mental Health, The University of Melbourne, Parkville VIC 3052, Australia

Mehta, Urvakhsh Meherwan Department of Psychiatry, National Institute of Mental Health and Neurosciences, Bangalore 560029, India

Meyer-Lindenberg, Andreas Department of Psychiatry and Psychotherapy, Central Institute of Mental Health, 68159 Mannheim, Germany

Nallur, Shreya V. General practitioner, Davanagere, Karnataka, India

Niell, Cristopher Institute of Neuroscience, University of Oregon, Eugene, OR 97403-1254, U.S.A

Nordentoft, Merete CORE–Copenhagen Research Center for Mental Health, Mental Health Center Copenhagen, University of Copenhagen, Faculty of Health and Medical Sciences, Department of Clinical Medicine, DK-2900 Hellerup, Denmark

Öngür, Dost McLean Hospital/Harvard Medical School, Belmont, MA 02478, U.S.A.

Patton, George C. Centre for Adolescent Health, Murdoch Children's Research Institute, University of Melbourne, Flemington Road, Parkville VIC 3052, Australia

Paus, Tomáš Bloorview Research Institute, Holland Bloorview Kids Rehabilitation Hospital; Departments of Psychology and Psychiatry, University of Toronto, Toronto, ON M4G 1R8, Canada

Reininghaus, Ulrich Department of Public Mental Health, Central Institute of Mental Health, Medical Faculty Mannheim, Heidelberg University, 68159 Mannheim, Germany; Centre for Epidemiology and Public Health, Health Service and Population Research Department, Institute of Psychiatry, Psychology and Neuroscience, King's College London, London SE5 8AF, U.K.; ESRC Centre for Society and Mental Health, King's College London, London WC2R 2LS, U.K.

Ruiz, Bernalyn Global Institute of Public health, New York University, New York, NY 10012, U.S.A.

Sabb, Fred Research and Innovation, University of Oregon, Eugene, OR 97403-1227, U.S.A.

Sawa, Akira The Johns Hopkins Schizophrenia Center, Johns Hopkins University, Baltimore, MD 21287, U.S.A.

Schoenbaum, Michael Division of Services and Intervention Research, National Institute of Mental Health, Bethesda, MD 20892, U.S.A.

Scott, Elizabeth M. Clinical Research Unit, Brain and Mind Research Institute, University of Sydney, Camperdown NSW 2050, Australia

Schumann, Gunter Centre for Population Neuroscience and Stratified Medicine, King's College London, London SE5 8AF, U.K.

Shah, Jai Department of Psychiatry, McGill University, Montreal QC H4H 1R3, Canada

Srihari, Vinod H. Department of Psychiatry, Yale University, New Haven, CT 06519, U.S.A.; Program for Specialized Treatment Early in Psychosis (STEP), New Haven, CT 06519, U.S.A.

Susser, Ezra Departments of Epidemiology and Psychiatry, Columbia University, New York, NY 10032, U.S.A; New York State Psychiatric Institute, New York, NY 10032, U.S.A.

Torous, John Division of Digital Psychiatry and Department of Psychiatry, Beth Israel Deaconess Medical Center, Harvard Medical School, Boston, MA 02115, U.S.A.

Uhlhaas, Peter J. Institute of Neuroscience and Psychology, University of Glasgow, Glasgow G12 8QB, U.K.; Charité Universitätsmedizin, Department of Child and Adolescent Psychiatry, 13353 Berlin, Germany

Verma, Swapna K. Department of Psychosis, Institute of Mental Health, 539747 Singapore

Woo, T. Wilson Department of Psychiatry, Beth Israel Deaconess Medical Center, Boston, MA 02215, U.S.A.; Laboratory for Cellular Neuropathology, McLean Hospital, Belmont, MA 02478, U.S.A.; Department of Psychiatry, Harvard Medical School, Boston, MA 02215, U.S.A.

Wood, Stephen J. Orygen and Centre for Youth Mental Health, The University of Melbourne, Parkville VIC 3052, Australia

Yang, Lawrence H. Department of Social and Behavioral Sciences, New York University, New York, NY 10003, U.S.A.

Yung, Alison R. Centre for Youth Mental Health, University of Melbourne, Parkville 3052 VIC, Australia; Department of Psychology and Mental Health, School of Health Sciences, Faculty of Biology, Medicine and Health, University of Manchester, Manchester M13 9PL, U.K.

1

Youth Mental Health

Toward a New Paradigm

Peter J. Uhlhaas and Stephen J. Wood

Abstract

Progress in science is frequently achieved when challenges are made to the dominant mode of thinking and novel paradigms begin to emerge, providing new frameworks to organize data and conduct empirical inquiry. To examine current thinking in the areas of youth mental health, this 28th Ernst Strüngmann Forum was convened to scrutinize early intervention and treatment for emerging mental disorders during youth. The multifaceted contributions in this volume argue that current approaches to research and intervention need to shift away from adulthood and focus on the predominant onset period for mental ill-health: youth, the period between 15–24 years of age. Wide-ranging implications emerged for diagnosis, treatment, and research. This chapter provides background to the topics addressed at this 28th Ernst Strüngmann Forum and highlights future prospects for a youth mental health paradigm.

The Challenge of Mental Health

Mental health disorders constitute a major challenge to both society and science. Syndromes such as schizophrenia, depression, anxiety, and personality disorders comprise some of the largest disease burdens worldwide, yet funding for research and treatment of these conditions is disproportionately small compared to other medical conditions (e.g., cancer, AIDS/HIV) (Woelbert et al. 2019). Moreover, the continued stigmatization of mentally ill individuals contributes to poor outcomes and barriers to help-seeking.

Currently, it is estimated that 1.1 billion people are affected worldwide by mental or substance use disorders. Moreover, in both high- and middle-income countries, significant gaps in treatment exist. For example, only one in five people from high-income countries and only one in 27 people from low- and middle-income countries receive minimally adequate treatment for depression (Global Mental Health Group 2007). For the vast majority of these people, limited availability of existing treatments is exacerbated by a lack of efficacy for some of the most disabling features of major syndromes, such as impairments in cognitive and functional domains. Despite the promises of genetics and translational neuroscience, insights into the causal mechanisms of major syndromes remain rudimentary, and the search for biomarkers to improve diagnosis and stratification has thus far been unsuccessful. Development of novel therapies, both pharmacological and psychosocial, has also largely stalled (Hyman 2013).

One reason for the absence of significant breakthroughs in improving mental health has been the way in which research and treatment have been framed. Over the last 100 years, a cardinal feature of the existing paradigm in mental health has been its emphasis on fully established disorders in adulthood. Diagnostic and therapeutic approaches constructed around the adult have resulted in a pervasive therapeutic pessimism, in particular in regard to syndromes such as schizophrenia. Fuelled by theories that neurodegenerative processes set a person on a course for life-long disability, this pessimism frequently has become a self-fulfilling prophecy.

Rethinking Mental Health

Over the last two decades, prevailing ideas about mental illness have started to change. Insel and Fenton (2005:591), for instance, stressed that "mental disorders begin in early life and are common and protracted," constituting "chronic diseases of the young." Out of the entrenched attitude from the past, a more optimistic outlook has emerged: one aimed at improving mental health, in particular in young people/youth, stimulated by the early intervention approach in the psychosis movement (McGorry et al. 2008a). These early pioneers realized that to improve outcomes in people with schizophrenia, which typically emerges during the transition from adolescence to adulthood, the duration of untreated psychosis must be reduced (Marshall et al. 2005). Specialized clinics set up to detect young people during their first episode of psychosis provided an initial impetus to improve mental health, followed by the concept of clinical high-risk for psychosis (CHR-P), which served as the first blueprint for a preemptive psychiatry approach (Yung et al. 2012).

CHR-P criteria define a group of young people (usually between the age of 15 and 30, the peak onset years for psychotic disorders) who are experiencing subthreshold psychosis symptoms and/or have a genetic liability combined with a functional decline (Fusar-Poli et al. 2015). An alternative approach to CHR-P diagnosis has been the basic symptom approach, which defines risk for psychosis based on the presence of self-experienced cognitive and perceptual anomalies, which are thought to represent the earliest indicators for the development of psychosis (Schultze-Lutter et al. 2016). Meta-analysis suggests that

CHR-P criteria confer a risk of developing psychosis within a two-year period at 10–30% (Fusar-Poli et al. 2013a).

The identification of behavioral and neurobiological predictors of transition to psychosis and functional outcomes in CHR-P cohorts is an ongoing endeavor. A critical aspect of the CHR-P approach has been the identification of interventions capable of reducing the likelihood of transition to psychosis. Overall, evidence suggests that psychosocial interventions, such as cognitive behavioral therapy (CBT), reduce the risk of transition (Fusar-Poli et al. 2013a). Evidence for pharmacological interventions, however, has thus far been mixed, and research is ongoing to identify more effective ways of modifying the course of emerging psychosis in young people.

Initially, the early intervention movement was firmly rooted in improving the outcome of psychotic disorders, especially in schizophrenia. Its scope has now been broadened to target emerging mental disorders of youth more generally, due to two important observations.

First, young people with CHR-P criteria rarely present solely with signs of psychosis. In the large majority of cases, they display a range of other symptoms that defy the idealized DSM-5 categories. Indeed, the CHR-P concept has been referred to as a "pluripotent risk stage" (McGorry et al. 2018a) for a range of mental health outcomes, of which psychosis is only one. This is supported by follow-up data which highlight that CHR-P individuals who do not transition to psychosis will, in the majority of cases, show nonpsychotic disorders that are associated with a significant impact on functional outcomes (Lin et al. 2015).

Second, emerging epidemiological evidence has pinpointed a crucial aspect of mental health: all major syndromes—schizophrenia, depression, personality disorders, and substance abuse, which constitute approximately 75% of mental disorders—begin before the age of 24 years (Kessler et al. 2005; Kim-Cohen et al. 2003), with a significant proportion of 15- to 24-year-olds affected by mental illness at any one time (McCrone et al. 2008). Prevalence has increased over recent decades (Collishaw et al. 2004; Rutter and Smith 1995) and is likely to continue to do so (McCrone et al. 2008). Data from the National Comorbidity Study Adolescent Supplement indicate that 40% of 13- to 17-year-olds in the United States had a mental disorder in any one year (Kessler et al. 2012). These findings are supported by large prospective cohort studies, such as the Great Smoky Mountains Study, which show that by age 21, 61% of participants had experienced a diagnosable mental disorder; this increased to 83% when subthreshold disorders (with functional impairment) were included (Copeland et al. 2011). Even when these disorders resolve, they can have lasting impacts on economic and social outcomes in later life (Gibb et al. 2010). Accordingly, these data emphasize that the time frame between 12 and 24 years of age constitutes *the developmental period* with the most pronounced manifestation of mental health disorders.

These findings have fundamental implications for the ways in which mental disorders are researched, diagnosed, and treated. To further the development of a youth mental health paradigm and establish trajectories for future research and intervention to pursue, we proposed this Ernst Strüngmann Forum to address collectively the questions and challenges in the field.

Core Themes

Three main themes, described below, provided a conceptual backdrop to this Forum and were used to focus our efforts. Any discussion of youth mental health, however, can easily be hampered when there is a lack of clear definitions. Terms such as *adolescence* or *youth*, for instance, are understood differently in different contexts (for an in-depth discussion, see Torous et al., this volume). Thus, qualifying these contexts proved important during our discussions. Now, as we prepare to pass along the results, we confront again the issue of terminology. Since there is no way to reconcile the multiple aspects involved, we have recommended that the WHO guidelines be used when reference is made to adolescents (10–19 years of age) and youth/young people (15–24 years of age). This was a pragmatic decision—one that we hope will not detract from the highly dynamic nature of this developmental stage of transition from adolescence to adulthood.

Rethinking Diagnostic Systems in Mental Health

Current diagnostic systems (DSM-5, ICD-10) have undergone extensive critique in recent years due to the lack of construct validity of major categories, the lack of biological markers, and high comorbidity for the large majority of disorders. One area that has received less attention, however, is the developmental aspect of psychopathology and the resulting challenges to current nosology. The clinical picture of emerging mental illnesses in young people is often complicated by mixed symptom patterns and frequent comorbid substance use (Sawyer et al. 2000). This may reflect the fact that the earliest manifestation of these conditions (in adolescence or youth) comes in the form of undifferentiated "subsyndromal" symptoms; that is, before a clear-cut diagnosable illness emerges.

This contrasts the long-standing assumption that mental disorders constitute categorical entities. It also highlights the limitation of current diagnostic systems, which are likely to reflect (artificial) end points of developmental trajectories. Indeed, research to identify genes that confer risk to individual syndromes have found instead that the genes are frequently shared across different DSM-5 categories (Owen 2014), consistent with long-standing evidence of comorbidity for most syndromes (Plana-Ripoll et al. 2019). While approaches that highlight the importance of comorbidity and transdiagnostic factors in adult mental health conditions are increasingly being recognized (Fusar-Poli et al. 2019), unclear diagnostic boundaries in emerging mental disorders are the rule, not the exception. This underlines an urgent need for novel approaches to define "disorders" and "caseness" in youth, as in clinical staging models that have been proposed to guide intervention (McGorry et al. 2006).

Rethinking Treatment

A fundamental implication of the emergence of the majority of mental disorders during youth is the importance of early intervention. Both at subsyndromal and threshold levels, mental disorders are costly, from personal and societal viewpoints. Disorders can lead to substantial disability, long-term morbidity, welfare dependency, and premature mortality (Butterworth and Berry 2004; Killackey et al. 2006) at a period when major developmental processes occur to determine the path that a young person follows, in terms of vocational and social milestones.

There is a growing recognition that a profound redesign of services and intervention is required. In 2010, early intervention for mental illness was established as a top priority in the U.K. Medical Research Council Mental Health Strategy (MRC Strategic Review Group 2010), which delineated the need to "identify individuals at risk in order to target intervention."

Despite the importance and high prevalence of mental disorders in young people, individuals with emerging mental disorders face major difficulties in accessing appropriate treatment (Singh 2009). This is partly due to the "gap" in care between child and adult mental health services as well as to a reluctance to seek help, stigma, and negative attitudes toward professionals (McGorry 2007; Rickwood et al. 2007). In the U.S. National Comorbidity Study, only a little more than one-third of adolescents with a mental disorder received mental health care, but this tended to be directed toward childhood-onset conditions, such as attention deficit hyperactivity disorder. Moreover, less than one in five adolescents with disorders of youth onset (anxiety, substance use disorders) received care (Merikangas et al. 2011).

Current treatment paradigms, at both the service and individual level, focus on diagnosis. Typically, official diagnostic systems, such as the DSM-4 and ICD-10, were derived from chronic samples, where the impression of stability and validity is enhanced (Cohen and Cohen 1984). Early clinical features are not differentiated from those that become apparent as a disorder persists. Such diagnoses are not useful in guiding early intervention or treatment of less severe cases, and do not further our understanding of the processes involved in the emergence of disorders.

It is essential that a different approach be developed. Diagnosis needs to be refined so that treatments can be selected in a safer, more effective manner, and prognosis must be accurately assessed. Such an alternative approach would allow for the array of biological disturbances at differing phases of the illness to be better defined and reappraised within an appropriate clinical-pathological framework.

Rethinking Research

The emergence of major mental disorders during youth highlights the need to identify the unique factors that contribute to their manifestation during this developmental period. Until recently, an essential dogma was the assumption that fundamental properties of cortical networks are sculpted mainly *in utero* and the early postnatal years. Accordingly, later developmental stages were assumed to have little or no effect on the functional characteristics and anatomical layout of large-scale networks. Recently, however, a range of disciplines from basic neuroscience to neuroimaging has provided evidence that the period between 15 and 24 years of age is associated with profound changes in behavior and cognition as well as the underlying neural processes, including modifications in neurotransmitter systems, reorganization of functional networks, and ongoing changes in anatomical parameters (Lee et al. 2014a).

While these processes have increasingly been described in detail, critical links to emerging psychopathology still remain to be established. Indeed, the close correlation between the onset of certain disorders, such as anxiety, and ongoing brain maturational processes, for instance in fear extinction (Pattwell et al. 2011), suggests that aspects of psychopathology may be directly linked to changes in neural circuits during youth. If true, such a framework could have wide-ranging implications for understanding the etiology of major mental disorders as well as treatment. Furthermore, monitoring normative developmental trajectories might provide opportunities to identify individuals at greater risk for mental disorders. Central to this effort will be research that links individual variability in these trajectories to clinical outcomes, and the extent to which multiple domains of cognitive performance and neurobiological assessment can be combined into a cogent risk score (Marquand et al. 2019).

Emerging evidence on the profound changes that take place in neural processing and behavior during youth carries important implications for interventions. Currently, the majority of psychosocial and pharmacological treatments that are applied to emerging mental disorders during youth were originally developed for adult populations. Accordingly, one important consequence of the youth mental health paradigm may be that interventions must consider developmental modifications to correct aberrant maturational processes so that therapeutic efficacy can be maximized. For example, interventions aimed at targeting social functioning need to recognize the specific developmental time course of social cognition across adolescence and adjust their contents accordingly (Bartholomeusz et al. 2011). Similarly, pharmacological therapies need to account for the ongoing maturational changes in basic circuit properties.

Our Approach

To "rethink" these core topics, experts from clinical research, neuroscience, health policy as well as developmental and social psychology worked collectively at this Forum to address the nature of psychopathology, its underlying causal factors, and mechanisms. Throughout, the overarching goal was to generate understanding that would move us further away from the current paradigm (i.e., diagnostic and therapeutic approaches designed to address fully established mental disorders in adults), toward one centered on the emergent nature of mental ill-health and the necessity for early intervention in youth. The results of this multifaceted dialogue are captured in this volume, organized around the following primary topics:

1. *Epidemiology, classification, and diagnostic issues.* The transition from childhood to adulthood is associated with the highest incidence of mental disorders across the life span (Costello et al. 2011), yet current classification frameworks were developed to fit the psychopathological presentation of adult populations. Thus, they perform poorly during early stages of mental illness. Several alternatives to the prevailing diagnostic approach have been suggested: the Research Domain Criteria developed by the National Institute of Mental Health (Cuthbert and Insel 2010, 2013), the Hierarchical Taxonomy of Psychopathology (HiTOP) (Kotov et al. 2018), network theory (Borsboom 2017), and the Psychopathology ("p") Factor (Caspi et al. 2014; Caspi and Moffitt 2018). Although all of these approaches embrace a transdiagnostic approach, they focus on different aspects of psychopathology, and none incorporates a longitudinal perspective or considers developmental context:
    - How can emerging psychopathologies best be characterized?
    - Are there early features that indicate trajectories toward mental disorders?
    - What are the temporal sequences and stages of the differential evolution of premorbid phases?
    - What is the relationship between normal functional trajectories and trajectories for psychopathology?
    - What are the best indicators of need for intervention during the unfolding course of mental disorders?
2. *Context for emerging mental disorders: biological, psychological, and sociocultural processes.* The transition from childhood to adulthood is a developmental period that is highly influenced by social and cultural context, but our understanding of the way these contexts interact with individual differences (e.g., genetic variation) to generate or moderate psychopathology is limited. Combined with known transcultural variation in mental health, there is a critical need to increase understanding of the general applicability of models in youth mental health. This is

likely to be important for the development of appropriate interventions and services as well as the identification of risk and resilience factors.

- Which key precursors are susceptible to contextual modification?
- Which contextual factors confer resilience and risk for emerging psychopathology?
- How can we characterize/quantify social and cultural context in the context of psychopathology?
- How do these precursors and risk and resilience factors evolve over time and interact?

3. *Biological mechanisms underlying risk for psychopathology*. A large body of evidence has accumulated over the years, from a range of disciplines, on the profound modifications in the anatomy and functionality of large-scale networks as well as basic circuit modifications during the transition from adolescence to adulthood (Lee et al. 2014a). Because of the temporal coincidence of these changes with the expression of major mental disorders during this period, we need to understand whether the developmental events at the neural and behavioral level constitute vulnerability for emerging psychopathologies. If so, this could point toward opportunities for understanding the etiology as well as possible interventions.
    - What are the core modifications to circuit properties during the transition from childhood to adulthood?
    - How might animal models guide our understanding of the development of psychopathology and interventions?
    - How do earlier risk factors interact with the expression of mental disorders in youth?
    - What are the implications for the development of biomarkers during this period?
    - How can these findings inform the development of interventions?
4. *Developing and implementing prevention and early intervention*. Given the clear evidence supporting the emergence of major mental disorders in young people, the continued division of mental health services along the same developmental lines (child vs. adult), as practiced in other areas of medicine, seems perverse. Actually developing and implementing services for young people has, however, presented a range of challenges across different cultures, communities, and health systems. Developing such services relies on decisions about boundaries between those who are well and those who have a disorder. Labeling and overtreatment are key concerns. Such boundaries also tend to be influenced by available resources, which vary by country and health system.
    - What political, economic, and systemic issues need to be addressed to deliver effective prevention and early intervention?

- How can translational basic science be used to improve assessment, treatment, and clinical decision making?
- What are the prospects of delivering interventions to young people through e-mental health and how might these be studied?
- What might be the optimal way to adapt and establish youth mental health services in current health systems?
- How might interventions consider the social, cultural, economic, and political contexts in which the transition from childhood to adulthood takes place?

Future Steps

Paradigmatic changes in science do not occur linearly: they follow a landscape of dynamic systems, characterized by local minima and bifurcations that can suddenly give rise to new system properties. So, too, may be the path that is followed toward a youth mental health paradigm.

We hope that the multifaceted exchanges from this Forum will contribute to shift attention away from the dominant paradigm in mental health toward a new approach: one focused on understanding emerging mental ill-health and early interventions in youth. Undoubtedly, this is an ambitious goal. Yet in the absence of significant advances and unfulfilled promises in the field, we are propelled forward by the urgent need to respond to the ever-increasing burden that mental health places on individuals and societies.

It is our sincere hope that the ideas and proposals outlined in this volume, as well as the open questions that remain, will provide a roadmap for research to follow over the next decade. Practices, perspectives, and methods need to be reconceptualized and reframed. This is a herculean task, reliant on vision, commitment, and collaboration.

Epidemiology, Classification, and Diagnostic Issues

2

The Utility of Clinical Staging in Youth Mental Health Settings

Ian B. Hickie, Elizabeth M. Scott,
Joanne S. Carpenter, and Frank Iorfino

Abstract

This chapter reviews a clinical staging framework that was developed for youth-onset anxiety, mood, and psychotic disorders. Used for over a decade in early intervention services in Australia, a more restricted version of this framework has been used internationally for specific diagnostic groupings, most notably among youth with psychotic or bipolar disorders. The validity of these different clinical staging frameworks is being assessed within longitudinal cohort, concurrent neurobiological, and specific intervention studies. Preliminary evidence suggests that (a) varying stages of illness are associated with predicted differences in a range of objectively measured neuropsychological, circadian, and structural brain imaging measures; (b) while earlier stages are considered subthreshold disorders from a diagnostic perspective, they are associated with significant reductions in educational, employment, and social participation as well as substantial comorbidity and suicidal thoughts and behaviors; and (c) as predicted by the Sydney model, earlier (subthreshold) stages of illness progress at lower rates to more severe (full-threshold), recurrent, or persistent disorders. Importantly, since approximately 15–30% of young people classified as "attenuated" (subthreshold) syndromes progress to more severe (full-threshold) disorders, this particular group is the most obvious focus for early clinical intervention and secondary prevention trials. The chapter concludes with a discussion of major issues that need to be pursued in future research.

Introduction

Internationally, there is widespread recognition of the premature death and disability attributable to major mental disorders (Bloom et al. 2011; Erskine et al. 2015; Gustavsson et al. 2011). This burden derives from their early age of onset, population prevalence, chronicity, and comorbidity with physical illness and the degree of resultant impairment (Gore et al. 2011; Gustavsson et al. 2011; Lopez et al. 2006). To reduce this burden, earlier identification, more effective and more personalized treatments, as well as enhanced long-term care for individuals at risk or in the early phases of developing life-threatening or chronic disorders have been prioritized (Hickie et al. 2013b; Insel 2007, 2009; Lopez et al. 2006; McGorry et al. 2014a; Scott et al. 2012a).

For the major mental disorders, a progressive illness trajectory typically has its onset in late childhood or early puberty and then recurs or continues progressively into adult life (Häfner et al. 2008; Merikangas et al. 2010; Paus et al. 2008). In a significant proportion of these individuals, earlier age-dependent clinical phenotypes will have been evident in childhood (e.g., attentional, anxiety, sleep-wake, somatic, autistic spectrum, or conduct disorders), reflecting significant deviations in brain or psychosocial development. Although 75% of major mental disorders begin before 25 years of age (Gore et al. 2011; Kessler et al. 2005), the diagnostic and research criteria currently being used to identify these subjects have been derived largely from the experiences reported by middle-aged persons with recurring or chronic illness. Often, these midlife phenotypes map poorly onto earlier and less specific phases of the illness experience (Hickie et al. 2013b; McGorry 2007, 2010; McGorry et al. 2008b). For example, young people who go on to develop bipolar disorder rarely present with mania as their first episode of illness. Typically, these young people will have experienced earlier depressive episodes, often with intercurrent periods of emotional instability, suicidal behavior, or brief periods of motor activation throughout their early and mid-adolescent developmental stages (Hafeman et al. 2016; Iorfino et al. 2018; Ratheesh et al. 2017; Scott et al. 2017).

Current diagnostic systems prioritize phenomena such as delusions and hallucinations for psychotic disorders; periods of elevated mood or increased energy for bipolar disorder; and psychomotor slowing, emotional blunting, or cognitive slowing for severe depression. Data from community studies that assess subjects longitudinally from childhood or adolescence emphasize the extent to which many of these phenomena are shared across diagnostic groups over this entire developmental period (Copeland et al. 2013; Kelleher et al. 2012a; Merikangas et al. 2008, 2010, 2012; Murray and Jones 2012; Ormel et al. 2015). A great clinical challenge is to derive new dynamic diagnostic systems that are not only consistent with developmental epidemiology and neurobiology but also useful when applied in everyday clinical practice.

A major response to this challenge has been to apply the general medical concept of clinical staging to the early phases of major mental disorders. In other areas of medicine, it is commonly accepted that it is inadequate to choose treatments, or plan health care, for persons who suffer from conditions that are likely to progress or recur, simply on the basis of broad illness categories (e.g., breast cancer or cardiovascular disease). An assumption of the clinical staging approach is that it is equally meaningless in mental health to plan personalized preventive or early intervention strategies or to select specific treatments simply on the basis of a diagnosis of broad categories, such as schizophrenia, bipolar disorder, or major depression. Indeed, a wealth of evidence indicates that subjects at different points along the illness continuum for all of these conditions show quite different patterns of response to various psychological or pharmacological interventions (McGorry et al. 2006, 2007a; Scott 2011; Scott et al. 2006).

Consequently, a range of frameworks for clinical staging have been proposed that can be applied either to all young people presenting for care (Hickie et al. 2013b; McGorry et al. 2006) or to a subset assigned to a "specific" disease category: staging models for major depression (Ruhe et al. 2012; Verduijn et al. 2015), bipolar disorder (Berk et al. 2007; Duffy 2014; Kapczinski et al. 2009), and psychosis-schizophrenia (Agius et al. 2010; Lieberman et al. 2001; McGorry 1995). In addition, staging models have included those who present for clinical care as well as those who may be asymptomatic but "at risk" due to another known risk factor (e.g., family history, prior neurodevelopmental disorder). These various models have been well summarized in the literature (for reviews see Hartmann et al. 2019; McGorry et al. 2018c; Scott et al. 2017).

When staging is applied to single diagnostic groups, the underlying assumption is that a unique pathway or pathophysiology underpins each "independent" or "clinical" category. This assumption is not readily supported by modern epidemiological, psychosocial, family, genetic, or neurobiological risk factor studies, where the same risk factors load on multiple disorders (Buckholtz and Meyer-Lindenberg 2012; Lichtenstein et al. 2009; Sullivan et al. 2012; Waszczuk et al. 2014). In addition, early-onset disorders, such as childhood-onset anxiety, conduct, and developmental disorders (i.e., clinically evident before age 12 years), do not predict specific "adolescent-onset" disorders but rather the full spectrum of later depressive, bipolar, and psychotic disorders (Kim-Cohen et al. 2003). When used in association with a transdiagnostic framework, which includes disorders with high known rates of comorbidity (e.g., anxiety, major mood and psychotic disorders), we propose that clinical staging is more likely to be useful in clinical practice, as it will more closely fit naturally occurring adolescent-onset clinical syndromes, and may prove to have closer links to those underlying pathophysiological processes that underpin these complex syndromes (Hickie et al. 2013c; McGorry et al. 2006).

Utilizing a Transdiagnostic Clinical Staging Framework in Youth Mental Health Services

The clinical staging framework, when applied to young people (12–30 years of age) presenting for health care, proposes that earlier (subthreshold) stages (as compared with more advanced stages) are characterized by lower rates of impairment and predict lower risk of progression to later, more severe, disabling, or persistent disorders. In Australia we have applied this transdiagnostic framework to young people who present for health care and clearly differentiate those in early phases (Stages 1a, nonspecific anxious or depressive symptoms or 1b, attenuated syndromes) from those who have reached a higher threshold for disorder (Stage 2 and above). Within the earlier (and assumed typically nonprogressive) Stage 1 disorders, we differentiate the attenuated syndromes (which often meet DSM-IV, DSM-5, or ICD-10 criteria for specific anxiety or mood disorders) from the more nonspecific anxiety and depressive syndromes. A more detailed description of these clinical stages is given in association with Figure 2.1, which outlines a simple and reliable decision tree for making such key distinctions. These decision processes have now been incorporated into our clinical practice systems. We have previously demonstrated the inter-rater reliability of this structured approach (Hickie et al. 2013b). Where there is uncertainty about the appropriate stage to assign, we rate down to the earlier and less severe category.

Importantly, this transdiagnostic approach (Hickie et al. 2013b, 2013c, 2013d; Scott et al. 2013b, 2014b) is consistent with the Research Domain Criteria (RDoC) proposed by the National Institute of Mental Health (NIMH) (Insel et al. 2010; Cuthbert and Insel 2013; Kozak and Cuthbert 2016). That is, clinical stages, in contrast to formal diagnostic categories, may map more reliably onto at least some independent neurobiological processes (and objective measures of those underlying processes). These approaches also place an appropriate emphasis on recognizing developmental trajectories and the active and bidirectional impacts of interaction with the environment.

From a health services perspective, this approach has the advantage of facilitating a more inclusive approach to recruitment. Clinical cohorts, however, are not representative of population-based cohorts as the process of "seeking help" is associated with a range of other demographic (e.g., female gender) and clinical (e.g., suicidal behavior) features. It is consistent, however, with the NIMH recommendation (Casey et al. 2013) that such clinical research should recruit cohorts from common service settings that are also likely to demonstrate appropriate variance along relevant dimensions of interest (e.g., neuropsychological function, cortical or subcortical brain structure).

Issues Related to At-Risk Populations: Stage 0

Clinical staging models variously propose a Stage 0 to be applied to specific "at-risk" populations. These may include young people *not already presenting for clinical care* but who may be at increased risk of developing one or more major disorders. When detected, these cohorts can then be subject to specific systematic evaluation (clinically or neurobiologically). These subgroups may be identified through a variety of strategies:

- Familial relationships with known probands with specific disorders (e.g., adolescent siblings of probands with major mood or psychotic disorders
- First-degree relatives of probands with major disorders

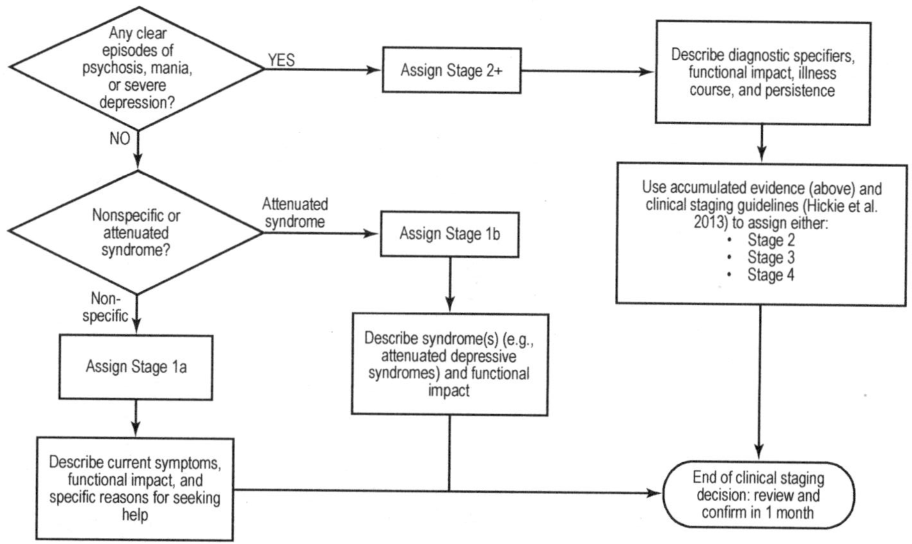

Stage 1a *Nonspecific Syndromes*	**Stage 1b** *Attenuated Syndromes*	**Stage 2** *Full-Threshold Disorders*
Mild or nonspecific symptons; mild functional impairment	Moderate anxiety, mood, or psychotic symptoms; comorbidity; moderate neurocognitive changes, and functional impairment (SOFAS <70)	First episode of full-threshold disorder with moderate to severe anxiety, mood or psychotic symptoms, neurocognitive changes and functional impairment (SOFAS 30–50)

Figure 2.1 Stepwise process taken in clinical services to assign those presenting for care to the appropriate stage. Stage 1a solely indicates nonspecific symptoms of anxiety or depression. By contrast, Stage 1b includes those with "attenuated" syndromes, who present more specific, severe, or comorbid mood or psychotic phenomena. Those who reach Stage 2 have discrete, full-threshold, and severe mood, psychotic, or comorbid syndromes. These disorders are assumed to justify specific clinical interventions and would also be at high risk of progressing to recurrent or persistent states in the absence of effective clinical interventions.

- Exposure to known developmental risk factors (e.g., maternal exposure to prenatal infection, low birth weight cohorts, childhood exposure to CNS infection)
- Concurrent medical at-risk groups (e.g., hormonal abnormalities including polycystic ovarian syndrome)
- Concurrent alcohol and other substance misuse cohorts

For adolescent-onset mood or psychotic disorders, cohorts consisting of individuals with prior but independent childhood-onset disorders (e.g., attentional, anxiety, or autism spectrum disorders) may be considered as at-risk populations. Further longitudinal studies of relevant developmental cohorts will assist the determination of actual transition rates from such at-risk states to adolescent-onset disorders.

Support for the Clinical Staging Framework

Cross-Sectional and Longitudinal Validation of the Clinical Staging Framework

We have reported extensively on the demographic, clinical (illness type and stage), disability, neuropsychological, brain imaging, and circadian characteristics of a Sydney-based transdiagnostic cohort evaluated over the last decade (see Table 2.1). This is one example of how clinical staging can be used within a cohort to address relevant clinical, neurobiological, and psychosocial issues. These Sydney-based studies have utilized both cross-sectional data with regards to social participation, educational, and employment status as well as longitudinal outcome data characterizing clinical course to test the construct and predictive validity of the transdiagnostic clinical staging model. With regards to levels of impairment, there is clear evidence that earlier stages are associated with lower degrees of functional impairment. This is not unexpected as the clinical phenotype used for staging purposes is, to some degree, inclusive of current levels of function.

Our preliminary longitudinal work using this clinical staging system among young people who present to our primary care services—typically with severe mood or anxiety disorders—indicates that in the short term, those initially classified as Stage 1b, attenuated syndromes, remain significantly impaired following ten sessions of treatment despite using more services and improving modestly (Cross et al. 2016). Within 12 months, approximately 17% of those rated as Stage 1b at initial assessment progress to a later stage (despite receiving clinical care) (Cross et al. 2018b). A significant proportion of these "clinical transitions" occur within the first three months, indicating the need for very close clinical supervision and monitoring following initial presentation. The transition rate varies between pathophysiological pathways: 11% for depression, 40% for psychosis, and 22% for bipolar (Cross et al. 2018b).

Regardless of the pathway, transition was found to be predicted by NEET (i.e., not in education, employment or training) status and negative symptoms—not by general psychological distress (K10) or positive symptoms. These data are consistent with findings from other studies (Fusar-Poli et al. 2010; Valmaggia et al. 2013).

To advance this work and, more specifically, to plan relevant early intervention and secondary prevention trials, we need to identify more accurately those who may be at particularly high risk of illness progression. Our related work (Scott et al. 2013a, 2014b), which focuses on identifying those subjects in the early course of bipolar disorder, indicates how difficult this is to achieve on the basis of clinical features or neuropsychological testing. Specifically, one study has highlighted the importance of family history of bipolar disorder, psychosis, or substance misuse in predicting this transition (Scott et al. 2013a).

Independent work, based on those at higher risk of developing psychotic disorders, has recognized similar difficulties. Consequently, there is a need to develop more refined clinical criteria to use in related neurobiological, longitudinal, preventive, or specific intervention studies. At this time, we propose that it is necessary to select for more specific phenotypic characteristics that are closer to the syndromal elements that would characterize transition to Stage 2 "full-threshold" disorders or beyond. The existing literature emphasizes that clinical features related to duration of illness, persistence, or recurrence of key symptoms and degree of current impairment may also be predictive.

Neurocognitive and Neuroimaging Evidence to Support Staging

We have conducted a number of studies to determine whether there are neurobiological features that distinguish key stages of illness. To date, these studies have utilized neuroimaging (Lagopoulos et al. 2012, 2013), sleep/circadian (Naismith et al. 2012; Scott et al. 2014a), and neuropsychological (Hermens et al. 2013; Tickell et al. 2017) measures. Across these studies, and consistent with a neuroprogressive model of illness, the data show that those with an attenuated syndrome (compared to controls) have reduced gray matter volumes, compromised white matter integrity, delayed sleep phase, and reductions in neuropsychological performance. By contrast, young people at later stages of illness (i.e., with "full-threshold" or discrete disorders) have significantly greater deficits across these domains. These varying levels of deficits were generally distinct from differences observed in other clinical (including diagnosis, clinical state) or functional (e.g., socio-occupational) measures. This suggests that the staging model may have utility in terms of distinguishing putative phenotypes, particularly with respect to underlying neurobiology. It should be noted that these studies focused on the two major stages of illness in our cohort: attenuated syndrome (Stage 1b) and discrete disorder (2+). The other stages within our model—that is, "nonspecific anxiety or depression" (Stage 1a) and persistent/unremitting disorders (Stage 4)—were intentionally

Table 2.1 Relationships between clinical stage and demographic, clinical (illness type), disability, neuropsychological, brain imaging, and circadian characteristics in a Sydney-based transdiagnostic youth cohort.

Sample (Stage, N)	Key Results	Other Relevant Information	Reference
	Clinical Studies: Cross-sectional		
1a = 293; 1b = 292; 2 = 121; 3+ = 133	Clinician-rated SOFAS strongly related to stages; later stages have more impaired role function	Stage 2 had highest levels of distress and role function impairment	Scott et al. (2012a)
1b = 286; 2+ = 289	Impairments in functioning and general behavioral disturbance were less marked in 1b compared to 2+	Interaction between stage and tripartite classification; 1b less common in developmental-psychosis	Hickie et al. (2013a)
	Clinical Studies: Longitudinal		
1a = 21; 1b = 112; 2+ = 53	Transition (median = 48 weeks): 11% of 1a; 19% of 1b; 33% of Stage 2	Those who remained within the same stage may have had persistent symptoms or dysfunction or responded to clinical interventions	Hickie et al. (2013b)
1a = 601; 1b = 257; 2+ = 31	Psychological distress (K10) and SOFAS improved over 1–6 to 10 sessions of care for both 1b and 1a	1b remained impaired after 10 sessions; 1a commenced with better SOFAS, less psychological distress	Cross et al. (2016)
1a = 579; 1b = 249	1b made and missed more appointments than 1a	Social functioning best predictor of female attendance; age and stage best predicted male attendance	Cross et al. (2017)
1b = 243	Ca. 17% transitioned to a major mental disorder; independent of syndromal diagnosis, transition more likely in NEET, females, and those with more negative psychological symptoms (e.g., social withdrawal)	NEET status and negative symptoms are modifiable predictors of illness trajectory across diagnostic categories and are not specific to transition to psychosis	Cross et al. (2018b)
1b = 243	Approx. 25–33% of individuals show reliable improvement; ca. 10% show reliable deterioration for both symptoms (K10 and BPRS) and functioning (SOFAS) over six months. Many individuals did not show linear improvement or deterioration.	Individual patterns of symptomatic and functional change are diverse in this group over time, highlighting the importance of routine outcome monitoring in treatment	Cross et al. (2018a)

Table 2.1 (continued)

Sample (Stage, N)	Key Results	Other Relevant Information	Reference
1a = 21; 1b = 112; 2+ = 53	Transition (median = 48 weeks): 11% of 1a; 19% of 1b; 33% of stage 2	Those who remained within the same stage may have had persistent symptoms/dysfunction or responded to clinical interventions	Hickie et al. (2013b)
	Neuropsychological: Cross-sectional		
1b = 94; 2+ = 100	2+ had most impaired neuropsychological profile; 1b had intermediate profile (cf. controls)	Greatest impairments in verbal memory and executive function.	Hermens et al. (2013)
	Neuropsychological: Longitudinal		
1b = 262; 2+ = 235	Baseline: 2+ worse than 1b in verbal learning, verbal memory, visual memory, set shifting. Both showed stability in processing speed, sustained attention, and visual memory at follow-up	Neuropsychological stability corresponded with stability in clinical and functional status, despite stage of illness	Tickell et al. (2017)
	Neuroimaging: Cross-sectional		
1b = 23; 2+ = 24	2+ had decreased GM in frontal brain regions cf. 1b	Cf. to controls, lb showed similar pattern of GM loss, albeit not to the same degree as their peers in 2+	Lagopoulos et al. (2012)
1b = 73; 2+ = 69	Both 1b & 2+ showed reduced white matter integrity in left ACR; 2+ had additional demyelination	ACR = junction point of 3 major long association fibers; impacts projections from thalamus to frontal lobes	Lagopoulos et al. (2013)
	Neuroimaging: Longitudinal		
1b = 28; 2+ = 16	2+ had markedly reduced levels of melatonin secretion cf. their peers in 1b	In 2+ only, reduced melatonin correlated with poorer verbal memory	Naismith et al. (2012)
1a = 18; 1b = 82; 2+ = 54	Delayed sleep phase (weekdays) increased progressively across illness stages	Older age, medication and later sleep offset strongest predictors of later stage	Scott et al. (2014a)

excluded from these studies because our aim was to determine the neurocognitive and neurobiological features that occur around the key major demarcation point in this model (i.e., Stage 1b vs. Stage 2+).

Hermens et al. (2013) examined the neuropsychological profiles between young people based on attenuated syndromes (n = 94) compared to those with discrete disorders (n = 100). The latter showed the most impaired neuropsychological profile, with the earlier Stage 1b group showing an intermediate profile compared to controls. Greatest impairments were seen in verbal memory and executive functioning. To address potential confounds created by diagnosis, profiles for those with a mood syndrome or disorder but not psychosis were also examined and the neuropsychological impairments for the Stage 2+ group remained. Thus, the degree of neuropsychological impairment discriminated those with attenuated syndromes from those with a discrete disorder, independent of diagnostic status and current symptoms. Our findings support the notion that neuropsychological assessment is a key tool of clinical evaluation in early stages of major psychiatric illness in young adults. Other studies from our group have illustrated the nature of neuropsychological functioning as a strong predictor of functioning longitudinally, over and above psychiatric symptomatology (Lee et al. 2013, 2014c, 2015). Additionally, more recent studies examining subjects at risk for schizophrenia identified neuropsychological dysfunction as a potential risk factor for illness onset/transition (e.g., executive function, verbal fluency, attention, visual memory, verbal memory, and working memory) (Lin et al. 2013; Maziade et al. 2011; Sumiyoshi et al. 2013).

As a follow-up to our first staging by neuropsychology study, we examined a larger sample (n = 497) of help-seeking young people (aged 21.2, ±3 years; 56% female) of whom 262 were rated as attenuated syndrome (Stage 1b) and 235 as "discrete" or "persistent" disorder (Stage 2+) at baseline (Tickell et al. 2017). Of this sample, 170 individuals (54% at Stage 1b) were reassessed neuropsychologically after 19.8 ±9 months (range: 3–51 months). At baseline, we found that the attenuated and discrete/persistent disorder groups differed significantly in four of the nine neuropsychological measures (verbal learning, verbal memory, visual memory, and set shifting). Despite this, both groups showed similar stability in neuropsychological functioning at follow-up, particularly in processing speed, sustained attention, and visual memory. Furthermore, longitudinal stability in cognition corresponded with increases in socio-occupational functioning. Importantly, we found again (Hermens et al. 2013) that the degree of baseline neuropsychological dysfunction discriminated those with attenuated syndromes from those with a discrete/persistent disorder. Furthermore, stability in neuropsychological functioning corresponded with stability in clinical and functional status, despite stage of illness. This suggests that neuropsychological functioning remains relatively stable in young people with a mental illness and may be a critical window for intervention.

We conducted two neuroimaging studies to examine whether attenuated syndrome and discrete disorder patient groups could be distinguished in terms of gray matter (GM) and white matter (WM) integrity. In a voxel-based morphometry study (Lagopoulos et al. 2012), compared to Stage 1b patients (n = 23) and controls (n = 33), Stage 2+ patients (n = 24) were found to have decreased GM volumes within distributed frontal brain regions. The greatest GM loss for Stage 2+ occurred within an overlapping region bounded by the superior and middle frontal gyri on the right side. Additional loss of GM volume was also observed in the inferior aspects of the frontal gyrus as well as the anterior cingulate and the orbitofrontal cortex on the right side and the medial prefrontal cortex midline. Of note, we did not find any evidence of GM loss that extended outside the prefrontal cortex. Overall the findings of this study suggest that, in terms of frontal GM changes, a major transition point may occur in the course of affective illness between early attenuated syndromes and later discrete illness stages.

In a subsequent study (Lagopoulos et al. 2013), we examined WM integrity—more specifically, fractional anisotropy in n = 74 patients in Stage 1b as well as in n = 69 patients in Stage 2+—and compared them with n = 39 healthy controls. Interestingly, we found a significant disruption in WM integrity in the left anterior corona radiata (in particular, the anterior thalamic radiation for both groups of patients) when separately contrasted with healthy controls. Our results suggest that patients with subsyndromal symptoms exhibit discernible early WM changes when compared with healthy control subjects and more significant disruptions are associated with clinical evidence of illness progression. Despite limitations (i.e., mainly cross-sectional studies, relatively small sample sizes, and the potential effects of medication), these studies are collectively consistent with a progression of illness model.

Sleep and Circadian Evidence to Support Staging

Abnormalities in the sleep-wake cycle and circadian rhythms are found across a range of psychiatric disorders and have been highlighted as potentially transdiagnostic factors (Benca et al. 1992; Dolsen et al. 2014; Harvey et al. 2011; Jones and Benca 2015; Karatsoreos 2014). Across adolescence and youth, developmental changes in sleep-wake and circadian systems typically result in delayed sleep and circadian rhythms (Carpenter et al. 2015a; Gradisar et al. 2011), which may predispose the circadian system to be particularly vulnerable to perturbations across this period. In our youth cohort, we have found that delays in sleep timing and increases in wakefulness across the night are found across multiple diagnoses (Robillard et al. 2015). We have also found sleep-wake delays to be particularly prominent in adolescents and youth (Robillard et al. 2014).

To examine sleep-wake cycles in young people at different stages of psychiatric illness, we used actigraphy monitoring to measure average rest and activity timing over multiple days of recording, comparing those with attenuated syndromes (n = 82) and those with discrete disorders (n = 54) to control participants (n = 21) (Scott et al. 2014a). We found delayed sleep timing in both patient groups compared to controls, with more severe delays in those with discrete disorders (Stage 2+) compared to those with attenuated syndromes (Stage 1b). The proportion of individuals with a delayed sleep-wake profile also increased across illness stages, with 9.5% of controls, 25.6% of Stage 1b, and 50% of Stage 2+ presenting with delayed sleep-wake. The potential confounding effects of medications (as they increase in complexity, dose, and duration with clinical stage or illness progression) on circadian measures also need to be considered (Robillard et al. 2016b).

In addition to being related to more established and severe illness stages, sleep-wake delays may also be indicative of a more bipolar type of illness, with our research finding delayed sleep phase to be more common in those with bipolar syndromes (over 60%) compared to those with unipolar mood disorders (30%) and controls (10%) (Robillard et al. 2013a). These findings suggest that sleep-wake delays may be an important feature to distinguish between stage of illness as well as being potentially indicative of a specific illness phenotype characterized by circadian dysregulation and bipolar type symptoms. We have also shown sleep-wake disturbances to be predictive of longitudinal outcomes in our cohort. Robillard et al. (2016a) report on 50 young people with sleep-wake assessment (actigraphy) followed up after 11 to 47 months (average 18.9 months). They found that lower sleep efficiency (i.e., more time spent awake during the night) was predictive of worsening of manic symptoms at follow-up, and both shorter sleep and poorer circadian rhythmicity of 24-hour activity patterns were predictive of worsening in verbal memory, demonstrating the utility of sleep-wake assessment in prediction of outcomes.

While disturbance of biological circadian systems is likely to underlie these delays of rest and activity behavior, the direction of causation of these effects is unresolved. In our studies we investigated circadian perturbation by measuring melatonin levels prior to habitual sleep in a subset of participants. While we found no difference in the timing of melatonin secretion across stages of illness, those at Stage 2+ (n = 16) had reduced levels of evening melatonin, compared to those at Stage 1b (n = 28), and shorter phase angles (time differences) between melatonin onset and sleep onset (Naismith et al. 2012). Abnormal phase angles indicate that internal circadian rhythms may not be optimally timed in relation to each other or the external environment, which may be indicative of severe disruption to the circadian system. Reduced evening melatonin secretion may also be a result of circadian misalignment or reflective of reduced circadian rhythm amplitude and weaker circadian signaling. These findings suggest that such disruptions are linked to stage of illness, and the circadian system may become increasingly disrupted with progression of illness. Notably, in this study we did not find any associations between melatonin measures and depressive symptoms, further suggesting that relationships with illness stage may be independent of current symptom levels (Naismith et al. 2012).

In concordance with the actigraphy findings, we also found reduced evening melatonin in those with bipolar disorders, compared to unipolar depressive disorders, as well as relatively delayed melatonin profiles in those with bipolar disorders (Robillard et al. 2013b). This provides further support for a distinct circadian profile with delayed rhythms and links to bipolar-type symptoms. However, it is important to note that while such a profile may be linked to bipolar-type symptoms, it likely exists across multiple psychiatric diagnoses, rather than being linked to the strict traditional diagnosis of bipolar disorder. In support of this, we used a data-driven technique to identify clusters of individuals in our cohort with similar sleep-wake profiles and found these profiles to be distinct from traditional diagnostic categories (Carpenter et al. 2017b; Carpenter et al. 2015b): those with a profile of delayed sleep demonstrated evidence of delayed biological circadian rhythms of melatonin and core temperature (Carpenter et al. 2017b), thus highlighting a biological basis for delayed sleep-wake presentations.

There is also evidence for interactions between sleep-wake and circadian abnormalities and neural structure and function in this cohort of young people with psychiatric disorders. We have observed links between sleep-wake and circadian disturbances and neuropsychological performance: one study found impaired visual memory in those with a profile of long sleep (Carpenter et al. 2015b) while another found that lower melatonin levels are related to poorer verbal memory functioning in those with discrete disorders (Naismith et al. 2012). An MRI investigation suggests that structural differences in the brain may underlie circadian outputs, with significant correlations between pineal volume and evening melatonin secretion (Carpenter et al. 2017a). We have also linked circadian disturbances with neurochemical changes, using proton magnetic resonance spectroscopy. These studies found that later sleep timing is associated with higher levels of glutamine in the anterior cingulate cortex (Naismith et al. 2014), and that later melatonin onset is associated with lower myo-inositol concentrations in the anterior cingulate cortex (Robillard et al. 2017). These various relationships suggest that observed abnormalities in sleep-wake behavior may reflect disturbed circadian and related neural systems, with potential transdiagnostic relevance to illness progression.

Designing Personalized Treatments Based on These Approaches

Internationally, there is an increasing move to manage actively in clinical settings adolescents and youth who present for care in the early phases of major mood or psychotic disorders. However, the symptom complexes presented are often an admixture of anxiety, depressive, hypomanic, psychotic, or substance misuse-related symptoms (Hickie et al. 2013b) and thus typically do not meet the diagnostic thresholds employed for more specific disorders. The evidence base for providing specific treatments for many of these subthreshold or first episode-type disorders is sparse. There is also an increasing desire to link interventions more closely to underlying developmental or specific pathophysiological pathways (Hickie et al. 2013b, c, d). While we have proposed the potential utility of adapting a clinical staging strategy to guide assessment and treatment selection for such early or less-differentiated cases of major mood or psychotic disorders, our view is that this approach is adjunctive to more conventional diagnostic practice. Consequently, we have developed preliminary approaches to plotting both clinical stage and major pathophysiological pathways, while proposing likely objective neurobiological markers that can be tracked concurrently (Figure 2.2).

We propose three major developmental trajectories, putatively linked with more specific (but not mutually exclusive) pathophysiologies: anxiety-depression, circadian-mania/fatigue, and neurodevelopmental-psychotic (Hickie et al. 2013a). These trajectories recognize preceding childhood-risk phenotypes and differential patterns of comorbidity, notably differential ages of onset of alcohol or other substance misuse. Within such a model, the majority of our work is located currently at the threshold between Stages 1b and 2, and it

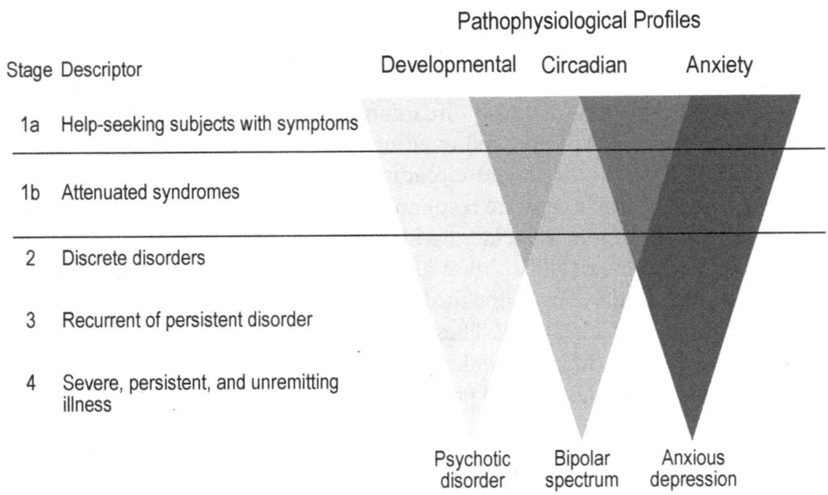

Figure 2.2 Clinical staging model for postpubertal onset and course of major mental disorders: developmental, circadian, or anxiety pathophysiological pathways progress from nonspecific to discrete syndromes. Overlap is evident between all three pathophysiological profiles in the early stages. Key neurobiological measures are neuropsychology (traditional, social cognitive, impulsive, and decision making), magnetic resonance imaging (magnetic resonance spectroscopy, diffusion tensor imaging, voxel-based morphometry, and cortical thickness), and circadian (dim light melatonin onset and actigraphy).

draws extensively from youth recruited uniquely through our enhanced headspace services and affiliated research clinics.

Complementary to this pathway model, we have commenced the development of a treatment selection model (Table 2.2), demonstrating the capacity to prioritize psychological, social, and behavioral approaches so that later pharmacological approaches can be chosen which may be most relevant to the underlying pathophysiological pathway (inferred from the observed phenotype or concurrent neurobiological testing). For example, 24-hour sleep-wake cycle behavioral interventions or melatonin-based antidepressants may be preferred for some depressive disorders in those who have phenotypic, actigraphic, or laboratory-based evidence of underlying circadian disturbance. This approach is the subject of ongoing clinical testing and refinement. Most recently, we have demonstrated that resolution of underlying circadian disturbance in response to circadian-informed psychological and medical therapies is strongly correlated with resolution of depressive symptoms (Robillard et al. 2018).

Table 2.2 Putative stepped-care therapies for relevant depressive subtypes. Cognitive behavioral therapy (CBT), interpersonal therapy (IPT), cognitive behavioral case management (CBCM), meta-cognitive therapy (MCT), selective serotonin reuptake inhibitor (SSRI), selective serotonin and norepinephrine reuptake inhibitors (SNRI), d-cycloserine (DCS), dialectic behavior therapy (DBT), transcranial magnetic stimulation (TMS), transcranial direct current stimulation (tDCS), individual placement and support (IPS).

Depression Type	First Line Therapy: Psychological or Behavioral	Second Line Therapy: Pharmacological	Experimental Therapies
Anxious depression	CBT, IPT, problem solving, e-health based anxiety management, exposure therapy, CBCM, MCT	SSRIs, SNRIs	Fish oils, DCS, oxytocin, ketamine
Circadian-fatigue depression	Behavioral regulation, physical activity, sleep-wake cycle/circadian-CBT, rumination-focused CBT, DBT, CBCM, MCT	Melatonin, melatonin analogues, lithium, pregabalin, lamotrigine	Sleep deprivation suvorexant, stimulants, modafinil, TMS, tDCS, ketamine, fish oils
Developmental psychosis	Problem-solving, social skills training, cognitive training, social recovery therapy, CBCM, MCT, IPS	Atypical antipsychotics	Ketamine, cannabidiol, oxytocin, novel neuropeptides, hormonal therapies, fish oils

Conclusion

Over the last decade, a variety of staging frameworks have been proposed for application in youth and early intervention mental health settings. In our Sydney-based studies, we have been able to test the clinical utility and predictive validity of clinical staging, when applied to young people presenting with anxiety, mood, or psychotic syndromes. The range of studies conducted to date provides a firm evidence base for further elaboration of a transdiagnostic model. The following are of greatest importance:

- longitudinal studies that evaluate the ongoing relationships between independent neurobiological correlates of clinical stage and illness progression,
- the design and implementation of stage-specific secondary prevention trials, and
- the testing of the clinical utility of stage-specific and pathophysiologically orientated treatment options.

Compared with practice based on traditional diagnostic systems, it appears that we can now use clinical staging to underpin the development of much more personalized and youth-relevant models of care. Major research questions, however, remain:

- *Longitudinal course*: Are there specific points along the staging continuum beyond which illness extension, progression, or enduring impairment is highly probable? Is it clear that interventions with lower risk of adverse effects, provided earlier in the course of illness, will actually result in prevention of illness extension or progression to later stages?
- *Alignment with existing diagnostic frameworks*: At present, there is poor concordance with current thresholds for formal (full-threshold) diagnosis or alignment with those entities that underpin clinical practice guidelines (e.g., major depression, bipolar disorder, schizophrenia as defined in DSM-5 or ICD-10).
- *Validation against independent neurobiological, interventional, and psychosocial measures*: To date, the literature remains largely cross-sectional and hence extremely limited. Most work has focused solely on individuals with psychotic syndromes. Longitudinal studies that utilize more heterogeneous cohorts of young people are required.
- *Relevance to clinical practice*: The extent to which new clinical staging systems result in better stratified guides to optimal and more personalized treatment selection, and prognostic statements, has not yet been clearly demonstrated.
- *Relevance to health system development*: Whether these systems can be used to facilitate early intervention for young people, and provide more effective health care, has yet to be demonstrated. The earlier clinical

stages within the frameworks are most relevant to at-risk populations and the development of new early intervention-style services. In these cohorts, traditional diagnostic concepts are less useful and choice of optimal interventions remains highly controversial.

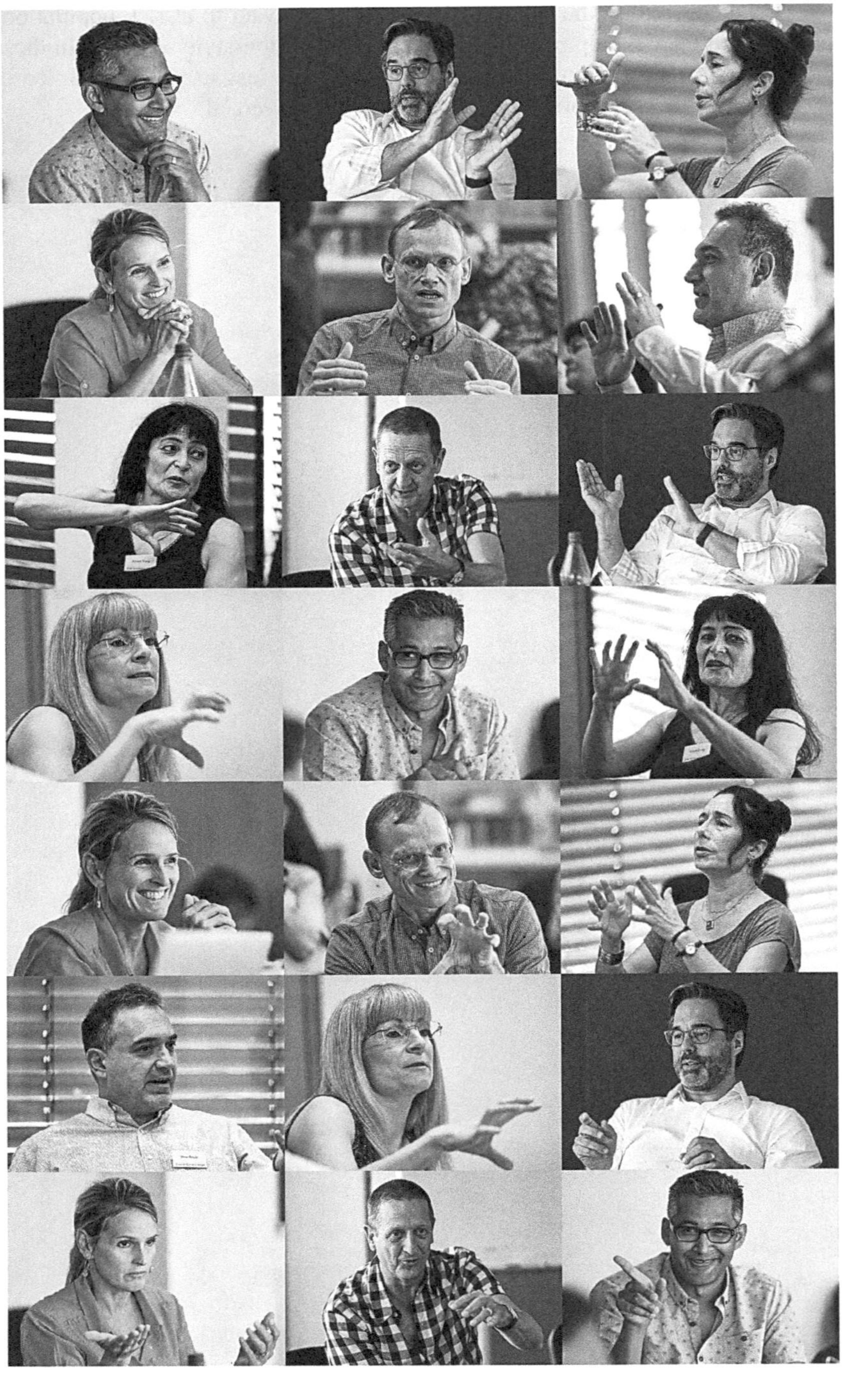

3

A Developmentally Informed Approach to Characterizing, Staging, and Intervening in Youth Mental Health Problems

From the Population to the Clinic

Jai L. Shah, Nicholas B. Allen, Shelli Avenevoli, Christoph U. Correll, Helen L. Fisher, Ian B. Hickie, Beatriz Luna, Dost Öngür, and Alison R. Yung

Abstract

This chapter articulates a framework for bringing together developmentally contextualized mental and physiological processes to guide the characterization, staging, and interventions necessary in treating mental health disorders in youth. This framework spans from population-level risk identification to individual-level clinical care, drawing on knowledge about developmentally informed trajectories and clinical systems. At a fundamental level, it necessitates appreciating the influence of both inherited and acquired factors on brain specialization and the setting of trajectories during periods of plasticity and risk, all of which delineate adult trajectories in multiple dimensions. More pragmatically, it requires us to track a range of salient mental/physiological systems during a dynamic developmental period that includes both vulnerability and risk, to contemplate their utility in identifying enriched groups that might benefit from further individual-level assessment in clinical or community settings, and to translate findings into planning prevention and intervention programs and to informing clinical decision making.

Group photos (top left to bottom right) Jai Shah, Nick Allen, Beatriz Luna, Shelli Avenevoli, Christoph Correll, Dost Öngür, Alison Yung, Ian Hickie, Nick Allen, Helen Fisher, Jai Shah, Alison Yung, Shelli Avenevoli, Christoph Correll, Beatriz Luna, Dost Öngür, Helen Fisher, Nick Allen, Shelli Avenevoli, Ian Hickie, Jai Shah

Introduction: The Need

Clinical and epidemiologic research over the past two decades has shown that approximately 75% of mental disorders emerge in youth (Kim-Cohen et al. 2003) and that one in five young people is affected by mental illness. Yet while prompt treatment of initial phases could improve outcomes, existing services often struggle to detect and manage them: there are substantial delays in identifying and intervening in these conditions, long waits to access care, and poor utilization of ineffective or inappropriate interventions (Kessler et al. 2005; Rubio and Correll 2017a, b). Paradoxically, when services are eventually accessed, current interventions are designed predominantly around end-stage, categorically defined mental disorders as they stereotypically appear during adulthood (McGorry et al. 2018a).

These treatment gaps are even more startling because the period during which early-phase mental health problems emerge plays a critical role in setting the trajectory of biological, psychological, and social milestones as well as achievements. Thus our mental health system organized around traditional categorical diagnoses in adults, instead of fundamental mental and/or physiological systems during youth, means that current approaches to classification have lacked a developmentally informed, longitudinal perspective that takes into account underlying pathophysiology and associated intraindividual variability (Fisher et al. 2018). Treatment and prevention would be far more effective if classification better reflected the naturalistic emergence and onset of mental health difficulties and disorders in youth. In other words, the design and deployment of prevention and early intervention approaches should be tied to relevant knowledge about the etiology, risk, onset, and course of early-stage mental illness (Vos et al. 2012; WHO 2014).

Fortunately, recent attention to early and distressing mental experiences in youth, aged 12–25 yr, offers opportunity for diverse forms of intervention to occur during windows as "close" as possible to the age of onset (McGorry et al. 2003). These developmentally aware approaches should ideally be informed by fundamental mental or physiological processes that increase vulnerability (or protection) for trajectories leading to youth-onset disorders in large populations or identified subgroups. This gap is not filled by alternative organizational systems, such as the research domain criteria (RDoC) from the U.S. National Institute of Mental Health's (Insel et al. 2010). Although RDoC acknowledges the role of development and environmental exposures as orthogonal assessments (Cuthbert and Insel 2010), it was explicitly developed as a research tool and is not intended to guide clinical diagnoses or decision making in its current form (Cuthbert and Insel 2013).

Accordingly, in this chapter we articulate a framework for bringing together developmentally contextualized mental and physiological processes—one that can ultimately guide characterization, staging, and interventions in mental health difficulties or disorders in youth, from population-level risk

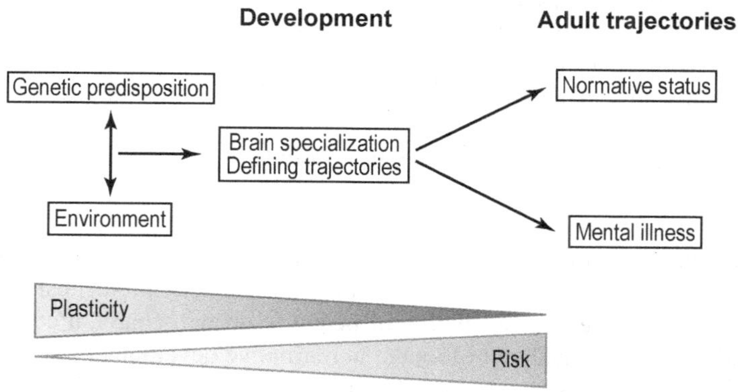

Figure 3.1 Conceptualization of a system to track developmentally salient, clinically meaningful mental/physiological systems and their translation from population-level risk to dimensions of mental ill-health. Any such schema must appreciate that there are complex relationships between these elements: etiologic factors, risk and plasticity, development, and their impact on adult trajectories.

identification to individual-level clinical care (Figure 3.1). Designing a framework and approach that draws on knowledge about developmentally informed trajectories and clinical systems to characterize and intervene in youth mental health problems involves a number of considerations. At a fundamental level, it necessitates appreciating the influence of both inherited and acquired factors (Figure 3.1, left) on brain specialization and the setting of trajectories (middle) during periods of plasticity and risk (bottom), all of which delineate adult trajectories in multiple dimensions (right). More pragmatically, it requires us to

- track a range of salient mental/physiological systems during a dynamic developmental period that includes both vulnerability and risk,
- contemplate their utility in identifying enriched groups that might benefit from further individual-level assessment in clinical or community settings, and
- translate such findings into planning prevention and intervention programs to inform clinical decision making.

Population-Level Differences in Mental and Physiological Maturation

The Framework: Identifying Vulnerable Youth

A developmentally informed approach must be embedded in appropriately contextualized population distributions as well as in knowledge regarding how an individual is progressing over time. As such, the tracking of trajectories in individuals (especially perturbations from normative trajectories), and the subsequent identification of youth at earlier (ideally preclinical) stages of distress and impairment represent key features of this framework.

An additional consideration is the choice of mental physiological systems that are themselves under development and therefore dynamically changing during adolescence. These should be purposefully selected to capture the full spectrum of relevant phenomena across an appropriate range of time points, bearing in mind variability in a range of individual- and group-level factors such as neurological and psychological developmental stage, exposure to adversity, family environment, gender identification, genetic predisposition, and cultural context. The analogy is that of pediatric growth charts, a commonly used and clinically valuable tool rooted in normative development and reflecting both physiology and external influences (Gardosi et al. 2018). A youth mental health (age 12–25 yr) analogue to growth charts could provide insight within the margins of a normative template but, importantly, would also provide information on individual-level developmental trajectories over time (Figure 3.2).

The selection of specific systems to track requires careful consideration, and an exhaustive examination of all possibilities is neither feasible nor practical given our starting point. Instead, we have identified examples of developmentally relevant, fundamental mental/physiological systems that might serve as initial systems to be investigated: sensory processing, circadian rhythm/activation, threat arousal, emotional regulation, reward salience, neurocognition, social cognition, and metacognition (sense of self). Figure 3.3 shows how the first four could be tracked over time, compared to normative trajectories. We selected these systems based on their face validity and known involvement in healthy and unhealthy mental operations: each system shows significant developmental change and growth during adolescence and has strong putative and

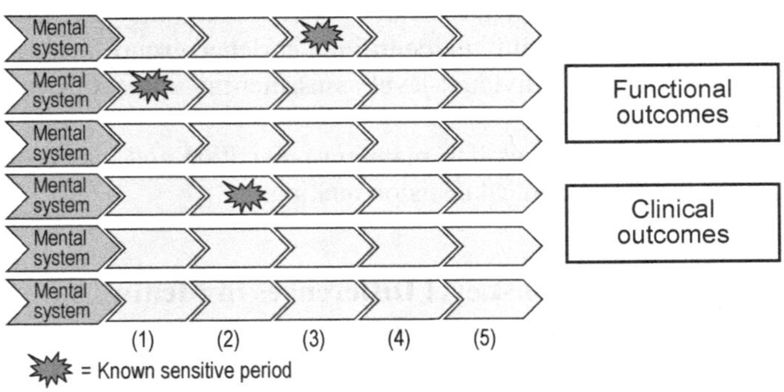

Figure 3.2 Visualization of developmental trajectories, maturation, and sensitive periods for tracking mental/physiological systems, developmental context, and clinical and functional outcomes for young people. The depicted developmental stages are (1) childhood (9–12 yr), (2) early adolescence (12–15 yr), (3) late adolescence (15–18 yr), (4) transition to adulthood (18–21 yr), and (5) early adulthood (22–25 yr).

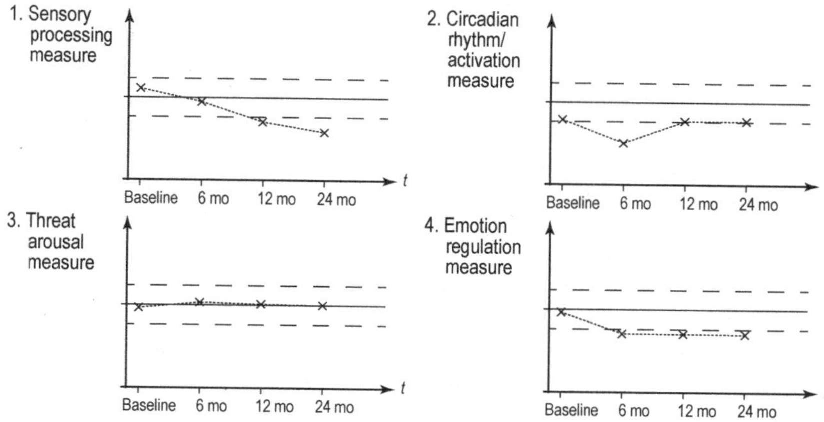

Figure 3.3 Graphical display of four proposed mental/physiological systems over time. The solid horizontal line represents the sex- and age-adjusted norm; dotted lines (above and below) represent its 95 percentile specific for each mental process domain. The line connecting each time point (e.g., baseline, 6 months, 12 months, 24 months) displays how an individual performs relative to the sex- and age-adjusted norm and relative to its own prior developmental state over time.

demonstrated links to the underlying psychopathology of emergent mental disorders in youth. Ideally, each system could be tracked in individuals over time, allowing early identification (and an offer of support) for persistent deviation from an expected trajectory.

For each of the proposed system domains, summary scores (and, possibly, subscores) on standardized measures (akin to weight percentile or BMI percentile) will need to be selected, tested, and agreed upon to enable the creation of such a multidimensional mental capacity growth chart. Ideally, all relevant dimensions would be tracked and visualized relative to each other to indicate (a) where an individual is located within normative development and (b) how any divergence tracked over time relates to the other dimensions. From a research perspective, this information would be useful to map individual and normative development across complex and interacting dimensions. For clinical decision making, it would help to identify areas of need for increased vigilance or monitoring in the context of emerging departures from normative development, low-risk preventive interventions when such departures begin to manifest clinically, or treatment of manifest abnormalities that are functionally relevant and/or lead to distress.

Contextualizing the Framework

Building on the notion of developmental trajectories, the framework presumes that there are critical or "sensitive" periods that serve as key time points at which mental/physiological "milestones" should be attained in order for optimal development to occur at the subsequent life stage. Such sensitive periods are generally timed to when important information is available and most useful to the development of the organism (Fawcett and Frankenhuis 2015). For example, molecular mechanisms of critical period plasticity markers are active throughout adolescence in association cortices (such as prefrontal cortex), indicating active specialization of systems that define adult trajectories and are involved in all psychiatric illnesses (Hickie et al., this volume; Larsen and Luna 2018). Similarly, mean performance in cognitive tasks improves through the adolescent period, with trial-to-trial variability decreasing with age (Montez et al. 2017); this suggests that processes underlying cognitive abilities are present early, but that engaging these processes in a controlled, reliable fashion is a function of development. There are also compelling examples of such sensitive periods with respect to vision (Hensch 2005b) and language acquisition (Doupe and Kuhl 1999; Werker and Hensch 2015) in early life. Failure to attain milestones in these systems may critically impair the achievement of subsequent ones. In general, however, the nature and timing of sensitive periods in adolescence for human cognitive, affective, and social development are not as well understood, yet these may be critical to understanding the developmental windows for the emergence of specific forms of psychopathology as well as for their most effective treatment modalities (Dahl et al. 2018).

Our conceptualization also assumes that an individual's departure from a normative trajectory can occur in more than one domain. Assessing such divergence across multiple domains is more likely to provide insight into the development of clinical distress, dysfunction, and disorders than if individual domains are considered in solitude. With appropriately large samples, processes may aggregate in combinations that have clinical relevance beyond that of current categorical diagnoses. For example, intraindividual variability in cognitive tasks has been commonly found to underlie schizophrenia, depression, borderline personality disorder (Kaiser et al. 2008; Millan et al. 2012), and ADHD (Munoz et al. 2003): neurocognition clearly does not define a specific disorder in its own right, but particular types of neurocognitive deficits may be found to cluster together in characteristic patterns with difficulties in other systems.

Based on the wealth of neurobiological and psychosocial evidence now available, the manifestation of non-normative trajectories in these systems during adolescence and young adulthood may be distinct from their manifestation during other periods. Specific exposures during or before youth may be especially salient in moderating risk or protective factors, particularly during the dynamic developmental period of adolescence. For example, the effects of socioeconomic factors on brain development are mitigated by exposure to positive parenting practices during early adolescence (Whittle et al. 2017). Similarly, during middle adolescence (typically 14–16 yr), developmentally relevant risk factors for a range of outcomes (e.g., peer stress, the breakup of romantic relationships, and substance misuse) may be modifiable (Bagge et al. 2013; Mirsu-Paun and Oliver 2017). Thus, environmental exposures may have at least some degree of developmental specificity that is potentially modifiable at either the population or individual level.

Finally, research is greatly needed into normal developmental trajectories for each system, so that we can delineate a threshold of trajectory divergence (and persistence) at which point individuals or families could be offered the option of closer monitoring or clinical intervention. While non-normative trajectories in individual systems may not in and of themselves reflect clinical caseness, they may (in combination with knowledge regarding sensitive or critical periods) represent the earliest signs of what could develop into one or more clinical conditions. Changes in expected trajectories may then return to the original trajectory either spontaneously or as a result of interventions; alternatively, the new trajectory may persist, accelerate, or arrest. Further research is needed to delineate thresholds of trajectory divergence and/or persistence, again in the context of knowledge regarding sensitive periods and relevance for outcomes. Once a threshold is reached, individuals or families could be offered the option of closer tracking, a more comprehensive assessment, or escalation to lower- or higher-risk clinical interventions by health services. A template for this may be found in measures of reading achievement, in which a lack of attainment of this important milestone following a known critical period signals a time-sensitive need to intervene in different ways (Kamil et al. 2016).

Techniques and Technologies to Assist Identification

Although growth charting has been a fundamental part of other areas of medicine, most prominently pediatrics, much remains unknown regarding developmentally informed charting of mental and physiological systems that might underpin youth (and ultimately adult) mental ill-health. As mentioned, the tracking of mental/physiological systems would benefit from focusing on longitudinal trajectories rather than individual snapshots; the former would emerge based on repeated outcome measurements that can be compared to a dynamically changing "normative" trajectory. A major investment in measurement development is thus required to demonstrate analytic capacity, reliability, and validity for each relevant system. Moreover, before widespread implementation, foundational work would need to be done to determine norms for each system across gender, cultures, and relevant clinical subgroups as well as for temporal variation of norms, for example, within a culture or subgroup over time.

To that end, a qualitative leap forward in the ability to track trajectories would be enabled by feasible, user friendly, affordable, and scalable passive sensing technologies that allow for continuous high-frequency sampling of a range of relevant behavioral and physiological systems (Mohr et al. 2017). Such approaches offer a unique opportunity to sample developmental changes with sufficient frequency to truly capture the dynamics of these phenomena. This high-frequency sampling may also be critical for revealing periods of greatest variability in behavioral and physiological functioning, which could correlate with plasticity during specific sensitive developmental periods. An exemplar approach increasingly used in research settings to obtain real-time fluctuations in mood and cognitive processes is the experience sampling method (ESM). This involves an individual systematically recording how they feel or what they are thinking about at multiple points across a day for several days in a row. Individuals receive a series of semi-random alerts via a beep from a mobile phone or wearable device during waking hours, and they are then tasked with completing a short questionnaire about their feelings, thoughts, social interactions, etc., at that precise moment in time. When taken together, these multiple recordings provide a more ecologically and time-sensitive assessment of a person's emotional and cognitive states and a picture of subtle fluctuations in these systems over time (e.g., 7 consecutive days) rather than a single cross-sectional snapshot (Reininghaus et al. 2016).

Clinical Application and Implementation of the Proposed Framework

Our focus here is on the potential use of the proposed system in youth mental health clinical settings, including for the purpose of decision making. Table 3.1 provides an example of an assessment tool that begins to characterize clinical correlates of each of the eight exemplar core mental/physiological systems (rows) at a single timepoint. To complete the tool, information acquired would first need to be indexed to data from developmentally informed representative population-level sampling (e.g., obtained using wearable and other mobile health technologies), as well as individual-level data that can be gathered in a clinical setting. In other words, the framework captures underlying markers that may relate to core features across a range of mental conditions and disorders, both requiring and allowing for clinical context.

The rows represent various features relevant to the characterization of each fundamental system, such as the symptom/sign manifestation, severity, duration, and developmental context. These will require clinical correlation between the raw data collected regarding mental/physiological systems and their functional impact on individuals' lives. For certain rows (e.g., the symptoms/signs and modifiable factors), free text can be entered to ensure that as much relevant clinical detail as needed is being collected. For example, in the portion, "Manifestations," clinical observations or potentially relevant factors can be added that might affect an understanding of etiology, ongoing exposures, or protective factors. In an era of patient-centered outcomes, self-rated

Table 3.1 Clinical assessment tool for the proposed framework and application for autism spectrum disorder (*) and bipolar spectrum disorder (+). The number of each symbols represents the putative severity of deviation from normative development.

	Sensory processing	Circadian system/ activation	Threat arousal	Emotional regulation	Reward salience	Neuro-cognition	Social cognition	Metacognition (sense of self)
Manifestations								
Trajectory:								
Symptoms, Signs,	+	+++	++	+++	++	***	***	*
Dysfunction	+		+	**		+		
Duration		+++		+++		**	**	
Severity		+++		+++ **		**	**	
Appraisal								
Functioning		+		+	+	**	**	
Developmental Context								
Other specific clinically relevant factors: To be completed across each domain as needed								
Childhood trauma								
Argument with spouse/peer								
Family history of bipolar disorder								
Clinician to add examples								
Interventions								
	Antisocial personality disorder	Sleep hygiene, circadian structuring, social rhythm therapy	CBT, selective serotonin reuptake inhibitors	Dialectical behavioral therapy	Addiction treatment, behavioral activation	Cognitive remediation	Social skills training	CBT, interpersonal therapy

scales and instruments should be used to make such data collection feasible in busy clinical settings. For most of the columns, data should eventually be available from developmentally appropriate standardized instruments, such as rapid neurocognitive testing batteries or high-frequency sampled physiological probes, as in circadian rhythms or threat arousal, via wearable or other new technologies.

Although the intended effect of the tool is to track mental/physiological systems in at-risk or affected individuals, Table 3.1 has been filled out for two examples: individuals with a prototypical autism spectrum disorder (*) and bipolar spectrum disorder (+)—to demonstrate relevance. There is some overlap between the two individuals, but the overall message is that each may present with non-normative features in relatively distinct systems, which in turn points to the need for different forms of early intervention that target specific systems rather than diagnoses. This example also illustrates how the system-based framework and approach intersects with clinically relevant information, and how current DSM or ICD diagnoses can transition to the targeting of system-level abnormalities that are graded in terms of severity, developmental relevance, and time trajectory (see also Figure 3.2).

Ultimately, the framework's utility at the individual level will emerge only as data in each cell in the table can be gathered easily and tracked over multiple timepoints. Although intra- and inter-individual variations in developmental timing velocity and milestone achievement may have a surprisingly wide range, we assume that clinically relevant departures from developmental norms would be traceable with sufficient sensitivity and specificity within the proposed framework by means of e-health-based and clinical longitudinal tracking across relevant individual systems. As mentioned, individual data must also be placed within the context of appropriate population norms once the latter can be appropriately contextualized across dimensions of age, sex/gender, race/ethnicity, culture, etc.

Refinement of the specific systems to be studied, or addition of novel systems, should also be investigated. Additional rows and/or columns could be added for individualized and qualitatively different sets of systems or markers, (e.g., insight). The information from Table 3.1 can also be used as a standardized means of documenting, visualizing, and communicating the collected information in clinical settings. Thus, a clinician has multiple options once they have identified a departure from a normative trajectory: they can attempt (a) to lessen the degree and impact of departure from normative development, (b) to bring system-level departures back onto a developmental track, or (c) to obtain critical information and additional data that recontextualizes the departure. This could establish opportunities and indicators of need for intervention, along with devising and validating the capacity of specific interventions (ranging from watchful waiting to increasing monitoring, to preventive measures or more intensive interventions).

Translation to Clinical Systems, Staging, and Interventions

Ethical Implications

If this framework is used for population-level screening, a persistent non-normative trajectory (or one that continues to "fall off the curve") may signify an enriched group at heightened vulnerability for a clinically relevant outcome, rather than identifying individuals with the outcome itself. Thus, as with traditional screening approaches in medicine, tools to identify potential non-normative trajectories may need to be biased toward sensitivity rather than specificity in order to capture enriched populations that can then be offered more detailed assessment. However, the move from systems of data collection based on large population studies, which utilize clinical assessments and various technologies, to the realm of health systems is fraught with challenges. Although elements of this approach have been attempted in the past, a systematic effort to bridge the public health perspective with clinical interventions and service design—from offering low-intensity interventions to groups at relatively low risk, to higher-intensity interventions for those enriched in various dimensions (e.g., family history, symptomatology, pathophysiology)—requires input from a range of disciplines, from epidemiology to ethics.

Perhaps the foremost of these challenges involves the implications of labeling individuals or vulnerable groups as "deviant" from developmental norms, along with societal or actuarial inferences that might be drawn from this. In the clinical realm, the extent to which population-level measures of mental/physiological systems map (or not) onto currently defined clinical disorders remains to be tested. This issue is intricately linked to the risk of prematurely identifying individuals as (false positive) clinical cases, based simply on raw data from mental/physiological systems. Such risk should not be taken lightly. Determining whether an individual's non-normative trajectories, dysfunction, distress, or other features meet threshold levels for "caseness" would depend, in part, on available interventions and context (clinical, local, and cultural). A clinical team might therefore suggest additional longitudinal tracking with more specific metrics and evidence-informed tools to differentiate "false positives" from those who have indeed transitioned to at-risk or early-phase clinical trajectories, bearing in mind the risk–benefit ratio of whatever preventative or other intervention is under consideration. In a public health context, the task may require identifying cases for indicated prevention programs in the community or in primary care, where issues of specificity may be less relevant. Depending on the circumstances, tracking could take place through passive data collection (via monitoring naturalistic patterns in behavior and physiological functioning) and/or more active sampling (e.g., in laboratory-based measurement of response to stressors or perturbation of the process under consideration).

With the multidimensional framework, attention to a vulnerable subgroup (e.g., those with a family history of specific mental illness) could be analyzed with regard to one or more mental/physiological systems. Specific individuals with non-normative trajectories on multiple processes could then be offered closer monitoring or even low risk–benefit interventions if they desired. A parallel example may be provided by the use of consumer smart watches to provide enhanced, continuous tracking of cardiac physiology in those at risk for cardiac disease (Koshy et al. 2018) . Similarly, relevant data and behavior could be collected via mobile, wearable technology to monitor risk of acute psychiatric crises. This could enable resources to be provided to those seeking immediate help as well as provide feedback to ameliorate symptoms, such as risk of suicide or relapse in psychosis, mania, or depression (Kennard et al. 2018; Torous et al. 2018).

Interface with Clinical Staging

A framework that overlaps with our approach, particularly once individuals are at the point of help-seeking, is that of clinical staging. In recent years, staging has been applied across the spectrum of major mood and psychotic syndromes in young people (Cross et al. 2014; Purcell et al. 2015). However, the mental/physiological systems and phenomena our framework highlights likely cut across traditional diagnoses (Table 3.1), as do presentations of youth experiencing the first phases of mental health problems or illness. Thus, clinical stages need to be more than arbitrary cutoff points on a single dimension of illness severity or duration. For example, circadian disturbance is likely to be relevant not only to those with bipolar-type disorders but in other mood and psychotic syndromes as well. Similarly, neuro- and social-cognitive processes are not only relevant to those with psychotic syndromes but are also likely to be strong predictors of social and other functional outcomes for those experiencing anxiety and mood syndromes.

In addition to its transdiagnostic parallels with our framework and approach, clinical staging can also help guide treatment selection on the basis of severity, characteristics, and personal choice rather than categorical diagnosis. Once individuals move from nonclinical to clinical settings, staging can be used to inform the entire range of decision making: from watchful waiting to invasive interventions, depending on combinations of stage, dysfunction, and distress as well as independent objective measures and other factors. In the arena of youth mental health, this implies greater use of less noxious (psychological and behavioral) approaches at early stages, reserving medications for those with more discrete syndromes or later stages of illness. It also implies that interventions are often being used for one or more purpose; that is, to treat the current syndrome and/or reduce the chance of progression to a later stage of illness.

The multidimensional framework proposed here will hopefully over time capture and map core components of biologically or clinically relevant systems onto clinical stages. In this way, it should assist the development of clinical staging, by promoting the move away from a strong reliance on either symptomatology, illness severity or duration.

Implications for Interventions

Aside from clinical staging, particular life phases (e.g., early, middle, or late adolescence as well as high school and postsecondary education) could be used to identify settings where interventions might best be situated. For example, education regarding sexual and romantic experiences has often been delivered in schools with the tone, content, and detail of delivery varying in accordance to the year of study. Similarly, studies could evaluate the effectiveness of interventions across different developmental stages, since plasticity is variable across systems and sensitive periods. This would help identify the potential for endogenous adaptation to environmental circumstances, as well as periods of particular sensitivity or those when interventions will be less effective. This, in turn, creates variable opportunities and challenges for intervention modification efforts: the proportion of individuals in certain settings (e.g., exposure to higher education) is increasing dramatically in the developed world, and may provide a more cost-effective option for interventions with high start-up costs but lower incremental costs.

This framework can also help us evaluate the impact of modifiable as well as nonmodifiable factors at differential developmental stages. For example, exposure to certain factors may cause deviations from normative development in specific systems whereas particular interventions may attenuate the impact of such factors. These exposures and stages should also be viewed in the context of sensitive periods, when particular exposures or endogenous processes may have a particularly perturbing or protective effect on one or more components. For example, childhood trauma may perturb a number of domains, including both physiological components as well as clinical measures. Alternately, factors present during the prenatal period may not be causative of a specific disorder in and of themselves. They may, however, place individuals at risk for the impact of other subsequent factors that contribute to departures from normative trajectories and mental conditions as we currently know them. Alternatively, they could be refined or redefined by using the proposed developmentally sensitive systems approach. In future work, the focus should be on understanding how certain risk and protective factors might contribute to the time of onset and subsequent course of developmental abnormalities that can culminate in mental disorders, and eventually whether relevant interventions can mitigate or supplement those factors.

Opportunities and Challenges

Our proposed framework should be viewed as a work in progress. It offers both an opportunity and a challenge, and will hopefully stimulate further research needed to clarify whether the eight initially formulated systems (along with additional dimensions) are able to yield insight into mental/physiological growth charting, and how this can best be achieved. Issues that need to be tackled to improve its impact include

- the identification and development of appropriate and scalable assessment tools for large cohorts seen and treated in real-world settings,
- the development of meaningful summary metrics, degree of integration of clinically and biologically relevant information, sufficient sensitivity, and specificity of clinically relevant thresholds for various levels of "caseness," and
- the utility for diagnostic formulation and treatment planning in clinical settings.

A further concern is that a research and implementation agenda organized around tracking mental/physiological systems over time could lead to stigmitization and discrimination of adolescents considered to be following "nonnormative" trajectories. A clear imperative, then, is to identify those at risk of future mental health problems and to offer them preventative assistance without characterizing them as being "different" or "deviant." Table 3.2 summarizes arguments for and against the proposed framework.

Setting the Course for a Future Research Agenda

This initial description of a developmentally informed approach to understanding mental/physiological systems that are indicative of emerging psychopathology during adolescence spans from populations to enriched (vulnerable) groups and to clinical or other service settings. Far from being finalized, it is a conceptual framework to be iteratively refined over time: improved knowledge regarding mental/physiological systems at the population-level will inform clinical decision making, which in turn can be utilized to further develop knowledge regarding systems at both individual and population levels. The framework also aims to contribute explicitly to the identification and validation of clinic-pathologic cutoff points, which could assist in defining both clinical stages and determining where and what kinds of interventions are required between cutoff points. The ultimate goal is to derive earlier, more specific, and personalized treatments.

Critical questions for future research of this paradigm are as follows:

- What are the most relevant, fundamental mental/physiological systems that need to be charted to best understand mental health and ill-health as it develops during childhood, adolescence, and young adulthood—the time frame when the majority of major mental disorders start to emerge?
- What are the normative trajectories of these fundamental maturational systems underlying mental disorders during adolescence?

Table 3.2 Arguments in favor and against the proposed framework and its application.

Pros	Cons
• Alternative to binary diagnostic labels, which integrates knowledge regarding normative developmental trajectories, phenomenology, and clinical staging. In doing so, it arguably promotes a more comprehensive and holistic view of the person at the center of care	• Based on assumptions about core underlying systems related to mental illness and their developmental anchoring, not all of which might be associated with clinically relevant phenomena and not all of which may be proven true by further research into the proposed mental/physiological systems
• Promotes a multidimensional understanding of individuals and their contexts that has an additional temporal quality	• Risk of being too complex and unwieldy and therefore not clinically useful
• Encourages thinking in developmental terms, with measurement of dynamic, high-frequency mental and physiological systems that might over time be found to aggregate	• Although one might see the framework's multidimensional nature as a strength, others might see this as overly dimensional, including clinicians who are trained in/used to binary classification and decision making
• Prompts health system planners, clinicians, and researchers to think jointly about the intersection of development with clinical staging for the purpose of prevention and early intervention	• Potential for providing a false sense of security for clinicians, whereby asking a larger number of questions ends up superseding the overall perspective of the patient and their social, familial, and vocational spheres
• Has the potential to evolve into precision medicine that is individualized and thus more effective	• In identifying individual systems/components, whether mental or physiological, the framework may be perceived to be reductionist
• Is sensitive to early markers of risk for mental illness or inability to thrive and could thus prevent a trajectory from veering into mental illness.	• Risk of overdiagnosing abnormal development given the large variations in normative development

- What combinations of mental/physiological systems during adolescence lead to risk for persistent distress and impairments, and in which contexts?
- How can normative and non-normative trajectories in the identified fundamental mental/physiological systems best be measured?
- To what extent could current or evolving technologies measure the systems identified in a mobile, unobtrusive manner with relatively high-frequency sampling?
- To what extent do mental/physiological systems vary depending on sampling frame (e.g., across time windows, cultures)?

- What meaningful summary metrics have clinical face validity and utility?
- How would one define "caseness" within the proprosed framework? To what extent does this vary across settings and for specific purposes?
- Are the analytic methods currently available to analyze such data (from intraindividual to vulnerable groups to youth populations) sufficient, or are further developments required?
- In individuals presenting for care, where are they in relation to their age, stage, and culturally normative trajectories, with regard to the mental/physiological systems identified?
- Do interventions that may improve mental/physiological systems lead to actual benefits in terms of reduced distress or functional impairment?
- What are the processes that best determine individual variability in impaired trajectories that would inform interventions (e.g., sex, genetics, trauma)?

Finally, it is critical to note that the success of our proposed approach and framework will not be measured by improvements in intermediate effects, such as population-level mental and physiological phenomena or systems. At its apex, the complex package of systems, methods, enrichment of vulnerable groups, clinical staging, and treatments that might be set in motion through this agenda would need to be seen through the lens of early intervention principles and implementation science. In other words, success down this path will only be realized through public campaigns to enhance mental health literacy, larger numbers of young people seeking low-threshold care voluntarily, substantial reductions in delays to care, improved delivery of stage-appropriate and developmentally sensitive interventions, reduced incidence of illness, and of course improved clinical and functional outcomes.

Context for Emerging Mental Disorders

4

A Developmental Science Perspective on Vulnerability and Intervention for Youth Mental Health

Nicholas B. Allen, Damien A. Fair,
Leslie D. Leve, Cristopher Niell, and Fred Sabb

Abstract

This chapter explores the ways in which developmental science can shed light on salient issues within developmental epidemiology and intervention science. The highly replicated pattern of typical age of onset for different classes of mental disorders suggests that these epidemiological patterns might be a result of periods of development when certain processes are highly plastic and more sensitive to environmental input (i.e., sensitive periods). Understanding the particular adaptive goals of each stage of development can thus reveal mechanisms associated with the characteristic forms of vulnerability during each life phase. Puberty appears to be a salient example of a developmental process associated with a sensitive period for social learning as well as with the emergence of a range of mental disorders that are particularly associated with social cognitive symptoms (e.g., depressive disorders). Developmental science also has implications for precision intervention. Developmental moderation of intervention effectiveness is commonly observed, but a mechanistic understanding of the processes that underlie these effects has received relatively little research attention. Although the integration of insights from developmental science into our approaches to understanding and treating mental disorders across the life span is just emerging, the prospects for greater understanding and more effective interventions appear to be promising.

Introduction

Developmental science is the study of the patterns and processes of biological, cognitive, and behavioral change that occur as an organism is growing and maturing. Our central thesis is that understanding the adaptive tasks that characterize different phases of development, and therefore the kinds of learning for which organisms are primed during these periods, offers a unique window into the mechanisms that increase vulnerability for the emergence of disorders at specific phases of life. This understanding, in turn, has the potential to inform us about how to fit treatments to individuals by matching interventions more precisely to the specific capabilities and forms of plasticity that are associated with their stage of development (i.e., developmentally informed precision medicine).

One of the striking features of the developmental epidemiology of mental disorders, especially the patterns of typical age of onset associated with specific disorders, is the consistency with which these disorders emerge at specific stages of development across multiple data sets (Jones 2013). For example, Kessler et al. (2005) reported data from the National Comorbidity Survey Replication study, a nationally representative epidemiological survey of mental disorders in the United States, and found that the median age of onset for anxiety (age 11 yr) and impulse control (11 yr) disorders was much younger than that for substance use (20 yr) and mood (30 yr) disorders. Moreover, Kessler et al. (2005) reported that half of all lifetime cases for these disorders begin by age 14 yr, and three-quarters by age 24 yr. In a subsequent review of the literature on the age of onset of mental disorders, which focused on the WHO World Mental Health Surveys, Kessler and Wang (2008) reported a very similar set of findings. Specifically, they found that the median and interquartile (IQR) range of onset age is much earlier for phobias (7–14 yr, IQR: 4–20) and impulse control disorders (7–15 yr, IQR: 4–35) than for other anxiety disorders (25–53 yr, IQR: 15–75), mood disorders (25–45 yr, IQR: 17–65), and substance disorders (18–29 yr, IQR: 16–43). They noted that although less data exist for non-affective psychoses like schizophrenia, evidence suggests that the median age of onset for these disorders is in the range of the late teens through early twenties.

These findings demonstrate that not only does each of the major classes of mental disorders have a specific and somewhat unique pattern of typical age of onset, but that the majority of individuals with a mental disorder experience the onset of the illness in childhood (< 10 yr) or adolescence (10–19 yr), which are particularly dynamic developmental periods in the life span. Although anxiety disorders are sometimes reported as a homogeneous category, it is important to note that some fear-based anxiety disorders (e.g., phobias and separation anxiety) typically begin in childhood. By contrast, other anxiety disorders that are characterized by more cognitive symptoms (e.g., worry), such as panic disorder, generalized anxiety disorder, and posttraumatic stress disorder, typically emerge after the early teens (Kessler and Wang 2008). As noted above, non-affective psychoses like schizophrenia typically begin in late adolescence or the early twenties, with males having a somewhat earlier age of onset compared to females (Häfner et al. 1989). It is also noteworthy that disorders with childhood or adolescent onset tend to be more severe, are less likely to be detected and treated, and are more likely to be associated with comorbidity, especially if untreated (Paus et al. 2008). All of this serves to emphasize the critical importance of understanding not only the underlying developmental processes that place individuals at greater risk for specific disorders during specific phases of maturation, but also how this information might inform early intervention and prevention programs.

The Emergence of Disorders during Development: The Role of Sensitive Periods

Although the patterns of typical onset age for specific disorders, described above, are well known and have been highly replicated, they are perhaps so familiar that we may forget to ask why a particular pattern, and not some other one, is observed. It is our contention that the key to understanding this is to characterize the specific developmental processes associated with each stage of the life cycle. By doing so, one can understand the nature of the particular capacities that are plastic (i.e., undergoing active growth and thus are sensitive to insult) during that phase of development. This, in turn, may help explain why, in some vulnerable individuals, these developmental processes go awry and lead to psychopathology. One approach to this set of questions, used extensively in developmental biology to characterize such periods, is the concept of *sensitive periods*.

Over time, evolutionary influences have shaped each species' development in order to regulate the timing of different forms of learning. Sensitive periods for learning are timed when important information is available and most useful to the adaptive development of the organism (Fawcett and Frankenhuis 2015). For example, humans and laboratory research animals have been found to share similar early sensitive periods in sensory regions, such as in binocular vision where there is a critical balance in the input from two eyes (Hensch 2005a). Humans also experience multiple early sensitive periods during the acquisition of language (Doupe and Kuhl 1999; Werker and Hensch 2015). Despite these compelling examples of developmental sensitive periods, the nature and timing that may exist in human cognitive, affective, and social development are not fully understood, and this may be critical to understanding the developmental windows that enable specific forms of psychopathology to emerge.

Consistent with these ideas, Ernst Mayr (1982:48) emphasized the "teleonomic" or goal-directed aspect of development:

> A physiological process or a behavior that owes its goal directedness to the operation of a program can be designated as "teleonomic"....All the processes of individual development (ontogeny) as well as all seemingly goal-directed behaviors of individuals fall in this category, and are characterized by two components: they are guided by a program, and they depend on the existence of some endpoint

> or goal that is foreseen in the program regulating the behavior….Each particular program is the result of natural selection and is constantly adjusted by the selective value of the achieved endpoint.

This approach suggests that we may be able to understand mental disorders as reflecting failures to achieve one or more of the goals of development (Costello and Angold 2016), which may provide a key to understanding why particular disorders are more likely to emerge during particular phases of life. This model, however, requires an understanding of which developmental goals are particularly salient at different developmental phases. Although there is no generally accepted taxonomy of such goals across human development, one compelling example by Sroufe and Rutter (1984) provides a series of developmental goals specific to phases of development:

- Age 0–1 yr: biological regulations, harmonious dyadic interaction, formation of an effective attachment relationship
- Age 1–2.5 yr: exploration, experimentation, and mastery of the object world (caregiver as secure base); individuation and autonomy; response to external control impulses
- Age 3–5 yr: flexible self-control, self-reliance, initiative, identification and gender concept; establishment of effective peer contacts (empathy)
- Age 6–12 yr: social understanding (equity, fairness), gender constancy, same-sex friendships, sense of "industry" (competence), school adjustment
- Age 13+ yr: "formal operations" (flexible perspective taking, "as-if" thinking), loyal friendships (same sex), beginning heterosexual relationships, independence from family, identity

Such a system has a number of potential implications for understanding the developmental epidemiology of psychopathology (Costello and Angold 2016). First, it suggests that if we want to understand the developmental vulnerability to, and prevention of, a particular disorder, we must understand the normal developmental processes involved in the emergence of a particular capacity. To understand the emergence and treatment of anxiety disorders, we need to characterize how organisms respond to threat as well as the various systems (i.e., affective, cognitive, social, and behavioral) that are most involved with regulating these challenges at different stages of development. For example, the emergence of fear-based anxiety disorders, such as phobia and separation anxiety disorders during early childhood, could be related to the developmental goals associated with exploration and mastery of the external world (i.e., discovering what is safe and what is dangerous) and the requirement of caregivers as a secure base to facilitate such exploration. The later emergence of worry-based anxiety disorders, such as generalized anxiety and social phobia (Kessler and Wang 2008), might be related to the later emergence of social understanding and formal operations; that is, the emergence of "if-then" thinking might be a prerequisite to the symptomatic processes of rumination and worry. Finally, the emergence of mood disorders, which involve prominent symptoms associated with social cognition (e.g., self-critical attitudes, concerns with one's social value), may be related to peripubertal developmental processes associated with social learning during the establishment of loyal friendships, sexual relationships, and personal identity (Allen and Badcock 2003).

Second, this developmental approach suggests that psychopathological conditions that present in various ways during different developmental stages may share similar underlying mechanisms. For example, anxious attachment in a one-year-old may be linked to the emotional liability in the same child at age five, as well as to an inability to form lasting intimate relationships during adulthood (Costello and Angold 2016). Accordingly, interventions designed to support secure attachments in infants may not only have benefits for anxiety in one-year-olds, but also prevent social dysfunction during adolescence and adulthood.

Puberty as an Example

Puberty appears to be a key inflection point in the developmental epidemiology of mental disorders, with a number of major mental disorders showing dramatic increases in incidence during the peri- and postpubertal period, including depressive disorders, eating disorders, and substance use disorders (Patton and Viner 2007). As such, to understand developmental psychopathology we need to understand the nature of the developmental processes that occur during puberty, and how this might influence developmental goals and sensitive periods of learning. Indeed, extensive cross-species work on puberty offers especially useful insights into the nature of the sensitive periods that occur during this phase of development, thus providing important evidence to support the proposition that puberty is a critical period of development for social learning in particular.

For example, human social learning during the pubertal transition may share some parallels with sensitive periods for the acquisition of song learning in songbirds (Dahl et al. 2018). Gonadal hormones are thought to regulate the neurobiology of song learning by altering both motor flexibility and the salience of social cues. Changes in salience are thought to ensure appropriate selection of the song to be copied (i.e., the correct species, time, and context) and selection of an appropriate mate (Bottjer and Johnson 1997; Marler et al. 1988; Matragrano et al. 2013). In mammals, frontal neocortical areas, which play a critical role in higher cognition, self-regulation, and social behaviors, develop late: from the time of pubertal milestones into early adulthood (Piekarski et al. 2017b). In laboratory mice, the onset of puberty has been found to alter frontal cortex neurobiology rapidly, changing inhibitory neurotransmission mechanisms previously identified as key regulators of sensitive periods in the neocortex (Piekarski et al. 2017a, b). Changes in frontal cortex inhibitory neurotransmission can also be connected to changes in learning, thus suggesting a causal link between puberty and adolescent shifts in social learning. Indeed, in rats, the adolescent period is characterized by social learning such as rough and tumble play and learning about sexual encounters. Interestingly, male rats need exposure to testosterone during adolescence to display rapid learning from sexual experience, and they do not recover this learning if testosterone is replaced in adulthood (Schulz and Sisk 2016). Thus, in rodents, as in birdsong, we see a repeated pattern whereby developmental signals (specifically, the pubertal rise in gonadal hormones) prime the brain's ability to learn during an adolescent sensitive period when the information is (a) available in the environment and (b) developmentally appropriate.

If comparable sensitive period processes occur in association with pubertal maturation in humans, this could inform developmental timing and targets for interventions. For instance, if pubertal hormones underpin distinct changes in social learning, leveraging these insights by designing interventions to target this window of opportunity could have large, positive effects on developmental trajectories. In fact, human studies have shown that the sharp rise in testosterone at the onset of puberty in human boys as well as girls is associated with shifts in social and affective information processing (Braams et al. 2015; Cardoos et al. 2017; Spielberg et al. 2014) and increased prioritization of social status feedback (Cardoos et al. 2017). In their review of decades of research into the behavioral effects of testosterone in animals and humans, Bos et al. (2012) concluded that testosterone increases the "motivation to gain social status." In humans, the process of earning status and prestige through prosocial actions may influence developmental trajectories in a manner that is separate from gaining status through aggressive dominance (Allen and Badcock 2003; Cheng et al. 2013). This may result in puberty being a sensitive period during which various experiences of earning prestige (e.g., through popularity, kindness, or aggression) may more powerfully influence learning, and thus ongoing trajectories of status-seeking behaviors (for good or ill), than at other stages of development (Dahl et al. 2018).

Implications for Intervention

Here we explore some of the implications of taking a developmental science perspective on psychopathology for intervention approaches. One of the key features evident in any intervention trial is the very significant variability in outcomes observed among participants. Consequently, there have been calls to understand the most salient moderators of intervention effects (e.g., Kraemer et al. 2002). Examining this issue has at least two major benefits: it facilitates precision medicine to ensure that treatments and interventions can be targeted to individuals who will benefit most (Collins and Varmus 2015), and it can help researchers to elucidate mechanisms of risk and disease.

The types of moderators that may exist for intervention effects can include both individual (participant) characteristics and intervention program features, such as content, provider, and design (Stice et al. 2009). Our focus here is on individual participant factors. Further, we address issues relevant to psychosocial intervention, as they are likely to be most informed by models of sensitive periods for learning.

There is a range of other individual moderating factors that have been studied in the context of intervention studies with children and adolescents. For example, sex is one of the most studied individual moderators of intervention effects. In general, females appear to benefit more from intervention and prevention programs that target psychological processes and risk factors (Stice et al. 2009). However, sex is clearly a relatively coarse measure of individual differences and needs to be supplemented by approaches that allow a more precise and fine-grained matching of individuals to interventions. Other moderators of intervention effects include socioeconomic disadvantage (Chen and Miller 2013) and genetics (Musci et al. 2014). Research is beginning to identify ways in which interventions can be matched to groups of individuals most likely to benefit. However, despite the fact that one of the greatest sources of individual variability among children and youth is their varying degrees of maturation, developmental factors have received relatively little systematic investigation as moderators of treatment effects. An extensive literature addresses the general question of which interventions are appropriate for children, adolescents, and adults as broad (and very developmentally imprecise) categories. However, little of this research has framed this question in terms of specific developmental *processes* that might serve to match individuals with treatments specifically designed to match their developmental capacities and/or critical inflection points in plasticity. In a recently published review on the developmental demands of cognitive behavioral therapy for depression in children and adolescents, Garber et al. (2016:208) concluded that "further research is needed to clarify the relations between specific skills taught to children in therapy and various developmental abilities, to determine the adequacy of existing assessment tools for creating a developmental profile for children entering therapy, and to identify the most effective strategies for tailoring treatment to a child's specific developmental level in the relevant domains."

Development as a Moderator of Intervention Effects

It seems plausible that older children and adolescents may be able to understand and utilize some of the concepts presented in psychosocial intervention programs better than younger adolescents or children, especially those that rely on complex self-regulation or decision-making skills based on executive cognitive functions. Consistent with this, a meta-analysis has shown that age was a significant moderator of depression prevention programs for youth, with older age predicting greater effectiveness (Stice et al. 2009). Another meta-analysis of eating disorder prevention programs found similar results (Stice and Shaw 2004). There have also been some failures to observe age moderation effects in treatment studies. For example, grade level was found not to be a moderator of the effect of a mindfulness intervention on self-regulation skills in primary school children (Alfano et al. 2009; Gould et al. 2012). It is unclear, however, whether these failures resulted from substantive (i.e., developmental processes are less relevant to these interventions) or methodological (e.g., low power to detect such effects) issues. Nevertheless, these findings suggest that some interventions might show stronger developmental moderation than others.

Developmental measures other than chronological age have also been known to moderate intervention effects in some cases. As noted above, one particularly salient developmental process during early adolescence is puberty, which may offer a better measure of maturation during this phase of life than chronological age. Indeed, pubertal development has been observed to moderate intervention effects. For example, an intervention designed to improve body self-esteem was found to be more beneficial among students who had already begun puberty (Cousineau et al. 2010), suggesting that those who had already experienced the developmental processes addressed in the program were more able to benefit.

What is missing in all of these studies is a mechanistic understanding of precisely *why* and *how* developmental differences determine differential responses to intervention. To achieve this, we need to take a more in-depth approach to understanding how specific developmental processes influence sensitivity to these environmental inputs.

Moderating Intervention Effects: Platforms and Plasticity

There are various ways in which developmental differences might interact to potentiate intervention effects. Some developmental differences, for instance, may be associated with the emergence of cognitive or self-regulatory abilities that provide a necessary *platform* to benefit from specific intervention techniques. One example might be an intervention that requires social perspective taking, often used in interventions for interpersonal aggression (Chalmers and Townshend 1990). Abilities associated with mentalizing and theory of mind are required for social perspective taking, yet they show significant developmental change across childhood and adolescence (Dumontheil et al. 2010). Still, without these abilities, the necessary cognitive platform will not be in place and the individual will be unable to utilize fully the techniques presented in the intervention. Such developmental platforms act primarily as moderators of treatment effects.

Periods of developmental change also involve significant *neural plasticity*. Environmental exposure can have a significant impact on sensitive periods (discussed above) as the brain is particularly susceptible to specific kinds of input during this time (Fawcett and Frankenhuis 2015). These periods of heightened plasticity may also act as moderators of treatment effects, by increasing the effectiveness of treatment during particular phases of development. They may also point the way to salient mediators (or mechanisms) by which interventions have such effects, by influencing trajectories via their enhanced impact on neural or psychological development during windows of high plasticity.

Defining Development: Limitations of Chronological Age and the Need for Developmentally Precise Measures

Typically, chronological age is used to define an individual's developmental stage or maturation. However, age is always, at best, an imperfect measure of maturation, a fact that has been recognized within developmental research for some time (Wohlwill 1970). This is particularly the case during adolescence, when developmental processes such as puberty and physical maturation can markedly vary between individuals of the same chronological age, even more so than at other developmental stages (Ellis 2004; Mirwald et al. 2002).

We need to develop ways of quantifying maturation such that there is a strong link between the maturational process being measured and the characteristics that act as proximal moderators of intervention effects (i.e., developmental differences in how cognitive, affective, and self-regulatory processes influence the ability to learn and utilize skills that enhance the management of mental health symptoms and risk factors). This will provide a platform to understand more fully the ways in which developmental variability might influence the impact of interventions. Given the neurodevelopmental processes that occur during the second decade of life, and the likely links between neurodevelopment and the emergence of capacities that will moderate intervention effects (such as executive cognitive functions), examining brain development may be an especially propitious way to advance our understanding of these issues. Indeed, developing reliable neurocognitive markers of adolescent development would be a boon to developmental science more broadly, as it would provide an important complement to other non-age-based measures of maturation that could have wide application.

Adolescent Brain and Cognitive Development

Adolescence is a particularly dynamic period of brain development, second only to infancy in terms of the extent and significance of neural changes that occur: neurobiological changes are observed in brain structure, function, and connectivity (Dahl et al. 2018). Overall, these brain changes are hypothesized to underpin growth in adolescent capabilities to engage in higher-order cognitive functions, including cognitive control and the regulation of behavior and emotion (Steinberg 2005). These normative developmental processes are required to prepare the brain to respond to the demands of both adolescence and future adult life, but they may also increase vulnerability for risk behavior and psychopathology (Paus et al. 2008).

Many changes in cognitive processing that occur during adolescence have been well established in the literature, suggesting that as adolescents develop, they show improvements in a variety of cognitive domains, including learning, reasoning, information processing, and memory (Kuhn 2006). In particular, cognitive control capabilities, which facilitate self-regulation of thoughts, actions, and emotions, continue to develop throughout adolescence in parallel with brain changes (Kesek et al. 2008). Cognitive control consists of distinct component processes that appear to be primarily supported by somewhat different cortical regions and to have distinct developmental trajectories (Dosenbach et al. 2006, 2008). For example, although the greatest developmental improvements in response inhibition and interference control are typically observed prior to adolescence, improvements in flexibility, error monitoring, and the updating of working memory are more likely to occur throughout the second decade of life (Crone and Steinbeis 2017). Those functions which do continue to show significant developmental change during adolescence seem to rely especially on the capacity for abstract representation, a capacity that increases distinctly during adolescence (Dumontheil 2014). The capacity for abstract representation can relate to both temporal (e.g., long-term goals, past or future events) and relational (e.g., higher-order relationships between representations rather simple stimulus features) processes (Dumontheil 2014). These increases in abstract thought lead to improvements in deductive reasoning, information processing, and the capacity for abstract, planned, hypothetical, and multidimensional thinking.

Recent research on cognitive development during adolescence has focused on both cognitive and affective processing, particularly in terms of how these processes interact and influence each other in the context of adolescent decision making. The capacity for abstract representation as well as for affective engagement with such representations (Davey et al. 2008) increases the capacity for self-regulation of affect (e.g., the capacity to initiate new or alter ongoing emotional responses) to achieve a goal (Ochsner and Gross 2005). Indeed, such capacities may specifically rely on the ability to represent and affectively engage with a longer-term goal to regulate a prepotent, stimulus-driven affective response. Short-term stimulus-driven affective influences on cognitive processing (including decision making, risk taking, and judgment) significantly change over adolescence (Hartley and Somerville 2015). The social and emotional context for cognitive processing during adolescence may also include factors such as the presence of peers or the value of performing a task, which are hypothesized to influence the motivational salience of specific contexts and the extent to which cognitive processing is recruited (Johnson et al. 2009). There is also increasing evidence that some of these changes in cognitive and affective processing are linked to the onset of puberty (Crone and Dahl 2012), and that flexibility of the frontal cortical network may be greater in adolescence than in adulthood (Jolles and Crone 2012).

These changes in cognitive functioning may have adaptive qualities that are part of normative adolescent development, but may also confer vulnerability to psychopathology in some individuals. Flexibility of cognitive control may result in an improved ability to learn to navigate the increasingly complex social challenges that are part of adolescents' social worlds. In addition, the ability to shift focus in a highly motivated way could allow increases in learning, problem solving, and the use of creativity (Kleibeuker et al. 2016). Of particular relevance here, such emerging abilities may also determine the degree to which an individual can take advantage of new learning opportunities, including mental health-promoting interventions.

A New Approach to Understanding Individual Differences in Development: Quantifying the Maturation of Neural Systems

Recent attempts to quantify brain maturation have most often utilized functional connectivity measures of the whole brain, whereby connectivity is calculated by correlating fMRI measurements between brain regions while subjects are "at rest" and not engaged in completing specific tasks (Dosenbach et al. 2010). Such measures offer significant advantages in terms of quantifying neural maturation: the task-free nature of the approach increases their generalizability (especially across development), there are no practice effects (facilitating repeated measurement within individuals), and resting-state measures generally show good test–retest reliability (e.g., Choe et al. 2015). Dosenbach et al. (2010) used multivariate pattern analysis (MVPA) methods to develop an estimate of each participant's functional connectivity maturation level, which explained 55% of the variance in chronological age; the cingulo-opercular and frontoparietal control networks showed the greatest changes. The pattern of MVPA feature weights indicated that functional maturation was driven both by the segregation of nearby functional areas, via the weakening of short-range functional connections, and the integration of distant regions into broader functional networks, by strengthening of long-range functional connections. These findings have now been replicated with new advanced techniques (e.g., Fair et al. 2013) in image processing and analysis. Moreover, deviation from normative growth curves in these maturational patterns has been associated with attentional control problems in youth. This suggests that maturation of these networks may critically underlie the development of executive control and abstract reasoning during adolescence.

These changes also have structural analogs. Networks of myelinated fibers, as measured through diffusion tensor imaging (DTI), gradually mature from local, proximity-based connectivity patterns to a more distributed, integrative pattern (Vertes and Bullmore 2015): a developmental shift that has also been proposed to support higher cognitive functioning. In a recent study, Baum et al. (2017) applied network analytic techniques to DTI data from a large sample of participants aged 8–22 yr and found that white matter networks become increasingly modular during adolescent development, but that targeted strengthening of hub connections also facilitated more global network integration. Importantly, these neurodevelopmental changes in patterns of structural connectivity mediated improvements in executive functioning during childhood and adolescence (specifically measures of attention, working memory, and abstraction/flexibility). Other recent reports from this cohort have demonstrated that abnormal patterns of neurodevelopmental change in connectivity, both in terms of the pattern and timing of these changes, are associated with increased risk for psychopathology (Alnæs et al. 2018; Kaufmann et al. 2017).

In sum, both functional and structural measures support models of increasing integration and segregation of networks across development. Although the principal focus in studies of adolescent brain development has thus far been on age-related changes, findings such as peaks in gray matter density, which coincide with timing of puberty onset, suggest that neurodevelopmental patterns align better with pubertal changes than with chronological age (Blakemore et al. 2010).

Developmental Consequences of Brain Network Maturation and Moderation of Intervention Effects

To date, no studies have applied these network-based measures of brain maturation to understand differential responses to intervention effects. However, there is a small literature that has explored the phenotypic and cognitive correlates of these neurodevelopmental patterns. As noted above, the current literature on structural and functional change associated with brain maturation suggests a model of tighter "integration" of some regions into long-range networks over development, while short-range connections between other sets of regions are segregated into separate networks. Crone and Dahl (2012) have proposed that because these long-range connectivity patterns are still maturing, it is likely that some aspects of executive function may be less automatic and more flexible during adolescence. This results in greater vulnerability on attentional and decision-making tasks under high demands (as the ability to integrate control is less automatic) and enables adolescents to respond in novel and adaptive ways. Dumontheil (2014) has proposed that the rostral prefrontal cortex (PFC) supports self-generated, abstract thought processing, and that the ability to attend flexibly to and process abstract representations develops in adolescence. Moreover, rostral PFC activation becomes more specific to relational integration during development. This may suggest that adolescence is a crucial time of development during which specific learning (or training) experiences may actively sculpt final connectivity patterns in some of these long-range executive function networks (i.e., plasticity; discussed above). In other words, this may be a particularly important period for the beneficial neurodevelopmental effects of psychosocial interventions, especially those that enhance self-regulatory abilities.

Integrating Neurocognitive Development into Precision Prevention and Early Intervention

Most psychosocial interventions aimed at treating or preventing mental disorders involve some combination of psychoeducational, cognitive, and behavioral techniques. The capacity of an individual to implement these techniques effectively relies on many of the executive functions that are thought to develop during adolescence. For example, many intervention techniques rely on the following cognitive skills (Garber et al. 2016):

- Metacognition: identifying thoughts or differentiating situations, thoughts, and feelings
- Recognition that thoughts can change
- Identification of different kinds of helpful and unhelpful thoughts
- Reasoning abilities: recognizing relationships between thoughts and feelings
- Cognitive flexibility

In addition, interventions often rely on social skills (e.g., self-reflection, social perspective taking, resistance to peer influence) and emotion regulation, especially the capacity to resist a strong prepotent, stimulus-driven affective response in service of a longer-term, temporally distant, goal. Critically, many of these capacities rely on the ability to represent, process, and affectively engage with temporally distant or relational abstract thoughts (Dumontheil 2014). However, there has been a dearth of studies in intervention science that have specifically studied the way in which developmental processes can act as salient moderators of an individual's capacity to benefit from these interventions. This opportunity to conduct such studies is particularly salient during adolescence, when the development of executive functions (especially those that rely on abstract representation) is occurring in concert with dramatic neurobiological changes. Adolescence is a key period in life that should be targeted for prevention and early intervention. Given the emergence of new insights into cognitive development, along with new methods for estimating neurobiological maturation based on characterizing both the functional and structural aspect of the neural connectome, such research programs need to be prioritized in the future. Ultimately, insights gained from these will advance developmental science, cognitive science, and intervention science.

Conclusion

Developmental science offers insight into salient issues within developmental epidemiology and intervention science, particularly early intervention and prevention approaches to mental health. It brings attention to the highly replicated pattern of typical age of onset for different classes of mental disorders and suggests that they should be interpreted in terms of the different patterns of vulnerability created by periods of development, when certain processes are highly plastic and more sensitive to environmental input. If we understand the particular adaptive goals of each developmental stage, we can generate plausible hypotheses about the underlying mechanisms associated with vulnerability to the mental disorders that show increased incidence during each stage of life.

Based on converging human and animal research into the effects of gonadal hormones on brain development and environmental sensitivity, we propose that puberty is a particularly sensitive period for social learning. A deeper understanding of the developmental process holds promise for precision intervention and may permit interventions to be matched to individuals who are most likely to benefit from them. Although developmental moderation of intervention effectiveness is commonly observed, these processes have received relatively little systematic attention as variables that can be used to tailor intervention to specific individuals. The usual methods of describing development and maturation in clinical settings (i.e., chronological age) are very imprecise, especially during adolescence. However, brain and cognitive sciences are rapidly developing alternative methods of conceptualization and measurement and may be able to advance our understanding of these issues. In sum, although we have just started to integrate insights from developmental science into an approach that looks at and treats mental disorders across the life span, our prospects for new learning and more effective interventions appear to be strong.

5

How Are Developing Social Relationships Relevant to Risk and Resilience in Youth Mental Health?

Kerstin Konrad and Hannah F. Behrendt

Abstract

This chapter provides a comprehensive overview of the impact of social context factors, conceptualized as both risk and resilience factors, on the emergence of youth (age 15–24 years) mental health problems. The influences of cultural background (i.e., individualism vs. collectivism) and recent societal developments (e.g., digital media use) are explored, as are innovative technological advances which may aid reliable measurement of such factors in future studies. It critically discusses the concept of a second sensitive period for social experiences to impact youth development starting in adolescence (age 10–19 years). It is argued that goals in social development may undergo systematic shifts across the life span and that social experiences in each developmental phase are interdependent insofar as their effects cascade into successive periods. To further understanding and improve treatment of youth psychopathology, conceptual models need to be broadened to include multiple, interdependent sensitive periods of social development. The timing of social experiences may play a central role in the efficacy of different types of interventions.

Introduction

The transition from childhood to adulthood is a developmental period that is highly influenced by social and cultural contexts. In addition to coping with dramatic changes in their physical appearance, adolescents must master changes in their social environment and accomplish a variety of social tasks as they prepare for adult responsibilities (e.g., productivity or fertility). In parallel, many mental disorders have their onset during this developmental period (Paus et al. 2008). Most adolescents, however, cope successfully with the transition from dependence on a caregiver to being a self-sufficient member of society, which demonstrates large individual differences with respect to adolescent vulnerabilities.

The adolescent transition period as well as the prevalence of mental disorders may also differ dramatically, depending on cultural context (Lund et al. 2018). An examination of how cultural and societal differences may impact adolescent development is thus crucial if we are to understand how social contexts and experiences may shape and impact youth mental health and well-being. To date, our understanding of how these social contexts influence individual development (i.e., interact with individual differences such as genetic variation) and generate or moderate the emergence of psychopathology is still limited.

In this chapter, we focus primarily on adolescent social and cultural contexts and explore how social experiences may influence youth mental health and the emergence of psychopathology. Specifically, we address the following questions:

- What are the most important social risk and resilience factors to youth mental health? Are these factors influenced by cultural backgrounds and recent societal change (e.g., digitalization, increased use of digital media)?
- How can we characterize and/or quantify social and cultural contexts of psychopathology?
- Is there really a (second) sensitive period for social influences during adolescence? Are the effects of social experiences particularly strong during adolescence?
- How do adolescent precursors, risk, and resilience factors to youth mental health evolve over time? How do they interact and what possible mechanisms underlie the associations between social risk factors and the development of psychopathology?

General Background

Eissler (1958) described adolescent patients as "neurotic at one time and almost psychotic at another." Although not literally true, this quote demonstrates the markedly fluctuating mental changes that are characteristic of individuals during this developmental period.

Many mental disorders emerge in adolescence. The earlier the disorders manifest in life, the worse the prognosis, its symptom chronicity, and the poorer the treatment response (Paus et al. 2008). Before the age of 25 years, 75% of individuals with mental illness experience their first symptoms (e.g., Kim-Cohen et al. 2003). According to the World Population Prospects, the estimated lifetime prevalence for any mental health disorder in this age group is around 45%, with a worldwide pooled point prevalence of 13%; this means that currently about 96 million youth worldwide are affected by mental health problems (Erskine et al. 2015). In addition, a higher prevalence of mental health problems is often reported for particular groups: for individuals with lower socioeconomic status or who belong to minority ethnic groups, as well as those living in more rural or remote areas (WHO 2012). Mental health problems in youth increase the risk of negative outcomes, such as lower educational achievement, higher likelihood of engagement in risky behaviors, higher rates of self-harm and suicide, as well as loss of productivity and reduced involvement in the community later in life. The most prevalent and impairing psychiatric diagnoses among children, adolescents, and youth are depression, anxiety, disruptive behavior disorders, attention deficit hyperactivity disorder, and substance use disorders. Risk-taking behavior (e.g., substance abuse, delinquent behavior) and self-harm—both considered early risk markers for psychopathology—are common among youth. In 2010, mental disorders were responsible for ~55.5 million disability-adjusted life years in individuals aged 0–24 years, thus accounting for ~5.7% of total disease burden in this age group (WHO 2012). Given the dramatic increase and chronic course of youth-onset mental disorders, together with the significant individual and societal costs (de Girolamo et al. 2012), it is critically important to enhance resilience and to increase youth mental health through preventive or early interventions. To date, however, appreciation of this increasing global burden of youth mental disorders has been based mainly on epidemiological studies conducted in Europe and North America. In developing countries, youth mental health issues have largely been neglected and the demographics of the global population poorly represented, yet up to 80% of youth worldwide live in low- and middle-income countries (see UN 2003; Atilola 2015).

The transition from childhood into adulthood involves a multitude of developmental tasks that are predominantly of a social nature. These age-specific developmental tasks vary according to the individual, the peer group, the family of origin, and the individual's role in society. Further, the formation of interpersonal relationships, individual interests, and ethical values shape personality development and may have long-term consequences on physical and mental health. Youth are confronted with social norms and societal (i.e., legal) rules that require decision making in accordance with individual goals and perspectives. Parents and the broader family context lose some of their significance as the peer group takes on greater influence. In Western societies, the peer group is particularly influential with respect to clothing, leisure activities, and attitudes toward school and education. Nonetheless, youth often join, at least initially, peer groups whose values resemble those of their parents. In addition, according to recent surveys in Germany, most youth reported that they had good relationships with their parents; only 9% reported that they could hardly get along with their parents (Herpertz-Dahlmann et al. 2013).

Social Risk and Resilience Factors in Youth Mental Health

What are the most important social risk and resilience factors to youth mental health? Previous research provides support for the premise that resilience may be protective against the development of mental health problems (Luthar and Cicchetti 2000; Dray et al. 2017). Despite recent growth in the field of resilience research, the terminology that is used to describe the concept of resilience, as well as the qualities and processes that may offer protection against negative outcomes, continues to vary greatly; to date, there is no universally employed operational definition (Luthar and Zelazo 2003; Davydov et al. 2010). Resilience is commonly referred to as a dynamic and multidimensional concept that comprises a collection of protective factors that are internal to the individual (e.g., personal resources, abilities and assets such as self-efficacy, coping skills, effective problem solving) as well as external. The latter include characteristics of the individual's broader social context, such as resources in the family, social, and community environments, family and peer relationships, support and meaningful participation within the home, school, and community environments. When these protective factors are strengthened and used by an individual during times of disadvantage or adversity, they promote a desirable outcome, such as the maintenance of or return to positive mental health or the prevention of a negative mental health outcome (Luthar and Zelazo 2003; Davydov et al. 2010).

In different studies, a number of nonspecific resilience and risk factors to mental health over the life span have been identified (for a comprehensive overview, see WHO 2012). Table 5.1 and Figure 5.1 provide an overview of nonspecific resilience and risk factors to mental health over the life span. In adolescence (age 10–19 years), key protective factors include supportive parenting, a secure home life, and a positive learning environment in schools. Overall, existing studies have found the presence of multiple protective factors (e.g., personal and social competence, perceived level of family cohesion, and social resources) to be associated with positive mental health outcome in adolescents, such as reduced symptoms of depression, anxiety, stress, and obsessive-compulsive disorder (Hjemdal et al. 2011). Adolescents with a parent who has a mental illness or substance use disorder, on the other hand, are at high risk of experiencing adverse social experiences, and thus more likely to have mental health problems themselves (Patel et al. 2007; Merikangas et al. 2009). Risk to youth mental health, more broadly, is related to similar adverse social experiences, conditions, and environments that impact mental health of children. Family violence or conflict, stressful life events, and a low sense of connection to schools or other learning environments constitute key risk factors (WHO 2012). Additionally, a number of other risks to youth mental and physical health are pertinent to emotional instability, which characterizes this formative developmental period in an individual's life. Emotional instability during adolescence is considered to be a continuum of normative development, yet out

Table 5.1 Overview of nonspecific risk and resilience factors to mental health over the life span (adapted from WHO 2012).

Context	Risk Factors	Resilience Factors
Personal	Low self-esteem Cognitive and emotional immaturity (e.g., difficulties in emotion regulation) Difficulties in communicating Medical illness, substance use	Self-esteem, self-worth, confidence Ability to solve problems and regulate stress and adversity Communication skills Physical health, fitness
Social	Loneliness, bereavement Neglect, family conflict Exposure to violence, abuse Low income or poverty Difficulties or failure at school Work stress, unemployment	Social support of family and friends, close confidants Supportive parenting (e.g., parental warmth), positive family interactions and relationships Physical security and safety Economic security Educational achievement Satisfaction and success at work/school
Environmental	Poor access to basic services Injustice and discrimination Social and gender inequalities Exposure to war, civil conflict, or natural disasters	Equality of access to basic services Social justice, tolerance, integration Social and gender equality Physical security and safety

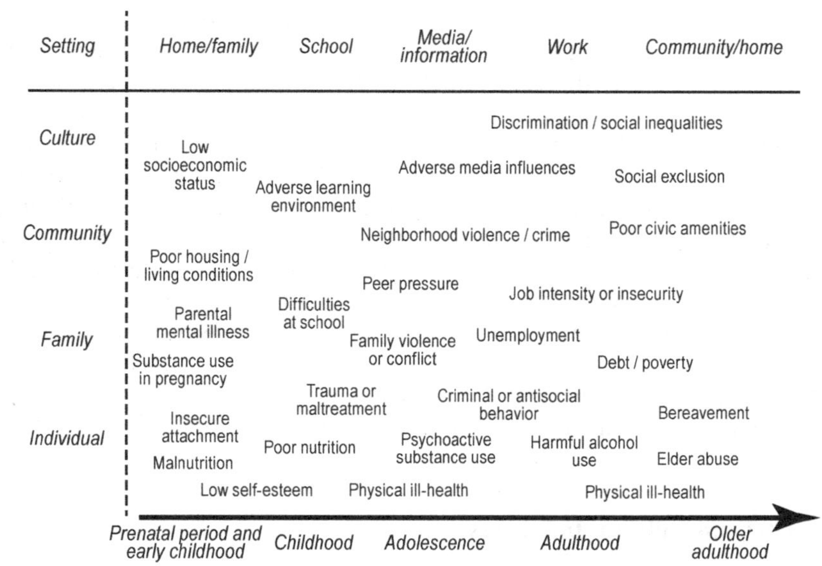

Figure 5.1 Schematic overview of risks to mental health over the course of the life span (used with permission from WHO 2012).

of the majority of adolescents who experience phases of emotional instability, only a few develop clinical psychopathology. The WHO report (2012) specifically highlights that adolescents tend to show an increased likelihood to engage in tobacco/alcohol/drug use and other risk-taking behaviors (e.g., related to sexuality, delinquency/criminality) and that the onset of substance abuse or substance-related mental disorders typically occurs during adolescence. At the same time, adolescents become increasingly susceptible to peer pressure and (social) media influences, which may promote substance use and risk-taking behaviors in general. Substance use is particularly dangerous as it can be harmful to neural and physical development. In addition, risk-taking behaviors, such as substance use, in adolescence are negatively associated with professional development trajectories, such as poorer educational achievement (WHO 2012).

In addition to nonspecific risk factors, the importance of disorder-specific factors needs to be stressed. Depression in adolescence—one of the most common mental health disorders that manifests during or shortly after adolescence (Merikangas et al. 2009)—is thought to arise due to the influence of both specific and nonspecific risk factors. Specific risk factors include a family history of affective disorders, a negative cognitive style, or a major loss experience (e.g., death of a parent, separation or divorce of parents, or household relocation). Negative cognitive styles are characterized by hopelessness, low self-confidence, and pessimistic attributions ("I'm no good at anything," "Nobody likes me"), among other features. Nonspecific risk factors include poverty, experience of violence, other negative life experiences (e.g., major conflicts in the home, neglect), and social isolation (Shaikh and Kauppi 2010). A review of disorder-specific risk and resilience factors for every psychiatric disorder that is prevalent in adolescents/youth exceeds the scope of this chapter. However, gender differences in the emergence of psychopathology during adolescence prompt the question as to whether risk and resilience factors may differ between genders (Dray et al. 2017). Moreover, the majority of existing concepts of resilience have failed to distinguish between different mechanisms that might underlie the capacity for, and process of, resilience as well as the use of protective factors. Lau and Waters (2017) offer an intriguing perspective on the context of the emergence of affective disorders (i.e., depression and anxiety) during childhood and adolescence. They find that proximal factors, such as information-processing mechanisms, could mediate effects of distal factors (e.g., genetic and environmental influences, temperament characteristics, and brain circuitry functioning) on symptomatology, and thus might account for an individual's increased risk for negative mental health outcomes (Lau and Waters 2017).

Societal and Cultural Influences

Are social risk and resilience influenced by cultural backgrounds and societal change (e.g., digitalization, increased use of digital media)? Although it has been broadly suggested that the Industrial Revolution caused adolescence to emerge as a concrete, formative period in development, ethnographic data from more than 170 preindustrial societies indicate that almost all societies possess a notion of adolescence. In many societies, the beginning of adolescence is marked by initiation ceremonies, or rites of passage, often celebrated as major public events and thematically consistent with eventual adult responsibilities (e.g., productivity or fertility). By contrast, in industrialized societies, few formal initiation ceremonies exist (cf. discussion on the universality of adolescence as a distinct life period in Chen and Farruggia 2002). Nevertheless, across societies many adults would agree, in retrospect, that adolescence was a challenging developmental period in their lives.

In line with Bronfenbrenner's system theory (Bronfenbrenner 1994) and more recent multisystemic concepts of resilience (e.g., Ungar et al. 2013), we argue that risk and resilience to mental health, in both childhood and adolescence, are impacted by context-dependent factors. Family and peer relationships as well as school, neighborhood, and community environments are deeply embedded within the local culture, practices, and policies (on multiple scales), and affect childcare and protection. These "macro-contexts" might affect the "micro-contexts" within which adolescents live out their daily lives—with their peers and their families, in their homes, at work settings, schools, and in local communities. This, in turn, can affect the mental health and well-being of adolescents. Importantly, adolescents are not only passive partakers in this process; they play an active role in selecting and interacting with the contexts in their immediate environment (Call and Mortimer 2001). However, experimental tests remain to be conducted on the capacity for, and process of, resilience. Since the use of protective factors embedded in these social contexts is at least partially culture specific (Lund et al. 2018), could this explain the putative differences in the emergence of psychopathology seen in adolescents across cultures? To date, cross-cultural research on this and related questions has been compromised by a predominantly Westernized understanding of the pertinence of different developmental periods, particularly childhood and adolescence, and universally applied to developmental tasks that ought to be accomplished during such formative periods (Atilola 2015). Importantly, cross-cultural research has yet to overcome methodological challenges inherent to the discussion on universality versus uniqueness of current (predominantly Westernized) definitions of mental health; left unaddressed, cross-cultural comparability and validity are reduced (Zheng 2013; Atilola 2015). Thus, findings from existing cross-cultural studies should be interpreted in the context of these limitations.

Aside from cultural influences per se, it is important to consider how more recent developments in modern societies impact adolescent mental health. Today, young people are growing up in contexts of rapid urbanization, increased educational demands, globalization, and access to worldwide information through the internet and social media (e.g., Blum et al. 2012). One recent societal change could be of great significance to risk and resilience processes in youth: digital communication. The shift from face-to-face to online communication may be one of the most obvious societal changes of the twenty-first century. Proximal to adolescents' everyday life, digitalization allows any individual to feel connected to others, independent of distance (e.g., Quinn and Oldmeadow 2012), yet powerful and harmful dynamics can arise in resulting social relationships (e.g., cyberbullying, harassment). Meta-analytic data provide compelling evidence that cyberbullying is associated with adolescent depression (Hamm et al. 2015). More recently, however, a study of British population-based data demonstrated that cyberbullying accounted for only a small share of variance in mental health outcomes in adolescents, when data were controlled for traditional forms of bullying and other covariates (Przybylski and Bowes 2017). In addition, time spent with digital media also appears to reduce physical activity dramatically in adolescents (Finne et al. 2013), which is considered an important protective factor for reducing stress and improving mood.

Social and Cultural Contexts of Psychopathology

How can we characterize and/or quantify the social and cultural contexts of psychopathology? Social development in adolescence is a process clearly driven by the maturation of specific social-cognitive functions, yet these functions do not develop in isolation: they are shaped by interpersonal relationships within an adolescent's social and cultural context. As research investigates the social and cultural influences on adolescent brain and behavior development, it faces a major challenge: How can assessment tools which adequately quantify complex environmental contexts and individual experiences within these contexts be integrated into studies grounded in neurobiology and neuroscience (see also Tost et al. 2015)? Recently, innovative methods have become available to permit better characterization of the changing social environments in adolescence, which we briefly describe below.

Ecological momentary assessment (EMA) is a promising technique that uses a smartphone app to obtain psychological data in real-time, real-life contexts. It allows for the assessment of social behaviors and social experiences in daily life without the bias that results from retrospective reflection. As adolescents are digitally savvy, smartphone-based assessments are generally well accepted. EMA studies can be broadly categorized according to time- or event-based sampling methods:

- A time-based strategy aims to acquire representative characteristics and patterns of behaviors as well as an individual's experiences across time through prompts at random points in time.
- An event-based strategy aims to examine antecedents and consequences of specific experiences through, for instance, self-initiated self-reports in response to specific events (e.g., an individual's location via GPS or physical activity via an accelerometer).

On the basis of the study rationales, different approaches to both methods of sampling have been used (see Ebner-Priemer and Trull 2009). EMA can also be combined with context-dependent social-cognitive tests or with psychophysiological assessments. Sliwinski et al. (2018), for example, demonstrated that electronic diaries combined with brief smartphone-based cognitive assessments in uncontrolled naturalistic settings provided measurements with a degree of reliability comparable to assessments collected in controlled laboratory environments.

Social network analyses provide another important tool that can be used to characterize and/or quantify social behaviors and experiences during adolescence. Individual attributes shape an individual's social network through a process called social selection. Conversely, characteristics of the network as well as an individual's position in the network influence individual attributes, such as attitudes or behavior (de Klepper et al. 2010). This occurs, for example, when individuals adjust their behavior to their close friends. Key network processes involved are homophily (the preference for relationships with individuals with similar characteristics), reciprocity (the tendency to reciprocate relationships), and transivity (the tendency for triads to form a closed network) (McPherson et al. 2001). Recent progress in statistical modeling of longitudinal network data (i.e., stochastic actor-based models) allows us to disentangle the effects of social selection and social influence (Snijders et al. 2010). Using this approach, longitudinal studies of networks and individual behaviors have revealed that selection is more important than influence in explaining similarity in adolescent smoking behavior, whereas both processes impact adolescent academic performance similarly (Mercken et al. 2010). One interesting study combined social cognitive tests and social network analysis in adolescents and found higher self-reported mirroring in adolescents to be associated with a more central network position (Wolfer et al. 2012). Social network data can be collected using surveys in which individuals nominate their friends or describe other relations.

Another exciting development is *mobile sensing*, which uses the ubiquity of mobile phones and their increasing functionality to study social relationships based on directly observable behavior in real time (Eagle et al. 2009). Using mobile sensing, social network data has been inferred from physical proximity and communication patterns. These data complement established survey methods.

Finally, *geographical maps* have become available that quantify certain environmental conditions (e.g., household income, ethnic diversities, average educational levels, air pollution, traffic noises). When combined with location tracking, geographical maps enable a more detailed characterization of an adolescent's socioenvironmental context on a daily basis. Such measures of neighborhood contextual factors, however, do not include an adolescent's perception or information on influential ongoing social processes. Nearly two decades ago, Tienda emphasized the importance of assessing the social impact of neighborhoods (Tienda 1991). More recently, the life sciences, in general, have acknowledged the importance of including more *participatory approaches* in quantitative research activities. This was recently done in a study by Landstedt et al. (2009), who investigated the gender-specific influence of social processes on adolescent mental health using a grounded theory approach based on focus groups with adolescents.

How, then, can the impact of complex social and cultural contexts be *reliably* assessed? Unfortunately, cross-cultural research lacks a thorough taxonomy of important cultural characteristics that might impact mental health.[1] Methods in cultural neuroscience vary across levels of analysis and include behavioral surveys, open-ended interviews, or ethnography to explore cultural values, practices, and beliefs. Such approaches could be combined with recent advances in *population genetics* that have indicated significant variations in allele frequencies across the globe as a function of population structure due to multiple evolutionary factors, including natural selection, genetic drift, mutation in gene expression, and gene flow (Chiao and Blizinsky 2013). With respect to adolescent social development, in particular, cross-cultural comparisons of societies that reflect more collectivist values (where self is defined as the connection to others or the social situation) versus individualistic values (where self is autonomous from others) might be particularly promising. The same holds for cross-cultural comparisons of adolescents who grow up in societies/cultures where there are large differences in initiation rites that mark the adolescent transition period, as well as comparisons of adolescents with and without experiences related to the promises and challenges of globalization (e.g., using data from current vs. historical cohorts).

Sensitive Period(s) for Social Influences during Adolescence

Is there really a (second) sensitive period for social influences during adolescence? Are the effects of social experiences particularly strong during adolescence? The sentiment "no man is an island," by the poet John Donne, offers a pertinent perspective. By nature, humans are social creatures, but throughout their development, are there particular periods that are sensitive or critical for social development to occur? Can we assume that adolescence constitutes a second sensitive period for social development, comparable to one when early caregiver influences shaped the maturation of infants' social-affective neural circuitries?

A sensitive period is defined as a period in which an organism "expects" to be exposed to a particular stimulus (Greenough et al. 1987). Originally referred to as "critical periods," this term is now used less often when referring to human development, as some recovery of functions may be possible outside of the time window of highest sensitivity (Takesian and Hensch 2013). Sensitive

---

1 An exception to this is Hofstede's cultural dimensions theory, which describes the effects of a society's culture on the values of its members, and how these values relate to behavior, using a structure derived from factor analysis (Hofstede 2015).

period models of brain development generally regard neural circuit maturation as a confluence of endogenous maturation and experiential sculpting. When neural systems begin to mature, they are weakly responsive to a wide scope of stimuli and generate diffuse patterns of activation within and across neural circuitries. Over time, brain responses become stronger, more efficient, and automatic as the boundaries of relevant stimuli become narrower and responses to non-experienced stimuli are dampened (Greenough et al. 1987; Werker and Hensch 2015).

As outlined above, adolescence has been proposed to be a time of particular environmental susceptibility, and the impact of puberty on the brain makes adolescents particularly sensitive to their social environments (Crone and Dahl 2012). Adolescents go through a period of social reorientation, as the opinions of peers become more important than those of family members. In one study, for example, adolescents aged 13 to 17 years reported that peer evaluations affected their feelings of social or personal worth (O'Brien and Bierman 1988). Although adolescents aged 10 to 13 years felt that peers provided companionship and support, they did not report that peer acceptance negatively impacted their self-evaluation. Blakemore and Mills (2014) suggest that increasing abilities of abstract thinking, together with an increasing motivation for positive peer acceptance, might account for peer influences on self-evaluations in adolescence. A recent behavioral study investigated the effects of social exclusion in the lab. After being excluded by other players in an online game (Cyberball), young and mid-adolescents (11–15 yr) reported lowered overall mood whereas young adolescents (11–13 yr) reported higher state anxiety compared to adults (Sebastian et al. 2011). In addition, Brumbach et al. (2009) showed that socioenvironmental conditions experienced during adolescence impact attitudes toward health and reproduction in young adulthood. Adolescents within socially unpredictable environments not only experienced decreased physical and mental health over the short term, they also showed decreased health and less sexual restrictedness over time.

Despite evidence for adolescence as a sensitive period for social processing from rodent studies (Marco et al. 2011; Foulkes and Blakemore 2016), it is critical to acknowledge that evidence for sensitive periods in human adolescence is scarce. A number of researchers argue that there is evidence for other periods of social reorientation beyond adolescence (e.g., Nelson et al. 2016). They suggest that there are at least five distinct social phases in development, each of which can be largely defined by the social target and type of social behavior expressed:

1. During infancy, sociality consists of engagement with the primary caregivers.
2. In the juvenile phase, between weaning and puberty, the caregiver–infant dyad is gradually replaced by peer-focused play behavior, but the caregiver is retained as a base.

3. In adolescence, between puberty and full maturity, social behavior becomes more important as individuals strive to become fully integrated into larger groups of peers.
4. The reproductive/intimacy phase is accompanied by social bonding and reproductive behavior.
5. The mature adult phase is characterized by social interactions within a relatively stable multigenerational group, along with expression of intimate relations and directed care of offspring.

Although this pattern of multiple phases in social development is not universal, it is widely expressed among most primates and in many socially living mammalian species (e.g., Zhang et al. 2012). Overall, this concept is in line with models that assume sensitive periods in social development to be related to changes in brain development; however, it broadens the concept of sensitive periods from one to multiple sensitive periods in social development across the life span. During these periods, although such social experiences are particularly important, there is as yet no evidence that they constitute sensitive periods for brain development, in which a specific input from the environment is expected. Each of these developmental periods, however, might sensitize neural structures to forthcoming social experiences. For example, it has been shown that individuals experience distress if a social target is absent: highly motivated social engagement is directed at caregivers in infancy, at playmates during the juvenile phase, at integration with peers during adolescence, at potential mates during early adulthood in the social intimacy phase, and at offspring and stable group members in the mature adult phase (e.g., Hostinar et al. 2015). Once new targets of social behavior emerge, motivational response to previous social categories typically diminishes. In a number of species, the duration and intensity of distress caused by maternal separation declines across infancy while play behavior increases (Zhang et al. 2012). Also, attention to a peer group becomes less important for adolescents once romantic engagements are established (Collins et al. 2009). Taken together, these data provide evidence for the idea that expected goals in social development undergo systematic shifts across the life span, and that these shifts are accompanied by changes in motivation to obtain or maintain specific types of social experiences. The social experiences in each phase are interdependent insofar as their effects spill over into successive periods. For instance, early experiences with a caretaker in infancy can moderate social behavior with peers in adolescence (Puetz et al. 2014), and parenting style can be redirected toward one's own offspring in adulthood (Olsavsky et al. 2013).

Precursors, Risk, and Resilience Factors to Youth Mental Health

How do adolescent precursors, risk, and resilience factors to youth mental health evolve over time? How do they interact, and what possible mechanisms underlie the associations between social risk factors and the development of psychopathology?

It has been suggested that the heightened vulnerability to mental disorders during adolescence is related to genetically or experientially preprogrammed neural development, triggered by acute stressors or adversities experienced in the current environment (Andersen and Teicher 2009). The desire to be accepted by one's peers and the importance of social reward and avoidance of social rejection could constitute particularly acute stressors in adolescence, and may result in extreme stress, if the desire is not adequately met. During adolescence, the cortico-striato-limbic circuitries are reorganized, and increases in pubertal sex hormones interact with the developing hypothalamic-pituitary-adrenal stress axis and glucocorticoids (for a review, see McCormick et al. 2017). Adolescents show increased sensitivity to stress-induced levels of glucocorticoids in parallel to an increase in glucocorticoid regulation in the prefrontal cortex (Perlman et al. 2007). Therefore, social isolation during this period, for example, may increase the likelihood of depressive-like behaviors as well as alterations in the structure of the prefrontal cortex (Leussis et al. 2008). Long-lasting effects of increased stress exposure in adolescence might disrupt social as well as reproductive behavior.

Recently, Suleiman et al. (2017) pointed out that the importance of sexual relationships during adolescence has been largely neglected. Rather than being sequential and distinct phases, the development of peer relationships, romantic relationships, and sexual relationships might occur simultaneously and interact. Early romantic and sexual relationships are shaped by the characteristics of the adolescent's peer group as well as by the quality of parent–adolescent relationships. At the same time, growing interest in sexual and romantic relationships introduces a new dimension to peer group dynamics. Suleiman and colleagues suggest that data from adolescent real-world experiences, especially those related to romantic and sexual relationships and behaviors, should be included in future studies to increase understanding of the social neuroscience of adolescence.

Furthermore, detailed study is needed into how social behaviors and experiences from earlier phases of development impact the responsivity of neural circuitries. Such experiences may have long-term effects on the organism's sensitivity toward risk and resilience factors present in subsequent phases in social development. Future models should thus consider incorporating interactive influences of changes in the adolescent social environment and adolescent neurobiology. Such models need to account for influences driven by stable individual traits (i.e., genetic variations) that determine timing, responsivity, and plasticity of neural network development. In addition, a better understanding of *genetic nurturing effects* (i.e., how nontransmitted alleles can still affect a child through their impacts on the parents and other relatives) is needed to improve understanding of social influences on adolescent development (Kong et al. 2018).

Interestingly, while the timing of the opening and closing of sensitive periods itself has generally been considered to be an internally mediated process with predetermined timing parameters, under some conditions, environmental experiences can also affect the timing and pace of sensitive periods. Several factors (e.g., body weight, life stress) influence the timing of puberty onset (e.g., Lee and Styne 2013). Recent findings suggest that the timing of neural circuit organization may also be susceptible to differences in environmental conditions, in particular in extreme variations, such as when brain maturation is accelerated by adversity (Gee et al. 2013).

Concluding Remarks

Broader concepts that assume "multiple sensitive periods of social development" may have important clinical implications for understanding and treating psychopathology. The phase of social development and the timing of social experiences may most likely play a central role in the efficacy of different types of intervention.

Although the extent to which environmental influences affect timing parameters of brain development has not been extensively tested, particularly in human development, existing data suggest that both timing and environmental influences should be considered in future studies. Advances in research on molecular effects in developmental plasticity may further inform our understanding of factors that contribute to the onset and offset of sensitive periods during early life and later development. For instance, recent studies indicate that changes in the plasticity of local circuits are dependent on the maturation of local inhibitory connections, which may regulate sensitive periods at a molecular level by shifting the local excitatory-inhibitory balance within local circuits (Takesian and Hensch 2013; Werker and Hensch 2015). Isolating regionally specific markers for heightened plasticity across sensitive periods in development may help us understand how neural organization influences specific social functions during different phases of development. This, in turn, may provide an avenue for pharmacologically based interventions, to allow previously closed critical periods to be reopened through targeted pharmacotherapy (Gervain et al. 2013). This might be particularly important for future preventive approaches, as the degree to which different experiences affect the developmental trajectory depends to a large extent on the timing of experiences (i.e., when during the course of development experiences occurred).

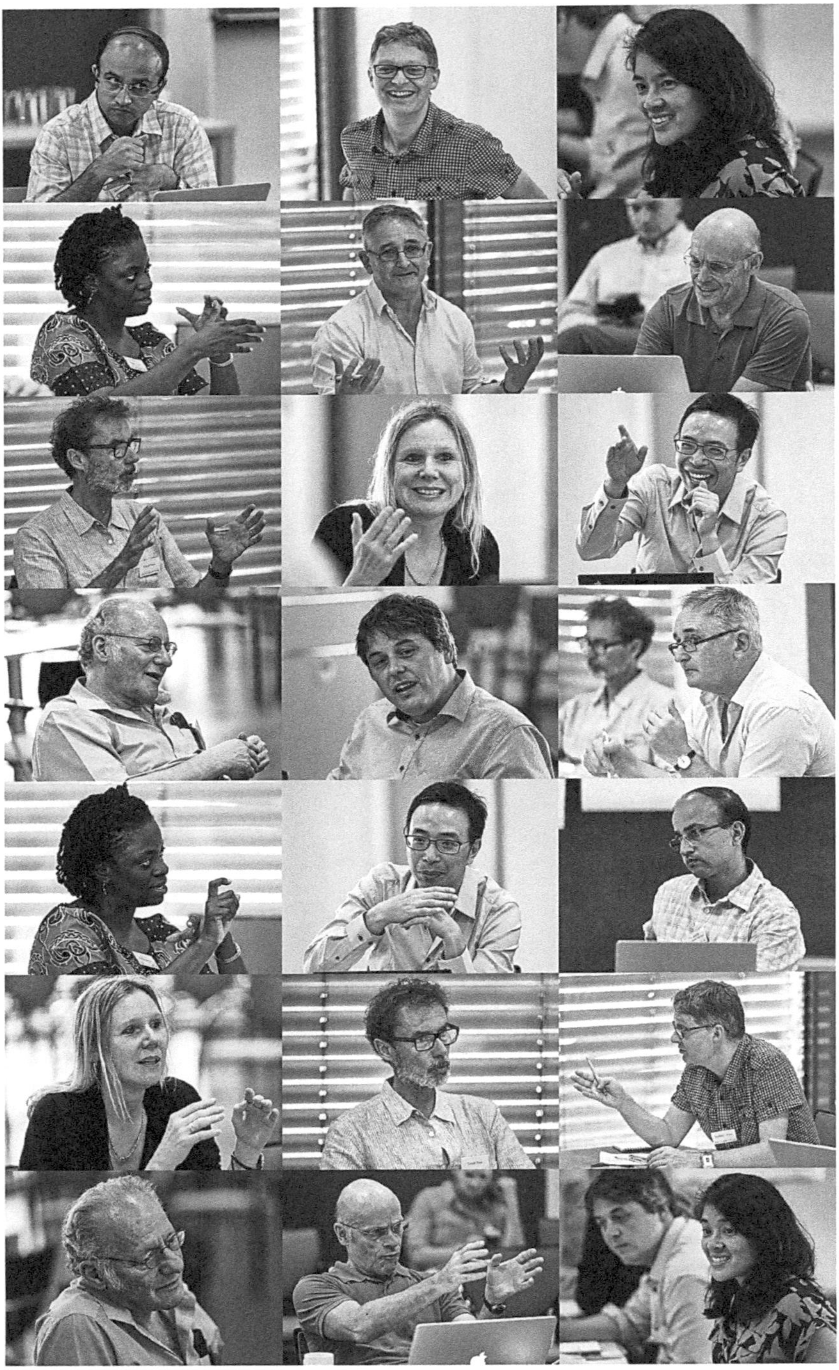

6

Biological, Psychological, and Sociocultural Processes in Emerging Mental Disorders in Youth

Urvakhsh Meherwan Mehta, Stephen J. Wood, Tolulope Bella-Awusah, Kerstin Konrad, Cindy H. Liu, George C. Patton, Tomáš Paus, Ulrich Reininghaus, Gunter Schumann, Ezra Susser, and Lawrence H. Yang

Abstract

Vulnerability for the development of major mental health conditions during the transition from adolescence to adulthood is highly influenced by social and cultural contexts, yet our understanding of the way these contexts interact with individual differences (such as genetic variation) to generate or moderate psychopathology is limited. Such contextual interactions are likely to be nonlinear, bidirectional, and potentially age sensitive, requiring complex modeling to disentangle the most significant factors that contribute to the onset of mental illness in youth. Combined with known transcultural variation in these contexts (and psychopathology itself), there is a critical need to better understand the general applicability of models of youth mental health if we are to develop appropriate interventions. This chapter identifies gaps in current understanding in terms of how an individual's interaction with the environment shapes the risks and vulnerabilities to develop major mental disorders, or their behavioral precursors, thus resulting in functional impairments and increasing the high global burden of disease.

Group photos (top left to bottom right) Urvakhsh Mehta, Stephen Wood, Cindy Liu, Tolulope Bella-Awusah, George Patton, Gunter Schumann, Tomáš Paus, Kerstin Konrad, Larry Yang, Ezra Susser, Ulrich Reininghaus, George Patton, Tolulope Bella-Awusah, Larry Yang, Urvakhsh Mehta, Kerstin Konrad, Tomáš Paus, Stephen Wood, Ezra Susser, Gunter Schumann, Cindy Liu

Introduction and Setting the Framework

The Youth Mental Health Burden

The dynamic and differential influences that the environment exerts on a developing individual, at multiple levels of confluence, can lead to the emergence of major mental disorders (e.g., psychotic, mood and anxiety, and substance use disorders) in youth and adulthood. Such disorders, which are often chronic, contribute substantially to disease burden, both directly and indirectly, through a high population attributable risk (Table 6.1). In 2010, the Global Burden of Disease Study found mental and substance use disorders to be the leading cause of disability in children and youth under the age of 25 yr globally, despite high probabilities of underestimating the full extent of the burden (Erskine et al. 2015). Although greater in high-income countries, burden estimates in low- and middle-income countries are likely to grow with the possible control of morbidity due to infectious disorders in the near future (Lozano et al. 2012). While identification and treatment of these disorders during childhood and adolescence is certainly desirable, effective prevention strategies most likely have the greatest capacity to reduce the burden (Erskine et al. 2015).

To develop, test, and implement effective preventive and early intervention strategies, a scientifically robust understanding of the etiology of these disorders is necessary. A range of etiopathogenic processes have been identified as risk factors for youth mental health problems, yet their complex nature and the interdependent relationships involved (e.g., genetics, parental mental illness, poverty, and childhood adversity) are not easy to modify and quantify.

Table 6.1 Population attributable risk (PAR) of adult disorders, having been diagnosed with other disorders during adolescence, based on a national survey of U.S. adolescents. Note: PAR is the proportion of the disease incidence in a population (exposed and unexposed) due to exposure. It is the incidence of a disease in the population that would be eliminated if exposure were eliminated (Kirch 2008).

Adolescent Disorders	Adult Disorders	PAR (%)
Anxiety disorder	Depression	17.95
	Schizophrenia	26.71
Depression	Depression	21.20
	Bipolar disorder	21.20
	Schizophrenia	42.82
Attention deficit hyperactivity disorder	Schizophrenia	23.34
Conduct disorder	Depression	20.96
Oppositional defiant disorder	Depression	32.38
Conduct/oppositional defiant disorder	Bipolar disorder	22.54
	Schizophrenia	25.88
Substance use disorder	Depression	15.51

Understanding these influences is necessary to identify key processes (as well as that which moderates and mediates specific outcomes), which in turn is needed to enable the early identification of vulnerable youth and the evaluation and initiation of scientifically informed corrective interventions in a scalable and sustainable manner.

A Conceptual Framework to Understand the Etiology of Youth Mental Disorders

Development encompasses various levels of biological (e.g., infancy, growth spurts, juvenility, puberty) and social (e.g., roles, responsibilities, interpersonal relationships) transitions—encountered and experienced by individuals within their unique environment—as well as neurobiological (brain size, white matter expansion, dendritic branching, myelination) and psychological (cognitive control and emotion regulation) changes. The developing child, with his/her own genetic endowment, progresses through these rapidly evolving phases of physiology and encounters along the way a range of environmental influences. The etiology and pathogenesis of major mental disorders in youth and adulthood cannot be comprehended without considering the various levels of milieus in which a developing child lives, and with which they transact (e.g., family, peers, school, and society), and the associated ethnocultural systems.

It is within this context that a life-course epidemiological perspective—one that focuses on the complex interplay of social and biological factors during gestation, childhood, adolescence, early adult life, or across generations in the production of mental disorders (Koenen et al. 2013)—appears to be an essential organizing paradigm to study the determinants of youth mental health (and disease). The population neuroscience approach is well suited to apply a life-course epidemiology paradigm to mental disorders as it acknowledges the complexity in time and space of *environmental* and *genomic* factors that shape the structure and functions of the human brain, best addressed at a population level (Paus 2010). Here, it is important to understand and apply the concept of *developmental cascades*, which is integral to population neuroscience approaches in appreciating how transactions at different timescales (e.g., perinatal, infancy, adolescence, early adulthood), constructs (cognition, mood, behavior), and levels (molecular, physiology, individual, and social) have a domino effect on subsequent development. Developmental cascades refer to the cumulative consequences of the many interactions and transactions which occur in developing children that result in spreading aftereffects across levels, among domains at the same level, and across different systems or generations (Masten and Cicchetti 2010). Therefore, efficient management of youth mental disorders and strategies to prevent them must consider this context to address the needs of children and families throughout the developmental trajectory. Effects of specific environmental exposures on the outcomes of mental disorders and their behavioral precursors can be potentially mediated or moderated

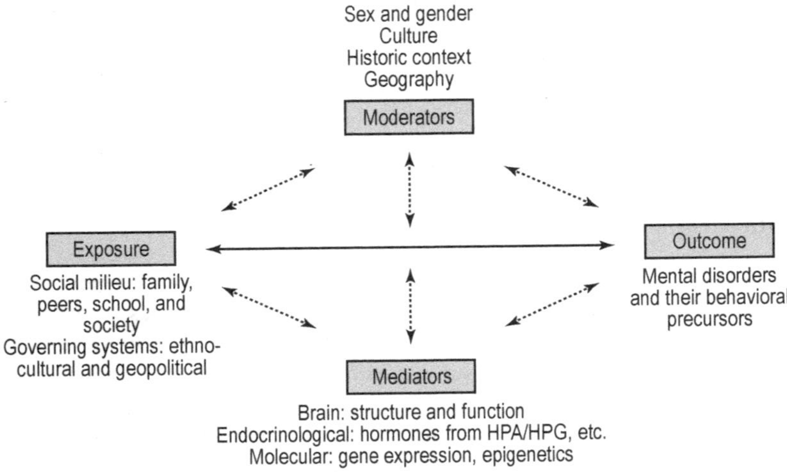

Figure 6.1 An illustrative model depicting how environmental exposures can impact behaviors across developmental cascades. Across exposures, mediators, moderators, and outcomes there is a dynamic fluid interchange, depending on where in the developmental cascade one is. HPA/HPG = hypothalamic pituitary adrenal/gonadal axes.

by a broad range of contextual, cultural, and biological factors, depending on the particular developmental epochs (e.g., periconceptional, perinatal, or peripubertal) during which the exposures occur (see Figure 6.1). A nuanced understanding of these developmental epoch-sensitive exposures and their mediators or moderators will reveal time-sensitive windows for therapeutic interventions that target remediation of the exposure, mediating, or moderating factors. This framework can elucidate the risks of environmental exposures in determining adverse mental health outcomes (Patterson et al. 1989) and may help identify protective factors (e.g., academic competency or sociability) during childhood that predict well-adjusted adult functioning, which can be harnessed during targeted interventions (Rutter 1999).

Environmental Adversities as Exposures

All complex human traits manifesting as personality, cognition, and psychopathology share varying causal contributions from the individual's genome as well as the shared and nonshared environment (Burt 2009; Plomin and Daniels 1987; Polderman et al. 2015). Emerging evidence from large-scale genomic initiatives reveal a finely distributed genetic influence of small effect sizes and low penetrance, spread across thousands of genetic variants (high prevalence), that are contingent on the environment and not specific to any single form of psychopathology (Brainstorm Consortium et al. 2018; Uher and Zwicker 2017). Similarly, several environmental exposures have now emerged that reveal low penetrance, high prevalence, and nonspecificity, resulting in ill-defined exposure-disease associations. Given the rapid advances in accurate and comprehensive measurement of variation across the entire genome, there is a pressing need to match similar progress in large-scale capture of potential environmental exposures as well as outcomes (Ioannidis et al. 2009). Concurrent measurement of such massive, large-scale data has the potential to yield novel etiologies and targets for intervention. This raises the following questions: How best can we characterize our environment? How can we improve measurement accuracy to account for the dynamicity, multiplicity, and collinearity of environmental exposures? Yet another challenge is to account for the cross-cultural variability involved in defining and measuring exposures. There have been strong proposals to improve the holistic measurement of environmental exposures within a developmental cascades framework in line with the exposome paradigm (Guloksuz et al. 2018; Wild 2005). When applied within a life-course population neuroscience framework, this will provide dynamic information about the total nongenetic component of psychiatric etiology as well as enable the study of interactions within and between the genome and exposome and lead to expression of the "phenome," the full set of phenotypes of an individual (Houle et al. 2010).

One step in improving the comprehensive and accurate measurement of the environment is to understand the levels at which it acts upon an individual. A developing child is not a mere solitary entity, but a social being that lives in and interacts with the environment (Hinde 1987). It is therefore important to identify the network of interpersonal relationships surrounding a child, as this dynamic network is a critical part of the environment that shapes the child's psychological and biological development. This context of social environment or ecological systems for the developing child ranges from a micro-level milieu of frequent direct interactions (e.g., with family, peers, and at school) to macro-level aspects of their broader milieu (e.g., available resources, infrastructure of their towns and cities, recreational and residential facilities, social support buffers, cultural practices), shaped and regulated by economic, geopolitical, and ethnocultural governing systems (Bronfenbrenner 1996). As depicted in Table 6.2, environmental exposures at micro- or macro-level ecological systems across critical developmental stages can trigger key processes with a potential cascading impact on subsequent development and psychopathology.

Influences of Micro-Level Environment Exposures

Peer–peer, peer–parent, or peer–teacher dyads are important contexts in which interpersonal relationships manifest in developing children. Secure attachment with a significant caregiver in childhood is linked to a reduced engagement in high-risk behaviors, higher prosocial behaviors, and healthy coping styles (Moretti and Peled 2004). In contrast, an ambivalent attachment has been associated with childhood anxiety (Colonnesi et al. 2011). Adverse

Table 6.2 Environmental exposures during crucial stages of development can trigger processes that compromise mental health. Built environment refers to natural and modified elements of the physical environment. After Uher and Zwicker (2017).

Environment	Domain
Periconceptional	Infections
	Malnutrition
	Environmental toxins
Perinatal	Preterm birth
	Season of birth
	Birth complications
Child developmental	Family
Social	Childcare and parenting
	Adolescence and peers
	Workplace
	Neighborhood
	Community and culture
	Poverty and violence
	Neighborhood amenities: housing, activity and recreational spaces, and measures of community design
Built environment	Lighting, parks, roads, sidewalks
Physical environment	Noise
	Water and air quality, pollutants

experiences encountered at various developmental stages are indeed one of the most compelling determinants of mental health problems throughout the life span (Garner et al. 2012; McLaughlin et al. 2012). Nevertheless, despite these observations, very little is understood about the dose-response relationship, specificity of these adversities to psychopathology outcomes, their mediators, the influence of culture and other moderators, as well as the role of timing paired to critical developmental epochs. Recent studies have begun to answer some of these questions by applying a life-course epidemiological framework. For instance, longitudinal data from the Avon Longitudinal Study of Parents and Children (ALSPAC; n = 7476) were tested for three potential theoretical models of how early childhood adversity (abuse and stress) predicted emotional and behavioral problems (Strengths and Difficulties Questionnaire) at the age of 8 yr. Recency (temporal proximity) and accumulation (cumulative repeated exposures) of childhood adversities predicted psychopathology better than sensitive-period (specific timing of exposure) effects (Dunn et al. 2018). Similarly, analysis of cross-sectional data from the National Comorbidity Survey Replication (Adolescent Supplement) revealed an association between exposure to childhood adversity (interpersonal violence) and adolescent psychiatric diagnoses, irrespective of the age at first exposure to violence (Dunn et al. 2017). This suggests that there was no particular sensitive period for the exposure to result in the outcome studied. In contrast, provision of a caregiving environment early (18–24 months of age) in the course of a deprived nurturing environmental exposure (raised from early infancy in institutions in Bucharest) resulted in normalization of the physiological reactivity to stress (cortisol and autonomic functions), thus highlighting the presence of a sensitive period during which the developing stress response system is strongly influenced by environmental inputs (McLaughlin et al. 2015).

The potential effects of global sociocultural variations on the relationship between childhood adversity in the family context and first-onset psychiatric disorders during adulthood revealed a striking similarity in associations across nationalities (21 countries) assessed during the WHO World Mental Health survey. This cross-sectional survey also highlighted the nonspecificity of the relationship between childhood adversity and mental health outcomes (Kessler et al. 2010). When studying the impact of childhood adversity on subsequent psychopathology, it is important to understand the context in which adversity manifests. For a developing child, these include the transactional relationships shared with parents and peers in family and school contexts (Aldridge and McChesney 2018; Darling and Steinberg 1993). Parenting styles (e.g., control) determine cognitive and behavioral outcomes in developing children as a function of "household chaos" (i.e., lack of structure and unpredictability in everyday activities), as demonstrated in longitudinal studies (Kim-Spoon et al. 2017). However, parenting styles and their subsequent determination of child behavior vary according to the culture in which they are manifest. For instance, while Japanese mothers focus on early mastery of emotional maturity and social courtesy in their children, American mothers promote early mastery of verbal competence and self-actualization (Bornstein 2013; Caudill 1973). Similarly, authoritative parenting styles in European American and African American children leads to positive mental health outcomes (Brody et al. 2008; Damon 1989). The peer environment is again shaped by the transactional relationship of the developing child with friends and manifests most commonly in the school context. Prospective studies reveal that adolescent friendship, but not family support, determines subsequent resilient psychosocial functioning one year later (van Harmelen et al. 2017). Similarly, a positive school climate determines better prosocial behaviors one year later in Colombian adolescents (Luengo Kanacri et al. 2017).

An additional approach to improve the measurement of environmental exposures is to identify distinct dimensions of the adverse experience and trace the differential brain pathways through which its outcomes are mediated. Drawing from animal experiments, one approach proposes that adverse experiences within the immediate family can have two dimensions: threat (e.g., physical, sexual abuse, domestic violence) and deprivation (e.g., lack of cognitive, social input). Adversities within the realm of threat may alter neural circuits underlying fear learning (e.g., amygdala and hippocampus), whereas those associated with deprivation may act via effects on the association cortices responsible for executive and social cognition abilities (e.g., prefrontal, inferior parietal, and superior temporal cortices) (Sheridan and McLaughlin 2014). A third dimension is that of rejection. Adolescents with adverse peer interactions (e.g., repeated rejections by peers) demonstrate exaggerated activity in the dorsal anterior cingulate, during a social exclusion (Cyberball) task, when compared to adolescents who do not experience adverse peer interactions (Will et al. 2016). These exaggerated neural responses are likely to mediate depression and social anxiety symptoms (Rudolph et al. 2016).

In summary, parenting and school climate provide a rich opportunity to study the influence of environmental exposures on psychopathology via engagement of specific neural systems. They also offer significant opportunities to intervene and remediate the exposures and their moderators early during the course of development (Aldridge and McChesney 2018; Ryan et al. 2017).

Influences of Micro-Level Environment Exposures (Virtual or Online)

To study these processes, we must address real-world as well as virtual or online interpersonal relationships. To date, however, the impact of this latter on emerging psychopathology is poorly understood. While some longitudinal studies report a strong negative relationship between virtual or online activities and adolescent mental health (Kim 2017), others hint at beneficial effects (Adachi and Willoughby 2013). Clearly, there is a gap in our understanding of how individual-, family-, and social-level factors influence the relationship between online social behaviors and psychological health. Fundamental questions are now beginning to be addressed, such as process-level differences in social interactions performed in the real and virtual worlds, and their impact on cognitive and behavioral functioning. For instance, the online environment permits interactions with audiences that are practically limitless by virtue of their sheer reach across spatial, temporal, and social distances (McFarland and Ployhart 2015). In contrast, real-world social interactions require moment-to-moment appraisals of social cues, which guide reciprocity during face-to-face interactions under certain sociocultural environmental constraints (Vlahovic et al. 2012). With increasing social media use, it is critical to examine this behavior as a potential psychopathological manifestation of an underlying diathesis (Bányai et al. 2017) as well as a potential environmental exposure that can have long-range effects on neural networks and behavior. The mechanistic basis of such positive or negative impact is also poorly understood and could operate in different ways:

- At a biological level, where frequency of use sensitizes specific social cognition and reward pathways (Meshi et al. 2015).

- At a psychological level, where newer anticipatory anxieties are an effect of maladaptive learning processes triggered by the immediacy and high expectancies of responses between peers.
- At a social level, where there is a false sense of secure virtual relationships at the cost of maintaining real relationships with peers and parents, as well as a negative affect secondary to having a constant external template of comparison and revising expectations based on fragile online peer relationships.

In contrast, online social networking, associated with psychological well-being, is perhaps mediated by a sense of greater "bridging" social capital. It enables "loose" connections between individuals, who may provide useful information or new perspectives to each other (Ellison et al. 2007).

Influences of Macro-Level Environment Exposures

Global variations in macro-level exposure to social phenomena can potentially elucidate the increasing rates of precise behavioral outcomes within specific cultural and geographical populations. Such complex social phenomena, with diverse underlying processes, include (but are not restricted to) migration (Cantor-Graae and Selten 2005), social and economic disparities (Weich and Lewis 1998), and population density (Colodro-Conde et al. 2018; Schweitzer and Su 1977). The concept of urbanization—a nonlinear process of population replacement or the global-scale reorientation of the social and environmental landscape across continents that results from population migration and natural demographic growth (Knox and McCarthy 2005)—encompasses these macro-level social phenomena and has been found to have varying associations with mental health morbidity (Dekker et al. 2008; Krabbendam 2005). These variations are likely to be a function of (a) the mental health outcome (e.g., psychotic vs. other disorders) being studied (Schifano 2008; Vassos et al. 2012), (b) the sociocultural variations and economic context (e.g., developed vs. developing societies) of the population being examined (de Vries et al. 2018; Paksarian et al. 2018; Wang et al. 2018), (c) the nature of urban exposure, such as green spaces, exposure to pollutants/toxins, built environment, dietary variations, population density, social capital (Bratman et al. 2015; Galea 2005; Wang et al. 2018), and (d) the study designs being implemented that determine the timing of exposure (Dekker et al. 2008; Paksarian et al. 2018). Moreover, specific aspects inherent to urban living can have disorder-specific associations, as in eating disorders, where a greater incidence of bulimia nervosa (but not anorexia) has been consistently tied to increased urbanization (Hoek et al. 1995; Van Son et al. 2006).

While urban living might confer potential causative influences on adverse mental health outcomes in a developing child, it also provides important benefits: greater employment and education opportunities, improved health-related knowledge, and better access to health-care facilities (Chen et al. 2017; Liu et al. 1999). Data are lacking, however, to determine if urban living yields greater overall health benefits or risks. It is thought that the strongest moderator of the effects of urban living on health outcomes is the economic disparity inherent to the urbanization process, which favors the rich over the poor (Dye 2008). Nevertheless, better observational data are required to understand risk processes across the life course, since we currently do not have definitive information about specific risk processes where we can intervene. One way forward is to have comprehensive cross-cutting quantification of environmental exposures based on existing risk ratios of specific exposures, as performed via polyenviromic risk scores (similar to the polygenic risk scores in quantifying genetic risk); this is likely to inform us about cumulative proportions of variance explained in the desired outcomes (Padmanabhan et al. 2017). In parallel, a more nuanced analysis of socially distributed exposures by age is needed to disentangle the complex interdependent effects of culture, ethnicity, and social class on specific environmental exposures and their predicted outcomes unique to specific developmental epochs; this will likely provide information about sensitive periods that may be targeted by appropriate interventions. Functional and morphometric brain changes (e.g., in the perigenual anterior cingulate and lateral prefrontal cortices), which mediate the impact of urban living and upbringing on the risk for youth mental disorders across the developmental cascades (Haddad et al. 2015), highlight the shared neurobiological mediators of micro- and macro-level environmental exposures. The translational utility of understanding such macro-level risk factors of youth mental health disorders is also illustrated in a novel prediction model that is applicable at the population level. Recently used to predict the annual number of new cases of psychotic disorders based on age, sex, ethnicity, population density, and socioeconomic deprivation, the PsyMaptic tool has potential in guiding us toward the appropriate allocation of resources (Kirkbride 2015).

Mediators and Moderators of Exposure–Outcome Interactions

A host of mediating factors can potentially drive the impact of environmental exposures on behavioral outcomes. These could be biological substrates that are engaged by environmental exposures in the process of generating adverse mental health outcomes: brain structure, function, and maturation; the endocrinological flux triggered by the hypothalamic-pituitary-gonadal/adrenal systems underlying the hormonal changes that drive puberty; immune and metabolic changes; the molecular-level gene expression changes and epigenetic factors that shape environment-related changes during sensitive periods of development. Yet, there are vast gaps in knowledge about this confluence of biological and environmental systems or "biological embedding," best understood as a process of experience getting "under the skin" and producing stable alterations in those biological and developmental processes that determine subsequent health and development (Hertzman 1999, 2012). The biological embedding of environmental exposures can provide us with a critical and mechanistic understanding about the pathogenesis of youth mental disorders. This, in turn, can provide targets that inform policy-making and preventive strategies and guide early and sustained interventions over the life course. Early life exposures are likely to be preferentially embedded due to a preponderance of sensitive developmental epochs that result in heightened brain plasticity (Berens et al. 2017).

Epigenetic alterations involve stable modifications of gene expression through attachment of chemical residues (e.g., methyl groups) to DNA or histones. These alterations may represent a biological vestige of early life environmental exposures, potentially transforming gene expression and thus, in principle, changing individual development trajectories. Emerging evidence suggests developmental epoch (e.g., infancy vs. preschool period) and gender-sensitive changes in DNA methylation of adolescents are triggered by maternal and paternal stress (Essex et al. 2013). Interestingly, epigenetic variations of neurodevelopmental genes at birth mediated the effects of prenatal maternal tobacco smoking on subsequent substance use behaviors during adolescence in a sample of 244 youth from the ALSPAC cohort (Cecil et al. 2016). These gene expression changes are likely to impact psychopathology via their effects on neural systems, as demonstrated in animal experiments (Jung et al. 2016). Novel efforts are underway to examine the impact of childhood adversity on behavioral outcomes and their epigenetic and neuroimaging mediators. One study on children and their families from an urban slum of Bangladesh reports preliminary data to suggest that adversity impacts neural systems, as measured using functional infrared spectroscopy and electroencephalography (Nelson 2017)—an impact seen at 36 months but not as early as 6 months of age. This suggests a potential window of opportunity for early interventions and reflects the benefits of intervening early (i.e., before the age of 2 yr) in deprived children (McLaughlin et al. 2015) highlighted earlier in this chapter.

Another promising model that can be examined using this approach is to examine the effects of urbanization on adverse mental and physical health outcomes as a function of exposure to artificial nighttime light (Cho et al. 2015). At an individual level, excessive artificial nighttime light exposure can trigger (a) circadian phase disruptions (Cho et al. 2015), (b) altered movement and activity patterns (Kurvers and Holker 2015), and (c) disruption of mood regulatory brain regions (e.g., medial amygdala and lateral habenula) via direct (stimulation of photosensitive retinal ganglion cells) and indirect (altered melatonin secretion and gene expression) effects on cortical physiology (Bedrosian and Nelson 2017). At a social level, this affects the frequency and duration of social interactions as well as the formation, maintenance, and size of social networks and social communication patterns (Kurvers and Holker 2015). In turn, this can have reciprocal influences on the individual's social brain, thus potentially increasing the risk for mood disorders (Bedrosian and

Nelson 2017). This hypothesis is partly supported by observations of a higher (dose-dependent) prevalence of major depression in individuals who work night shifts, which predisposes the individual to greater exposure to artificial night light as well as disturbed circadian rhythms (Scott et al. 1997). Animal studies reveal a more nuanced understanding: a wavelength-dependent effect of nighttime blue-light is mediated by alterations in circadian rhythm (Bedrosian et al. 2013), and directly effects depressive behaviors via stimulation of the intrinsically photosensitive retinal ganglion cells, independent of circadian rhythms and sleep architecture (LeGates et al. 2012). If the latter is true for humans, then redesigning our nighttime light environment using a different wavelength (e.g., red light) could be an effective preventive strategy (Bedrosian and Nelson 2013).

The process of biological embedding socioenvironmental exposures must also account for changes in brain architecture throughout specific developmental epochs (e.g., juvenility and puberty). We do not yet understand if, and how, environmental risks operate differently before, during, and after the pubertal transition, information that is crucial for development of interventions across this period. Adult health outcomes in later life (e.g., general mortality, obesity, type 2 diabetes mellitus, cardiovascular disease, low bone mineral density, and major depression) have been linked to early puberty (Charalampopoulos et al. 2014; Day et al. 2015). In late childhood and early adolescence, more advanced pubertal stage has been associated (independently of age and school grade) with depression, anxiety, eating disorders in females, pain syndromes, self-harm, and substance use; this suggests that puberty marks the point of transition in risk for many early-onset mental disorders (Patton and Viner 2007). There is interest in knowing whether early pubertal timing may be associated with higher rates of emotional and behavioral problems, particularly in girls (Copeland et al. 2010). Puberty can be considered a sensitive phase, especially for LGBTQ (lesbian, gay, bisexual, transgender, queer) children and adolescents for whom the pubertal transition presents a higher risk for psychopathology. It appears to be a period when socioemotional strategies adapt to the prevailing social environment. Emerging research suggests that pubertal development is a sensitive phase and that interventions during this stage may have the ability to change the trajectories of health risks, and perhaps also mental disorders (Del Giudice et al. 2009). More research is needed, however, to characterize juvenility and measure the social environment during this life phase, as pubertal transition might provide a second chance for social and emotional development in children who have suffered early life psychopathology. Timely, effective interventions could modify the developmental trajectory and mitigate adverse behavioral outcomes.

Additional factors to consider include gender differences, the prevailing culture, dynamicity of social roles with development, and the vicarious transferability of behavior based on social learning and modeling. The latter includes positive (aspirations, self-identity, coping with adversity) as well as negative (substance abuse, restrictive eating, self-harm, and maladaptive coping) behaviors that can potentially be transferred, peer–peer, parent–peer, and teacher–peer. While gender norms that determine peer–peer affiliations are not well defined, the type and impact of negative interactions (e.g., bullying) is different in boys (shorter lasting physical bullying) than it is in girls (longer lasting social bullying) (Björkqvist et al. 1992; Carrera Fernández et al. 2013; Iossi Silva et al. 2013). The translation of these effects in the context of cyberbullying is poorly characterized (Wolke and Lereya 2015).

Cultural processes—the symbolic apparatus of meaning-making, representation, and transmission—are dynamic and grounded in local contexts; they diverge significantly from the experiences of other groups and result in the cultivation of collective and individual identity (Kleinman 1999; Kleinman and Benson 2006). Culture also influences how risk factors interact with social support and protective psychological factors that determine youth mental health outcomes (Kleinman 2004). Directly or indirectly, culture may even provide unique milieus for gene expression and physiological reactions that are reflected in regional secular trends of youth mental health disorders and their behavioral and pathogenic precursors (Thirthalli and Jain 2009). Cultural norms and expectations may also have transformative influences on the enactment of social roles in developing children and adolescents. For instance, cultural norms that define social responses to puberty shape the rate of social role transition (e.g., early marriages and early parenthood in developing countries) and hence impact psychological well-being. Cultural differences may also exist in the dynamics of peer–parent relationships (e.g., degree of affection being displayed, parenting style). Cultural processes and contexts also influence migration, especially from underdeveloped and developing to developed societies (Ali 2007; Caira 2008). Migration and the associated cultural bereavement and cultural identity confusion are significant risk factors for a broad range of mental health outcomes (Bhugra and Becker 2005). Cultural contexts are therefore important and complex dynamic moderators of environmental exposures on mental health outcomes, from a risk as well as a resilience perspective. There is, in fact, scant empirical data on the impact of different child-rearing beliefs and practices that are culturally grounded on early brain development. There is also limited data to determine which interventions have a significant impact on child well-being across a variety of political and cultural contexts, thus limiting policy reforms (Shonkoff 2010).

In the process of determining appropriate mediators and moderators of the effects of environmental exposures on disease outcomes, it is critical to acknowledge that these relationships are by no means unidirectional. In fact, there is a dynamic fluid interchange across exposures, mediators, moderators and outcomes depending on one's genetic endowment and where in the developmental cascade one is. At the macrolevel, secular time trends in global variations of exposures, mediating influences, and outcomes should be studied as moderating factors which are likely to shed light on increasing rates of particular behavioral outcomes within specific cultural and geographical populations. The changing megatrends in adolescent development, nutrition, inequality, economic globalization, migration, and urbanization are examples of such processes in need of future research.

Social Cognition as an Exemplar of Key Processes

Social cognition is the application of mental operations in social interactions (Brothers 1990). This broadly includes domains of mentalizing or theory of mind, emotion processing, social cue identification, and attributional styles (Green et al. 2008) that subserve a whole range of complex higher-order cognitive abilities (e.g., perspective taking, deception detection, empathy, trust). Illustrations from clinical vignettes (Penn et al. 2008) and extensive factor analytical studies demonstrate that the latent variable which best supports social cognitive processing is one related to (but significantly differs from) general cognitive processes (e.g., attention, concentration, and memory), which are utilized in both nonsocial (e.g., remembering a shopping list) and social (e.g., responding to an arrogant colleague) situations; further, it is relatively affect neutral (Mehta et al. 2013). In contrast, social cognition represents the interface between emotional and cognitive processing; it has an intersubjective quality, requiring reflective (metacognitive) and social inferential abilities (Dimaggio et al. 2008). The brain networks that support these diverse streams of cognition and behavior are also, understandably, overlapping yet distinct. The social brain network overlaps the mentalizing network (medial prefrontal and temporoparietal cortex), the affect-sharing and motor-resonance networks (premotor, inferior frontal, inferior parietal, and insular cortices), as well as the social cue detection network (fusiform gyrus, amygdala, and superior temporal gyrus) (Green et al. 2015).

Social cognitive processes follow a typical ontogeny during development, are key elements required for successful social functioning, and map on to the development of distinct structural and functional brain networks (Kilford et al. 2016). The development of these social brain networks happens distinctly from the development of motivational affective and cognitive control processes. Since the developing child socially transacts with most of his/her environment, there is a constant experience-based reciprocal shaping of the processes involved in this triangulation of social cognition and behaviors, their underlying social brain network structure and function, and the social environment (family, school, society). Social brain network structure (e.g., amygdala volumes) and function (e.g., intrinsic amygdala-cortical connectivity) are found to relate to social network size as measured using the social network index (Bickart et al. 2011, 2012). In addition, there is a bidirectional, probably causal, relationship between mental disorders and social network size in adolescents (Hill et al. 2015; Rosenquist et al. 2011). General intelligence, the prevailing school climate, cultural influences, environmental stimulation and enrichment, recreational opportunities, pubertal stage, parenting, mental ill-health in parents, and chronological age can all moderate how environmental exposures engage the social brain in driving specific social-behavioral outcomes during adolescence. The successful transition to adulthood requires a rapid refinement and integration of these processes. In the transition of childhood to adolescence types of behavior, dynamic interactions (e.g., peer influence, sensitivity to social exclusion) take place between these systems. The environmental factors that can alter these brain and cognitive processes include adverse social experiences (in the context of family and school transitions) as well as migration and urbanization, which bring about critical social role transitions for developing youth. These environmental factors, as discussed earlier, are not uniform; they vary across cultures.

Culture also has a substantial scaffolding impact on shaping social brain processes and their behavioral outcomes. For instance, perceiving and expressing emotions seem to be governed by prevailing cultural folk schemata (Uchida and Kitayama 2009); emotion recognition abilities are better between members of the same (rather than different) national, ethnic, or regional group (Elfenbein 2002). Developmental studies have demonstrated that while there is synchrony in the age at onset of social cognition abilities across cultures (Callaghan et al. 2005), culture-specific principles strongly influence the subsequent shaping of these abilities across the life span (Lillard 1998). Developmental plasticity is responsible for this, mediated through immediate and delayed probabilistic-epigenetic processes, with an emphasis on bidirectional interactions among genes, neuronal activity, behavior, and environment across developmental epochs and generations (Li 2003). Indeed, neuroimaging studies demonstrate how culture influences differential neural responses in the amygdala to fearful faces and gaze direction in the processing of fear (Adams et al. 2010; Chiao et al. 2008). Neural correlates of theory of mind abilities may also differ depending upon cultural background (Kobayashi et al. 2007). Some researchers propose different levels of processing socially relevant information. The immediate responses of premotor mirror neurons may be independent of culture, but the inferential responses of the medial prefrontal cortex are culture dependent (Vogeley and Roepstorff 2009).

In summary, social cognition and social connectedness (which themselves are influenced by genetic, epigenetic, brain maturational, and sociocultural factors) foster resilience or amplify the risk (from multilevel social environmental exposures) for mental health outcomes during adolescence (Lamblin et al. 2017). Within the developmental cascades framework, social cognition includes processes that (a) are related to specific social brain networks, (b) drive an individual's multilevel social interactions that form a major component of the environment and (c) are mediated by the developmental stage, gender, and culture. These key processes can be studied in laboratory as well as within population-level epidemiological settings, thus enabling large-scale measurements and identification of specific intervention targets to be delivered at specific points in time.

Measurements and Study Designs

As we pursue the expansion of our knowledge of these multilevel contexts in which the environment can shape emerging psychopathology, we face significant gaps in defining and measuring the exposures and outcomes, especially at a larger scale (comprehensive coverage at a population level of a broad range of exposures/outcomes), with sufficient accuracy and at a critically dense time frequency. How does one measure, for instance, the robustness of a social network? A healthy social network could be defined by the *number* of individuals (MacCarron et al. 2016) that are part of one's social network (e.g., the Dunbar number or layers) or by a "happy medium" that characterizes the peer–peer interaction quality as assessed using ethnographic methods (Morgan-Trimmer and Wood 2016). Modeling of social networks in the real and virtual worlds by implementing *graph theory approaches*, traditionally used by social scientists (Wasserman and Faust 1994), is already being implemented in health sciences (Hogan et al. 2016). When used in conjunction with digital technology, such a framework promises the acquisition of important social engagement data, at a much larger scale and better frequency than can be collected using traditional assessments (Zhang et al. 2015). *Experience sampling methodology* (ESM), or ecological momentary assessment, is a structured self-report diary technique used to assess moment-to-moment variation in cognition, emotion, and behavior in the real world and in real time, outside the laboratory (Myin-Germeys et al. 2018; Shiffman 2009). ESM typically requires participants to complete a momentary assessment questionnaire several times a day over a number of days. Given its superior veridicality, ESM lends itself to more accurate investigations of the effects of social contexts (e.g., family, peers, school, work) on individuals and their interaction with these contexts at the micro level. The informed pairing of ESM with (a) *digital data streams* (Giles 2012; Insel 2017), mapping individual and group behavior via sensor, keyboard, location, voice, and speech data from smartphones, and (b) *novel artificial intelligence guided language and behavior processing algorithms* (Bedi et al. 2015) can provide a template for acquiring ecologically accurate social behavioral data at unprecedented scales, measurement densities, and levels of detail. Another method of improving accuracy in the measurements is to examine collaborative behaviors under specific conditions in the laboratory by focusing on dyadic stranger interactions (Weinstein et al. 2010); this permits process-related outcomes not influenced by past experience to be identified, independent of social interaction quality (partner closeness and responsiveness). These innovative but more definitive approaches can be further modified for application in large-sample population studies and combined with other deep phenotyping assessments in longitudinal designs.

Holistic capture of puberty during adolescence presents another gap in contemporary knowledge and measurement practice. Existing studies have done little to examine the speed of transition through puberty or the relationships between the different elements in pubertal development (Dorn 2015). Moving beyond the timing of pubertal completion and focusing on the critical pubertal transition stages of adrenal and gonadal maturation, as well as the pubertal growth spurt, are likely to yield clues to sensitive periods during which environmental exposures can manifest as adaptive or maladaptive outcomes.

Similarly, recent studies have begun to better characterize and define components of urban living that play a role in influencing mental health. Green spaces, artificial nighttime light, and built space, for example, can now be accurately mapped using geographical information systems. An illustration of its application is the demonstration that exposure to natural environments (e.g., greenery) might have a role in reducing suicide mortality (Helbich et al. 2018). A related novel method is to use satellite imagery in conjunction with convolutional neural networks, a deep learning technique used to extract features of the built environment and examine their influence on health outcomes, as was carried out for obesity prevalence rates (Maharana and Nsoesie 2018). These methods can be similarly applied to mental health outcomes across massive population samples and geographical boundaries, and offers the potential to guide region-specific environmental modification policies which, in turn, could affect mental health outcomes.

A combination of dense time series assessments at critically defined intervals (sufficient time for effects of exposure to manifest) throughout the developmental trajectory will reveal necessary data which can then be modeled using complex computational approaches. To harness the naturalistic course of adolescent development, study designs need to be both flexible and creative to yield sufficient data points and data depth in studying these influences. To help minimize costs and increase the yield of potentially new information needed to disentangle the complexities of developmental cascades across large population-based samples, we recommended (a) using samples from ongoing prospective birth-cohort studies and (b) performing nested randomized trials that incorporate some of the collection methods described here (e.g., ESM and digital phenotyping) within a collaborative framework. This will certainly help us overcome the limited length and breadth of measurement and shed more light on how early developmental factors relate to child psychopathology.

Using Newer Computational Approaches in Modeling Complex Systems

Given the tremendous amount of information that is likely to emerge from an in-depth acquisition of genomic, environmental, and brain connectomics data, parallel advances in statistical methods and data science techniques are imperative. In our efforts to tease out the effects of environmental exposures and behavioral health outcomes relevant to the developmental cascading context, we are likely to encounter not only direct and indirect linear relationships that can be understood using mediation models, but also more complex *nonlinear dynamic systems*, which encompass a more holistic rather than reductionist approach without sacrificing scientific and mathematical rigor. These models take into account the nonproportional exposure-outcome relationship, whereby "minimal" initial variations in exposure may produce "massive" unanticipated outcomes later, thereby being amenable to explore the dynamic environmental exposures on youth behavioral outcomes within the developmental cascading framework (Crutchfield et al. 1986). One important unanswered question concerns the timing of risk exposures in the development of behavioral and mental health problems. One possibility is that exposure to adversity in critical or sensitive periods is more likely to be followed by disorder. Alternatively, cumulative exposure over a longer period is the major determinant of risk. The adoption of sophisticated modeling techniques paired with appropriate measurements and study designs should provide more definitive answers to a question that is crucially important in designing prevention strategies.

Several efforts are already underway using advanced computational and analytical tools to identify hidden patterns in physiological (Drysdale et al. 2017), behavioral, phenomenological (Bedi et al. 2015; Clementz et al. 2016), real-world (Lee 2008), and virtual-world (Lazer et al. 2009) interpersonal exchanges, underwritten by both behavioral and neural responses and a broad range of macro-level environmental exposures (Maharana and Nsoesie 2018). Once identified, generative models of mental health outcomes can be tested by integrating these interactive levels of description (Huys et al. 2016; Stephan and Mathys 2014). Such models, when examined in prospective studies with dense time series data acquisitions, help to capture more accurately the relations between latent factors and observations, thereby facilitating theory building and empirical testing. This, in turn, can enable a more nuanced mechanistic interpretation of the data, ultimately permitting the identification of patient-specific combinations of various model parameters and model evidences for genetic and environmental disease mechanisms, as well as their mediators and moderators (Reiter et al. 2017).

Interventions

Despite the importance of the early childhood and adolescent periods as watershed developmental epochs in the manifestation of major psychiatric disorders of young adulthood, the availability of preventive and treatment services during these developmental phases is limited (Bailey and Dolan 2004). Based on the developmental cascades framework, strategies aimed at primary prevention and early intervention can be targeted at specific timescales (sensitive developmental epochs) and at specific levels of exposure, mediation, or moderation.

At the developmental timescale level, a valid example of a time-sensitive intervention that can inform potential translations to the field of mental health is borrowed from studies in youth to prevent polycystic ovarian syndrome—a complex endocrinological disorder of genetic origins prevalent in ~7% of women of reproductive age (Dunaif 2012) that has significant associations with anxiety and depressive disorders (Blay et al. 2016) —as well as neurodevelopmental disorders such as autism spectrum syndrome (Cesta et al. 2016; Cherskov et al. 2018). It has been demonstrated that if girls vulnerable to develop polycystic ovarian syndrome (low birth weight and precocious puberty) were administered metformin early (8–12 yr) as opposed to later (13–14 yr) in life, a distinct change in their phenotypes (e.g., taller, low central fat) occurred at age 15 yr. In addition, the early-treated girls had a two- to eightfold lower risk of developing polycystic ovarian syndrome than later-treated girls (Ibáñez et al. 2011). These are certainly encouraging examples of time-sensitive interventions that can potentially alter the developmental cascade.

At the micro, social, and environmental level, schools are ideal for intervening across diverse developmental timescales, as large populations of children can be targeted who spend significant amounts of time in a controlled setting, learning as well as interacting with peers and teachers. Primary or secondary prevention school-based interventions also offer scalability across regions and sustainability over time if found to be effective. HealthWise is one such comprehensive life skills program. Developed for use in South Africa to encourage positive free-time behavior and reduce the prevalence of unhealthy or risky behaviors (Wegner et al. 2007), HealthWise has shown promise in preventing substance use in school children (Smith et al. 2008). In this context, it is also important to consider who provides the intervention. Although teachers may be an ideal choice because of their availability in schools, lay counselor-guided interventions may have a more far-reaching impact, due to responsibility and time constraints in both professions. This was recently demonstrated in a recent pilot skills training intervention in the state of Bihar, India (Shinde et al. 2017). Given the impact of peer group influences on an individual during early adolescence (Sawyer et al. 2012), peer-driven interventions need to be explored for acceptability and effectiveness in promoting youth mental health.

One youth-friendly way to disseminate an intervention on a large scale to targeted populations is through the use of digital technology and online social networks (Biagianti et al. 2017). Both can complement existing youth mental health support systems and, if found to be feasible and effective, can be used as separate interventions. Apart from providing platforms for educative discourse, digital technologies can integrate individuals into online networks to increase levels of perceived support and belonging. It is crucial that general practitioners and other primary care workers be trained to not simply recognize mental and substance use disorders, but to deliver simple treatments as well, including supportive counseling, cognitive behavioral therapy, and psychotropic medications (Patel et al. 2007). Digital technology can facilitate this through skill development modules and "on-consultation" training provided through collaborative video consultation modules (Manjunatha et al. 2018).

Conclusion

Understanding how the environment interacts with genetically shaped human behavior along the developmental cascades over time, systems, and levels in the presence of several moderating and mediating mechanisms, to determine precursor symptoms that lead to severe mental illness in later life, requires a complex framework. Several micro- and macro-level influences—ranging from interpersonal relationships with parents, peers, and teachers to the rapidly changing social, economic, political, and environmental landscapes of our larger environment (e.g., urbanization)—have a dynamic interplay within the prevailing cultural and developmental (e.g., early brain development, puberty) contexts. This can lead to possible changes in epigenetic regulation of gene expression, neuronal circuits, and, through an iterative process, the generation of protective and risk states that determine mental health later in life. Here, we have highlighted several challenges and gaps that exist in piecing together this complex jigsaw puzzle and offered ways to address them:

- Definitions and measurements of key dynamic processes need to be improved.
- Study designs require refinement.
- Novel computational approaches need to be implemented to enable the identification of hidden (perhaps nonlinear) patterns across various levels of analyses, and to model these patterns more accurately and efficiently.

Advances in the field of genomic sequencing and gene expression studies, nuanced and comprehensive characterization of the *envirome*, untangling of the structural and functional brain connectome, and the applications of novel computational tools that integrate clinical, social, and basic neurosciences suggest that we are at the threshold of being able to make the leap toward creating specific maps of symptoms, vulnerability, and resilience with respect to environmental risks. Hence, we should soon have an outline of sensitive phases during development where targeted interventions can work. This confluence of multidisciplinary scientific questioning of human development has implications for our ability to enhance the life prospects of children and to strengthen the social, intellectual and economic fabric of society.

Biological Mechanisms Underlying Risk for Psychopathology

7

Dynamic Elements and Aspects of Neural Circuitry in Relation to Developmental Psychopathology in Youth

Byron K. Y. Bitanihirwe and T. Wilson Woo

Abstract

The journey from youth to adulthood involves a dynamic neurodevelopmental agenda which governs a series of intricate molecular and cellular events in the brain that ultimately affect the maturation of neural circuitry and cognitive properties. These neurobiological changes confer the ability to transition from parental guidance or guardianship to self-sufficiency. Adolescence represents an important inflection point on this journey: each person's unique experience during this distinct neurodevelopmental period is linked to positive and negative gradients of mental health as well as to vulnerability to mental illness. Despite significant technical achievements and advances in neuroscience, gaps still remain in our understanding and knowledge of the mechanisms that guide brain development and their relevance to the onset of psychiatric disease in youth. To contextualize the emergence of psychopathology in youth, this chapter outlines the neurobiological mechanisms underlying the development and maturation of neural circuitry in the brain during this critical period of life. Emphasis is placed on examining neural circuitry reorganization in response to physiological and pathological influences in relation to the emergence of developmental psychopathology. Controversial and open questions are discussed regarding developmental psychopathology in relation to youth. Unsolved problems, knowledge gaps, and the neurobiologically inspired notion of preventing psychopathology during this delicate period of neurodevelopment are also addressed.

Introduction

Youth is a phase of the life span that includes puberty, adolescence, and young adulthood. It is a distinct period of life when important neuronal developments and maturational refinements take place in the brain. Some of the key maturational processes known to occur in the brain during this period include synaptic pruning and myelination (Barnea-Goraly et al. 2005; Huttenlocher 2002). These neurodevelopmental changes lay the cognitive and emotional foundations for the individual to make the transition from parental guidance or guardianship to social and personal responsibilities associated with adulthood, such as starting a family, working, and contributing to one's community (Dahl et al. 2018).

While the brain maturation process has long been tied to hormonal fluctuations during puberty and adolescence (Sisk and Foster 2004; Vigil et al. 2016), genetic, environmental, and experiential phenomena are also known to provoke neuroplastic changes, which in turn can modulate the connectivity and communication between neurons and within and between individual neural circuits and brain regions (Tau and Peterson 2010). Notably, youth marks a critical period of life when the brain is particularly vulnerable to environmental, psychological, and physiological stressors that may disrupt the neural circuit architecture of the developing brain, culminating in the emergence of psychopathology (Lockhart et al. 2018; Paus et al. 2008). Indeed, it has been estimated that approximately 50% of all mental disorders emerge before the age of 15 yr and 75% before the age of 18 yr (Kessler et al. 2005). Hence, successful diagnosis and early intervention of major mental disorders in young people (e.g., schizophrenia, bipolar disorder, anxiety disorders, depression) will alleviate and perhaps even prevent lifelong detrimental consequences in terms of personal, family, economic, and societal cost (Holmes et al. 2018; Merikangas et al. 2009).

Here, we outline the key neurobiological mechanisms that govern the postnatal maturation of neural circuits in the developing brain. We also examine circuit reorganization in response to physiological and pathological influences in relation to the emergence of developmental psychopathology. Beyond the onset of psychopathology in youth, we discuss controversial and open questions as well as unsolved problems regarding the neurobiologically inspired notion of preventing psychopathology during this distinct period of neurodevelopment.

A Narrow Glimpse into Neural Circuitry Development in the Brain

Human brain development is a protracted, highly complex, and metabolically expensive process that begins during the second week of gestation and spans throughout adolescence and into adulthood (Kuzawa et al. 2014; Stiles and Jernigan 2010) (Figure 7.1). At birth and during early postnatal development, the brain is comprised of a surplus number of neuronal connections. As the brain develops during infancy and childhood, these connections afford benefits that are formed and strengthened; those that are "noisy" are eliminated

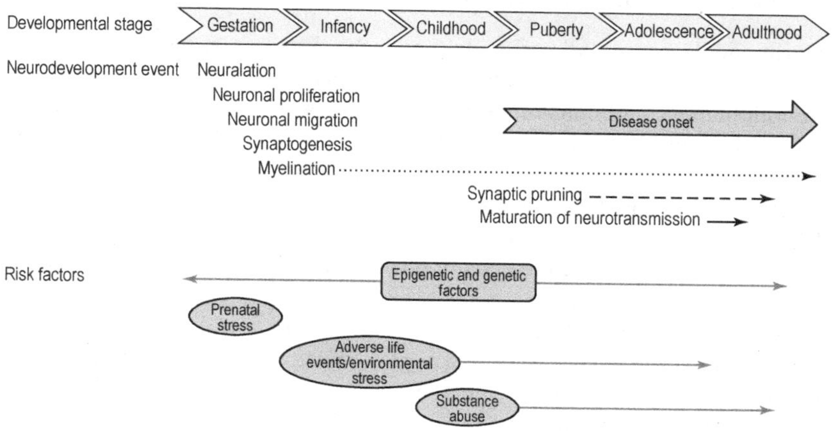

Figure 7.1 Timeline of neurodevelopmental processes involved in brain maturation in relation to onset of psychopathology in youth.

(Budday et al. 2015). The specificity of synapse connections involves a series of neurodevelopmental processes, including dendritic growth, axonal guidance, synaptogenesis, and synaptic elimination, which all ultimately contribute to the generation of a blueprint for neural circuits (Colon-Ramos 2009). Through the dynamic process of synaptic reorganization, which results in a net loss of the number of synapses, as well as the myelination of axonal fibers linking these cortical circuits and the maturation of neurotransmitter systems (e.g., the inhibitory circuitry within the cerebral cortex and dopaminergic innervation of the cerebral cortex), this blueprint is eventually sculpted into mature networks of functional neural circuits during the period of adolescence and early adulthood. This blueprint provides the neurobiological substrates that support higher-order cognitive and emotional abilities: decision making, executive planning, reasoning, problem solving, impulse control, and affective regulation, all of which are vital for an individual to navigate adulthood (Barnea-Goraly et al. 2005; Greiff et al. 2015; Stiles and Jernigan 2010; Tau and Peterson 2010).

Indeed, it is speculated that the pathophysiological underpinnings of major mental disorders stem from aberrations from the normal trajectories of maturation that take place during youth (Giedd et al. 1999; Paus et al. 2008). Here, we consider and summarize these dynamic neurobiological processes as they are thought to be particularly susceptible to both intrinsic (e.g., increased oxidative stress due to genetic vulnerability) and extrinsic (e.g., stress) perturbations that could derail their trajectories of maturation, and hence lead to psychopathology.

Maturation of Cortical Excitatory Circuits through Synaptic Pruning

During adolescence and early adulthood, the densities of glutamatergic synapses and dendritic spines on pyramidal neurons in the prefrontal cortex (PFC), in both humans and nonhuman primates, decrease by ~50% (Anderson et al. 1995; Goldman-Rakic et al. 1997; Huttenlocher 2002). Synaptic pruning can extend into the third decade of life in the human PFC (Petanjek et al. 2011). Other evidence has shown that in the monkey PFC, neural circuits furnished by layer 3 pyramidal neurons undergo large-scale pruning of axonal arbors (Woo et al. 1997). In contrast, the density of inhibitory synapses of γ-aminobutyric acid (GABA)ergic terminals is believed to be largely unaffected during this period of development (Kuzirian and Paradis 2011).

Imaging studies have shown that gray matter in prefrontal, parietal, and temporal cortices undergoes volumetric reductions through the period of late adolescence and early adulthood (Gogtay et al. 2004; Shaw et al. 2008; Sowell et al. 2001). This finding is generally thought to reflect, at least in part, the pruning of synapses, dendritic spines, and axonal terminals. Functionally, the establishment of the mature, large-scale neural networks of pyramidal neuronal circuits within and between brain regions is a prerequisite for the maturation and emergence of the highest level of cognitive and emotive regulations that, in many cases, are uniquely human.

Dysregulation in this developmental process has been associated with a number of neuropsychiatric conditions, perhaps most notably in schizophrenia and autism spectrum disorders (ASDs). While children with ASD have been posited to possess an excess number of synapses due to a deficit in pruning (Hutsler and Zhang 2010; Neniskyte and Gross 2017), patients with schizophrenia are thought to exhibit reduced synaptic connections as a result of exaggerated pruning (Feinberg 1982; Keshavan et al. 1994; McGlashan and Hoffman 2000; Woo and Crowell 2005).

Consistent with these hypotheses, the temporal window for synaptic overproduction commences around the age of onset for ASD. Although the onset of the synaptic pruning process temporally coincides with the decline in the prevalence of these disorders, the conclusion of this pruning process occurs at around the typical age range of onset for schizophrenia. In the case of schizophrenia, an alternative but not necessarily mutually exclusive hypothesis, is that pathophysiological events or insults (e.g., infection or hypoxia) which occur during the earlier stages of brain development (e.g., *in utero* or perinatal development) may result in "subthreshold" synaptic deficits, whereas the peri-adolescent synaptic pruning process magnifies these preexisting deficits, resulting in an alteration of synaptic numbers beyond the critical threshold. As such, the functional integrity of neural circuitry becomes compromised and ultimately contributes to the expression of the psychiatric phenotypes (Lewis and Lieberman 2000; McGlashan and Hoffman 2000; Weinberger 1987). Regardless, understanding the neurobiological mechanisms that govern synaptic pruning and dendritic and axonal remodeling during adolescence is likely to provide important insight into the pathophysiology of several neuropsychiatric conditions (Forrest et al. 2018).

Maturation of Cortical Inhibitory Circuits Mediated by Parvalbumin-Containing Neurons

Converging evidence of recent preclinical studies suggests that the maturation of inhibitory neural circuits regulates the onset and possibly the duration of the critical period for synaptic plasticity of excitatory pyramidal neurons (Berardi et al. 2000; Di Cristo 2007; Hensch 2003; Huang et al. 1999; Jiang et al. 2005; Kirkwood et al. 1995). For example, evoked GABA currents gradually increase postnatally, which temporally coincides with the critical period for synaptic plasticity (Berardi et al. 2000). In addition, the $GABA_A$ alpha 1 subunit, which is preferentially localized to synapses formed by basket cells—a subset of inhibitory neurons that express the calcium-binding protein parvalbumin (PV) (Gao and Fritschy 1994; Gao et al. 1993; Klausberger et al. 2002)—is necessary to initiate the critical period (Fagiolini et al. 2004). The notion that PV cells play a key role in regulating the critical period is also supported by the observation that dark rearing, which prolongs the duration of the critical period and delays the functional maturation of the visual cortex, is associated with a downregulation of the expression of the mRNA for PV (Tropea et al. 2006). Interestingly, these effects of dark rearing can be rescued by the overexpression of brain-derived neurotrophic factor, or BDNF (Gianfranceschi et al. 2003). Furthermore, in transgenic mice in which BDNF is overexpressed, the functional maturation of PV neurons is accelerated and accompanied by the precocious termination of the critical period (Hanover et al. 1999; Huang et al. 1999). Likewise, in the mouse barrel cortex, the maturation of PV neurons coincides with the time course of critical period and their maturation is arrested in BDNF (-/-) animals (Itami et al. 2007). Finally, it has been directly demonstrated that optimization of somatic inhibition provided by basket cells, many of which are PV-containing cells, is essential for critical period onset (Katagiri et al. 2007). Altogether, these observations indicate that inhibitory circuits mediated by PV neurons play a central role in the postnatal maturation of pyramidal neuronal circuits in the rodent cerebral cortex by regulating developmental synaptic plasticity, which subsequently affects excitatory/inhibitory synaptic balance.

At present, virtually nothing is known about the neurobiological mechanisms that govern adolescent synaptic pruning in the primate cortex; however, it appears that mechanisms similar to those identified in rodents may be involved. For instance, in both monkeys and humans, expression of BDNF in the PFC increases during postnatal development and peaks during the adolescent period (Huntley et al. 1992; Webster et al. 2002), when PV neurons gradually achieve maturation (Anderson et al. 1995). In addition, the expression of the $GABA_A$ receptor alpha 1 and 2 subunits, which are preferentially localized to synapses formed by PV-containing basket and chandelier neurons, respectively, undergo significant changes during adolescence (Cruz et al. 2003; Hashimoto et al. 2009). Together these observations suggest that similar inhibitory mechanisms that underlie the critical period for synaptic plasticity in the rodent cerebral cortex may also regulate the final maturation of the primate PFC during adolescence until young adulthood.

One aspect of the functional properties of PV neurons that is of particular interest is their preferential expression of the N-methyl-D-aspartate (NMDA) class of glutamate receptors: activation of these receptors plays an essential role in sustained neuronal activation during working memory (Durstewitz and Gabriel 2007; Wang 1999, 2001, 2002). Conversely, ablation of NMDA receptors on PV neurons impairs oscillatory synchrony of excitatory circuits in the gamma frequency band and working memory (Korotkova et al. 2010), which is an emergent property of gamma. Furthermore, in the rodent PFC, NMDA neurotransmission on PV neurons undergoes maturation during adolescence (Wang and Gao 2009), providing a physiological foundation for the maturation of working memory. Disturbances involving PV neurons at either the pre- or postsynaptic end are known to affect excitation-inhibition balance and have the potential to disrupt synaptic homeostasis, synaptic plasticity, and the maturation of gamma-band oscillations. These neurophysiological changes are known to lead to information processing and working memory deficits, in addition to other impairments in cognitive operations that require gamma, hence contributing to some aspects of psychopathology.

Microglia and the Complement System Sculpt the Maturation of Cortical Circuits

Increasing evidence implicates components of the neuroimmune system (e.g., certain proteins and microglia) as major players in the elimination of synapses during normal brain development (Paolicelli and Ferretti 2017; Schafer and Stevens 2010). While complement proteins play a role in the recognition and opsonization of pathogens, microglia serve as sentinels of the central nervous system (CNS). In contrast to all other elements of the brain, including other types of glial cells, which are derived from the neuroectoderm, microglia arise from the embryonic endoderm, which gives rise to cells of the blood and immune system.

Over the past few years, there has been a steady growth in knowledge about microglia and the complement system in the physiology of the CNS (Aguzzi et al. 2013; Kettenmann et al. 2013; Paolicelli and Ferretti 2017). Indeed, a burgeoning body of evidence indicates that these immunomodulatory components play a central role in many aspects of neurodevelopment (Mallya et al. 2018; Paolicelli and Ferretti 2017; Reemst et al. 2016; Tay et al. 2017). Specifically, in the context of the current discussion, microglia and the complement cascade have been shown to be involved in synaptic formation, elimination, and maturation (Hoshiko et al. 2012; Miyamoto et al. 2016; Ueno et al. 2013). Notably, a recent study of the PFC in rats during critical periods of postnatal development has found microglia to engulf glutamatergic elements on both the presynaptic end—identified by vesicular glutamate transporter 1 (vGlut1) immunoreactivity—and the postsynaptic end—identified by postsynaptic density-95 (PSD-95) immunoreactivity (Mallya et al. 2018). Thus, in conjunction with other processes discussed in this chapter, it appears that the immune system plays a key role in the final maturation of cortical circuits (Mallya et al. 2018).

Given the apparent roles of microglia and the complement cascade in the critical processes of circuitry refinements that sculpt the eventual maturation of the cerebral cortex, one may speculate that any deviation from the functional homeostasis of either of these immunoregulatory systems during brain development could contribute to the onset of neuropsychiatric disorders as a result of dysmaturation of synaptic connectivities. Indeed, Sekar et al. (2016) recently reported that diverse alleles of the *complement component 4* gene promote altered expression of the *complement component 4* gene in the brain of patients with schizophrenia. Given that the complement 4 protein is located at neuronal synapses, dendrites, axons, and cell bodies, anomalies in *complement component 4* expression may influence synaptic pruning and stability, thus contributing to the synaptic and neural circuit deficits observed in schizophrenia patients (Sekar et al. 2016). Similarly, published evidence suggests that microglial dysfunction exists along with deficits in synaptic connectivity reported in schizophrenia and ASD (Monji et al. 2009; Morgan et al. 2010). Findings using animal models have mechanistically linked microglia to some of the behavioral phenotypes that resemble deficits associated with these conditions (Bilbo and Schwarz 2012; Blank and Prinz 2013). For example, in mouse models of maternal immune activation, in which animals are subjected to infection *in utero*, offspring are observed to develop a constellation of behavioral deficits, such as deficits in prepulse inhibition and social interactions as well as cognitive impairments associated with schizophrenia (Bitanihirwe et al. 2010b, 2010c; Meyer 2014; Vuillermot et al. 2010). Beyond the changes in cognition and behavior observed in these animal models, the number and the activational state of these cells in the brains of these animals are also drastically altered (Bilbo et al. 2007; Giovanoli et al. 2013; Williamson et al. 2011). Perhaps most interestingly, these effects are especially prominent in those animals that are further exposed to stress later in life (Giovanoli et al. 2013). These findings, therefore, support the concept that *in utero* insults, such as maternal infection, can "prime" microglia such that exposure to subsequent challenges later in life elicits an exaggerated neuroinflammatory response mediated by these cells; this may then lead to aberrant maturation of brain circuits and thereby contribute to the onset of neuropsychiatric disorders in youth.

Perineuronal Nets Consolidate the Maturation of Cortical Circuits

Perineuronal nets (PNNs) are lattice-like structures comprised of extracellular matrix molecules, including chondroitin sulfate proteoglycans, hyaluronan, tenascin-R, and link proteins (Wang and Fawcett 2012). These structures are commonly found ensheathing various neuronal and neuritic elements, including the soma and proximal dendrites of PV neurons (Hockfield et al. 1990; McDonald et al. 2018). Although the exact functions of the PNN remain to be elucidated, a number of studies suggest that they may play a contributory role in neuroprotection (Cabungcal et al. 2013b), ion homeostasis (Morawski et al. 2015), synaptic plasticity (Pizzorusso et al. 2002), as well as regulating the excitatory-inhibitory balance of neural circuits (Cabungcal et al. 2013b; Donato et al. 2013; Liu et al. 2013a).

Together with the maturation of inhibitory neural circuits involving PV neurons, as described above, the progressive formation of PNNs during the postnatal developmental period increasingly restricts cortical plasticity, hence marking the end of the critical period of adolescent neurodevelopment (Sorg et al. 2016). Notably, enzymatic removal of PNNs in the adult brain, such as by chondroitinase ABC, is known (a) to reinstate a juvenile state of experience-dependent plasticity, such as restoring ocular dominance plasticity in the visual system (Pizzorusso et al. 2002) or reestablishing auditory relearning capacity that is normally lost after the adolescent period (Happel et al. 2014) and (b) to erase fear memory, which is normally only possible in the juvenile brain within a critical period during postnatal development (Gogolla et al. 2009). Further, PNN removal resets neural network activity to the juvenile state by readjusting excitatory-inhibitory balance (Lensjo et al. 2017), hence providing a neurophysiological mechanism for enhanced plasticity that is otherwise not possible in the adult brain.

Expression of PNN components around PV neurons is modulated by the homeoprotein orthodenticle homeobox 2 (OTX2) (Sugiyama et al. 2008), which is produced and secreted by epithelial cells of the choroid plexus (Spatazza et al. 2013a, 2013b). OTX2 is then taken up by PV neurons and subsequently promotes their functional maturation. Recent research has shown that OTX2 uptake into PV neurons is dependent on the structural maturity of PNNs in terms of the sulfation pattern of chondroitin sulfate proteoglycans, resulting in a positive feedback loop (Beurdeley et al. 2012; Lee et al. 2017; Miyata et al. 2012).

Given the integral role of PNNs in the regulation of postnatal experience-dependent maturation of brain circuits and the maintenance of their functional integrity in the mature brain, aberrant formation of PNNs during development can, in theory, contribute to developmental neuropsychiatric disorders by disturbing these processes. Indeed, deficits in structural components of PNNs have been reported in postmortem entorhinal cortex, thalamic reticular nucleus, amygdale, and PFC in people affected by schizophrenia and bipolar disorder (Mauney et al. 2013; Pantazopoulos et al. 2010; Steullet et al. 2017). In addition to the postmortem evidence linking PNN disruption to developmental psychopathology, evidence from preclinical work using a rat model of prenatal immune activation, which captures some aspects of the pathophysiology of schizophrenia, found a reduction of PNNs in the PFC and amygdala in offspring exposed to maternal immune activation during pregnancy (Paylor et al. 2016). Other research has shown that mice lacking the NR2A subunit of the NMDA receptor exhibit alterations in redox status that results in the delayed maturation of PNNs (Cardis et al. 2018). Interestingly, a reduction in NR2A mRNA expression was previously observed in the cerebral cortex of subjects with schizophrenia (Woo et al. 2004), and this reduction occurs preferentially, if not selectively, in PV neurons (Bitanihirwe et al. 2010a). Furthermore, redox regulation is increasingly recognized to be altered in this disorder (Do et al. 2009, 2015). Thus, it appears that NR2A reduction together with redox dysregulation may represent one of the possible mechanisms that underlie PNN deficits in schizophrenia.

Ventral Tegmental Area Dopaminergic Projections Sculpt the Maturation of Cortical Circuits

A number of specific and unique brain connections that are established during early to mid-adolescence may influence a variety of behaviors (e.g., such as risk taking) as well as affective and cognitive abilities (Crone and Dahl 2012). For example, dopaminergic projections from the ventral tegmental area (VTA) to the cortex exhibit marked postnatal maturation (Goto and Grace 2007; Rosenberg and Lewis 1995; Tseng and O'Donnell 2007). Until young adulthood, the concentration of dopamine and the density of fibers immunoreactive for tyrosine hydroxylase (the rate-limiting enzyme in the synthesis of dopamine from tyrosine) continue to increase in the PFC (Lambe et al. 2000; Rosenberg and Lewis 1995). Aside from the PFC, dopaminergic neurons within the VTA also project to the medial and ventral parts of the caudate putamen, nucleus accumbens, hippocampus, and amygdala (Goto and Grace 2007). These projections from the mesolimbic dopaminergic system are not fully mature until after adolescence. The late maturation of these dopaminergic connections has been proposed to influence the development and integration of normal and abnormal emotional behavior and cognition during adolescence (Goto and Grace 2007). Consistent with the observations of adolescent maturation of dopaminergic fibers, distinct developmental trajectories have also been reported in other components of the dopamine system, including dopamine receptors (D1, D2 short and D2 long isoforms, D4, D5), catechol-*O*-methyltransferase, and monoamine oxidase (A and B) (Roudi and Moser 2014).

PV neurons are a principal recipient of dopaminergic inputs to the PFC (Sesack et al. 1998). In monkeys, PV neurons preferentially express the dopamine D1 receptor (Muly et al. 1998). Furthermore, dopaminergic innervation of the monkey PFC undergoes a process of overproduction followed by pruning during adolescence (Rosenberg and Lewis 1995). The expression of the D1 receptor follows a very similar time course of postnatal maturation (Lidow and Rakic 1992), although how the neuronal localization of the D1 receptor is developmentally regulated is unknown. As the D1 receptor plays a critical role in working memory by mediating sustained neuronal firing (Williams and Castner 2006), the maturation of D1 expression in PV cells may be one of the key players in the emergent ability of PFC circuitry to engage in gamma oscillatory synchrony during postnatal development (Uhlhaas et al. 2009, 2010), which may provide the temporal structure within which experience-dependent synaptic pruning is possible (Woo et al. 2010). Disturbances in gamma-band oscillations may therefore interfere with developmental synaptic reorganization processes. Such disturbances may, in turn, contribute to the behavioral symptoms and cognitive deficits observed in neurodevelopmental conditions such as schizophrenia and ASD (Uhlhaas 2013; Uhlhaas and Singer 2015; van Diessen et al. 2015).

Myelination Consolidates the Maturation of Cortical Networks

One of the final steps involved in brain maturation is myelination. Within and between brain regions, it facilitates neural circuit communication by allowing myelinated axons to transmit electrical signals much more rapidly than unmyelinated axons, hence maximizing the fidelity and efficiency of information processing and cementing the final functional maturation of the entire cerebral cortex (Picton and Taylor 2007; Weil et al. 2016). The timing of myelination is dependent upon the region of the brain. For instance, while sensory and motor regions tend to be myelinated during brain development in childhood, myelination of the PFC is not completed until early adulthood (Sousa et al. 2017). Interestingly, the period in which the normal maturation of myelinated pathways involving the PFC takes place coincides with the common age of onset of many neuropsychiatric conditions, such as psychotic disorders (Kroken et al. 2014; Mighdoll et al. 2015). It is of interest to note that in metachromatic leukodystrophy, a dysmyelination disorder with a wide range of ages of onset, patients who develop the disease during the adolescent period, but not during childhood or adulthood, are most prone to develop psychosis (Hyde et al. 1992). Perhaps because myelination is a temporally discordant process in which different brain regions follow specific temporal trajectories of myelination, dysmyelination that occurs at different developmental times may lead to the emergence of distinct constellations of clinical symptoms and cognitive deficits by disturbing information processing mediated by different brain circuits and networks. Thus, unraveling the pathophysiological basis that explains the propensity of adolescent dysmyelination for the emergence of psychosis would be instructive in deepening our understanding of the neurobiological substrate of psychosis.

Normally there is an age-related increase in the numerical density of oligodendrocytes, consistent with greater myelination of the major fiber tracts that link areas of the associative cortex, such as the PFC and the anterior cingulate cortex, with the temporal regions throughout adolescence (Benes 1989). Beyond the neuroimaging studies that have played an integral role in delineating the developmental trajectories of white matter (Lebel and Deoni 2018), further evidence supporting the progressive increase of myelin observed during neurodevelopment comes from protein and mRNA studies evaluating 2′,3′-cyclic nucleotide 3′-phosphodiesterase (CNP) and myelin-associated glycoprotein (MAG), markers for mature oligodendrocytyes. Indeed, it has been found that both MAG and CNP expression appear to increase with age (Miller et al. 2012).

In addition to the genetic program that dictates the developmental time course of myelination, neuronal activity has also been shown to play an important role in fine-tuning the myelination process and thus axonal conduction velocity, which can directly affect the precision of information-processing dynamics within neural circuits (de Faria et al. 2018; Tomlinson et al. 2016). Aberrant oligodendrocyte differentiation has been suggested to underlie myelin deficiencies in schizophrenia (Mauney et al. 2015) and may also contribute to the development of other neuropsychiatric conditions, such as depression, bipolar disorder, or obsessive-compulsive disorder (Marlinge et al. 2014; Miyata et al. 2016; Nissen et al. 2016).

Hormonal Changes

The surge in hormones that takes place during puberty is known to play an influential role in neurodevelopmental changes (Blakemore et al. 2010; Peper and Dahl 2013; Sisk and Foster 2004; Sisk and Zehr 2005; Vigil et al. 2016). These have been linked to risk taking as well as social and exploratory behavior (Crone and Dahl 2012). While the exact endocrine mechanisms underlying the onset of puberty continue to be unraveled, it is widely appreciated that a key event that signals the beginning of this transitional period is the activation of the hypothalamic–hypophyseal–gonadal axis, which is maintained in a dormant state during prepubertal years through what has been defined as an "intrinsic CNS inhibitory mechanism" (Vigil et al. 2016). The "release" of the hypothalamic–hypophyseal–gonadal system from the dormant state involves gonadotropin-releasing hormone secretion, which leads to gonadal maturation and the awakening of the reproductive system through the production of sex steroids (testosterone in boys and estradiol in girls).

These hormonal influences have been categorized as either activational or organizational (Arnold and Breedlove 1985). Activational effects are transient, occur throughout life, and can facilitate sex-typical physiological processes or behavior. Organizational effects are permanent and are believed to occur during early development. For instance, when testosterone is transiently elevated in males, it is believed to masculinize the brain (Celec et al. 2015). Similarly, when ovarian hormones are released into the system, they are believed to program sex-typical physiology and behavior (Arnold and Breedlove 1985). Interestingly, brain developmental studies applying imaging techniques have reported the effects of sex steroids on cerebral gray matter morphology, and these differences are believed to underlie the risk for sex-biased psychopathologies. Indeed, a recent study by Koolschijn et al. (2014) reported that sex-specific differences in testosterone can influence the volume of the anterior cingulate cortex. This cortical region, which has been linked to developmental psychopathology (Lichenstein et al. 2016), is a neural hub that integrates cognitive, affective, and social information so as to guide self-regulation across domains and support adaptive development of self-regulation during adolescence. In another study, ovarian hormones at the onset of puberty were shown to exert organizational effects in the PFC via increased GABAergic neurotransmission, thus contributing to its functional maturation (Piekarski et al. 2017a). While the inhibitory neuronal cell type mediating this observation was not identified, Piekarski et al. speculate that PV neurons are the likely candidate by virtue of the preferential expression of the estrogen β receptor in these cells, compared to any other neuronal types. Furthermore, manipulating puberty onset by altering the levels of ovarian hormones can directly influence the maturation of PFC-mediated functions, providing a possible link between sex hormones, maturation of inhibitory circuits mediated by PV neurons, and the onset and emergence of psychopathology in youth.

Effects of the Microbiome on the Maturation of Cortical Circuits

The human microbiome represents an ecosystem comprised of bacteria, archaea, viruses, and eukaryotic microbes that reside in and on our bodies, resulting in a unique symbiotic relationship (Eloe-Fadrosh and Rasko 2013). These microbes have tremendous potential to impact physiology, and their composition is now known to change throughout life in response to physiological and environmental cues (Rodriguez et al. 2015). Increasing research has shown the microbiome to modulate a number of key metabolic aspects, such as the immune and endocrine systems (Dickerson et al. 2017; Zeevi et al. 2016). Beyond these aspects, increasing and provocative evidence has linked the microbiome to processes related to the development of brain circuits, including myelination, neuronal maturation, and neuromodulation, such as that mediated by GABAergic, glutamatergic, serotonergic, or dopaminergic pathways (Lu et al. 2018). Additional evidence suggests that a plethora of external challenges and events to which adolescents are exposed (e.g., diet changes, sleep patterns, psychological stress, alcohol and drug use) have all been suggested to result in alterations to the composition of the intestinal microbiota (Shreiner et al. 2015). These changes in microbiome homeostasis may affect neural pathways and circuits and contribute to the emergence of neuropsychiatric disorders (Dickerson et al. 2017; McVey Neufeld et al. 2016; Tognini 2017). Using mouse models and intervention studies involving fecal microbiota transplantation, a series of recent translational studies, for instance, have linked a dysfunction in the microbiome with neuropsychiatric conditions such as ASD (De Angelis et al. 2015; Li et al. 2017; Williams et al. 2012), schizophrenia (Castro-Nallar et al. 2015; Olde Loohuis et al. 2018; Yolken et al. 2015), and affective disorders (Castro-Nallar et al. 2015; De Angelis et al. 2015).

Other evidence linking the microbiome to psychopathology stems from studies that evaluate the effects of antibiotic treatment and intestinal microbial dysbiosis in germ-free animals. These studies not only identified alterations in brain neurochemistry typically associated with psychopathology, they report changes in behavioral phenotypes relevant to psychiatric illness, including increased anxiety- and depression-like phenotypic traits (Clarke et al. 2013; Desbonnet et al. 2014; Moloney et al. 2014; Neufeld et al. 2011). Against this background, targeting the microbiota–gut–brain axis during adolescence in individuals at high risk for psychopathology may represent a preventative approach to protect the brain from undue physiological stress and improve mental health outcome (McVey Neufeld et al. 2016).

Aberrant Maturation of Cortical Circuits in Youth

Impact of Neuroinflammation on Emerging Psychopathology

The CNS had long been considered to be "immune privileged," neither susceptible nor contributing to inflammation (Klein and Hunter 2017). Increasingly, however, it has been appreciated that the immune system and its associated inflammatory processes may play a crucial role in various aspects of normal and aberrant brain development, such as synaptic organization and function. Neuroinflammation can be broadly defined as a complex set of orchestrated biochemical processes in the brain in response to a wide variety of intrinsic (e.g., oxidative stress, autoimmune condition) or extrinsic (e.g., infection, environmental stress) events or insults involving the activation of microglia and the increased release of many molecular signals (e.g., cytokines, chemokines, growth factors, and immune components such as complements) by microglia as well as other cell types (e.g., astrocytes, neurons).

Pre- or perinatal insults (e.g., infection, poor maternal health, malnutrition) can trigger inflammatory and immune responses, which may compromise or alter the course of *in utero* brain development. These insults have been associated with an increased incidence of developmental neuropsychiatric disorders, the onset of which occurs during childhood (e.g., ASD, obsessive-compulsive disorder) or youth (e.g., schizophrenia, bipolar disorder, borderline personality disorder) long after the occurrence of the insults.

What mechanisms account for the delay between the occurrence of these insults and the actual onset of psychopathology a decade or two later? It has been hypothesized that the immune system is "primed" or "sensitized," especially in individuals who may be genetically predisposed, by the initial inflammatory events, and that subsequent exposure to insults (e.g., psychological stress, infection), during postnatal brain development, triggers the same or an exaggerated response at a lower threshold—the second hit. In other words, the individual becomes more vulnerable to developing psychopathology at the second hit because these insults nonlinearly magnify the resultant neuroinflammatory response, thus disturbing the brain circuits that are undergoing maturation at the time of the second hit. This leads to impairment in cognitive, emotive, or perceptual functions that are normally supported by these circuits.

Immune proteins and cytokines, such as IL-1 β and IL-6, have been found to be elevated in the serum of patients suffering from various neuropsychiatric conditions, including depression, schizophrenia, or bipolar disorder (Goldsmith et al. 2016). Moreover, postmortem studies in schizophrenia and depression implicate immune cell activation in the disease process (Shelton et al. 2011; Trepanier et al. 2016). These findings, however, are inconclusive due to the wide variability in results and factors associated with death. Recently, a series of positron emission tomography studies evaluated neuroinflammation in psychopathology by using a ligand for translocator protein (TSPO), which is greatly induced in activated microglial cells (Albrecht et al. 2016). Studies conducted in schizophrenia and depression, for example, revealed differences in the levels of TSPO in distinct neuroanatomical regions of the brain known to be associated with the clinical symptoms of these disorders (Hafizi et al. 2017a, 2017b; Holmes et al. 2018) and support the role of neuroinflammation in psychopathology.

Within the concept of neuroinflammation contributing to psychopathology onset, the potential roles of oxidative stress have attracted increasing attention (Do et al. 2009, 2015; Mahadik and Scheffer 1996). Neuroinflammation and oxidative stress are inextricably linked to one another, with events such as infection or stress inducing proinflammatory cytokines, which in turn evoke free radical formation that result in oxidative damage to DNA, proteins, and lipids, possibly contributing to the pathophysiology of a number of psychiatric disorders, such as depression, anxiety, and schizophrenia (Edlow 2017; Najjar et al. 2014; Neier et al. 2015; Xanthos and Sandkuhler 2014). In fact, oxidative stress is thought to lead to an increase in the expression of the matrix metalloproteinase MMP-9, which in turn promotes the proteolysis of receptors for advanced glycation end products (RAGE) 55-kDa type I membrane glycoprotein of the immunoglobulin superfamily, resulting in the shedding of a soluble ectodomain, which then promotes neuroinflammation (Dwir et al. 2017). In addition, MMP-9 was shown to be involved in brain structural and functional plasticity (Murase et al. 2017). For instance, increased expression of MMP-9 during neuroinflammation and oxidative stress may disrupt the postnatal maturation of brain circuitry in part through the degradation of PNNs (Gray et al. 2008; Wen et al. 2017). Given that PNNs play an integral role in capturing OTX2 (Beurdeley et al. 2012), the availability of which is necessary for modulating cortical plasticity by promoting and sustaining the functional integrity of PV neurons, MMP-9-mediated degradation of PNNs would negatively impact, if not overtly derail, the maturation of brain circuits in youth by disrupting excitatory-inhibitory balance (Takesian and Hensch 2013), hence contributing to the developmental pathophysiology of neuropsychiatric disorders (Chauhan et al. 2010; Lepeta and Kaczmarek 2015; Vafadari et al. 2016; Wen et al. 2017).

Impact of Stress on Emerging Psychopathology

The dopamine system is known to undergo remodeling and maturation during adolescence (Wahlstrom et al. 2010). Exposure to stress during early life has been hypothesized to interfere with the maturation of the dopamine circuitry in the brain, with subsequent implications for adolescent onset of psychiatric disorders (Syed and Nemeroff 2017). Indeed, synaptic perturbations within dopaminergic circuitry of the nucleus accumbens have been suggested to provide the neural substrate for the altered hedonic state often observed in depression (Russo et al. 2012; Russo and Nestler 2013). Recent work has found an elevation of dendritic spine density and increased glutamatergic postsynaptic currents on nucleus accumbens medium spiny neurons in mice following chronic social defeat stress—a paradigm that induces a depression-like phenotype (Christoffel et al. 2011; Golden et al. 2013). It is also known that medium spiny neurons within the nucleus accumbens contain both D1 and D2 type receptors, which play distinctive roles in stress-induced depression-like behavior. Thus, mice which display depression-like behavior following the chronic social defeat stress paradigm exhibit a decrease in excitatory synaptic input to medium spiny neurons expressing the D1 receptor and an increase in medium spiny neurons that express the D2 receptor. Furthermore, using cell-specific optogenetic techniques, it has been directly demonstrated that activation of D1 neurons can promote resilience, whereas activation of D2 neurons promotes susceptibility (Francis et al. 2015). These findings are consistent with other recent studies which suggest that similar circuit mechanisms may play a role in depression-like phenotypes (Bruns et al. 2018; Heshmati et al. 2018; Hodes et al. 2015). Further work is necessary to establish and understand the specific circuitry that undergoes plasticity after stress, as well as to test their functional role in regulating depression-like behavior.

In addition to the nucleus accumbens, the VTA represents a key dopaminergic region involved in affective regulation. Utilizing a two-hit stress mouse model, which combines early life stress from maternal separation with chronic social defeat stress later in life, Pena et al. (2017) recently showed that stress during an early postnatal sensitive window can increase susceptibility to depression in adulthood via long lasting transcriptional programming in the VTA in an OTX2-dependent fashion. Thus, OTX2 may be a key regulator of developmental neural circuit plasticity that transcends sensory and functional domains.

Impact of Cannabis on Emerging Psychopathology

Based on the increasing literature linking exposure to cannabis with psychotic illness (Murray et al. 2017a, 2017b; Sami and Bhattacharyya 2018), this psychoactive drug remains an integral model for understanding the neurobiology of psychosis (Burns 2013; Shrivastava et al. 2014). Given recent activities to legalize recreational use of cannabis in the United States and Canada, this is a most relevant issue. These studies suggest that several factors moderate the link between cannabis and psychosis, including age of exposure, amount of cannabis use, potency of the substance, and a family history of psychotic illness (Murray et al. 2017b). However, because of a lack of clear information in the published studies regarding the potency of the cannabis evaluated, recall bias in the individual's pattern of cannabis consumption, as well as a clear definition of the cannabis consumer in terms of frequency and duration of use, straightforward conclusions are difficult (Burns 2013).

Neurobiologically, the potential mechanistic link between cannabis and psychosis remains unclear, although research studies do point toward alterations in dopamine neurotransmission. Preclinical evidence has revealed that tetrahydrocannabinol, one of the main psychoactive constituents of cannabis, increases dopamine levels and dopamine firing in the VTA, nucleus accumbens, and striatum (Cheer et al. 2004; Ginovart et al. 2012; Tanda et al. 1997), which in turn can modulate striatal endocannabinoid release (Giuffrida et al. 1999). In the cerebral cortex, the cannabinoid 1 receptor (CB1), the principal cannabinoid receptor expressed in the brain, is widely distributed across layers especially in the upper layers (i.e., 2–4), which furnish corticocortical and thalamocortical connections (Eggan et al. 2010b). Furthermore, the CB1 receptor appears to be preferentially localized to the presynaptic terminals of the population of basket cells that express the neuropeptide cholecystokinin (CCK) which, along with those basket cells that contain PV, regulate perisomatic inhibition of pyramidal neurons (Soltesz 2005).

Activation of CB1 is thought to suppress GABA neurotransmission between CCK and pyramidal neurons. In schizophrenia, the density of the mRNA for CB1 receptor and that of CB1-immunoreactive profiles have been found to be decreased, which may represent a compensatory mechanism to restore the perisomatic inhibition that is diminished as a result of a deficit of PV neurons (Eggan et al. 2008, 2010b). These findings provide a neurobiological pathway through which cannabis can affect perisomatic inhibition of pyramidal neurons via their binding to the CB1 receptor and, through this mechanism, may influence higher cortical functions by affecting gamma synchrony.

Can the Emergence of Psychopathology in Youth Be Prevented?

Youth represents a distinct developmental period of brain circuitry associated with resilience and vulnerability. It is also a period during which many mental disorders tend to emerge. We have provided a conceptual framework derived from the latest understanding of the neurobiology of aspects of postnatal brain maturation. Specifically, many elements of the brain undergo profound changes during postnatal development: the excitatory circuits furnished by pyramidal neurons, the inhibitory circuits involving PV neurons, which regulate the maturation of the excitatory circuits, and the PNN which, in turn, regulates and consolidates the maturation of both the PV inhibitory and pyramidal neuronal circuits. Additionally, hormonal changes, neurotransmitter systems (e.g., the dopamine and the cannabinoid systems), and the microbiome can further modify the maturation of these circuits. Finally, myelination represents perhaps one of the last steps to solidify the functional maturation of the brain by "insulating" the communication between and within neural circuits to ensure the efficiency and fidelity of information processing. It is important to note, however, that all of these processes are developmentally and mechanistically intertwined. Thus, any perturbation at any point in time in development can affect one, some, or all of these processes.

Within this framework, it may be possible to begin to develop theoretical models that may explain the developmental pathophysiology of psychopathology. Nevertheless, there are many unanswered questions. For example, neuroinflammation appears to be one of the possible mechanisms that can affect all aspects of the entire developmental processes—from prenatal development to the final maturation of the cerebral cortex during youth and early adulthood—although the precise molecular pathways that mediate these pathophysiological mechanisms are poorly defined. How and why can the same mechanisms (e.g., stress) influence the pathophysiology of a wide range of clinically distinct neuropsychiatric disorders? Is this due to the timing of the occurrence of the specific events or the nature of the events themselves? What determines whether (and if so how) some individuals are more or less vulnerable (or susceptible) to identical insults? What are the protective mechanisms that mitigate the potential detrimental effects of these insults? In other words, which neurobiological elements confer resilience? Perhaps the most provocative question is: Can psychopathology be prevented?

The goal of preventive interventions is to reduce the impact of established causal risk factors, affect the availability and/or influence of known protective factors, and reduce the likelihood that adolescents will develop or progress toward psychopathology (Costello 2016). Realizing this goal requires a multipronged approach to identify the pathogenetic variables at the genetic, epigenetic, genomic, molecular, cellular, circuit, physiological, behavioral, and even psychosocial levels, and to understand how these variables may drive the onset of psychopathology in youth by causing aberrant or maladaptive neural circuit development. Despite the knowledge outlined in this chapter, substantial gaps remain as many of these variables have yet to be identified and elucidated. Ultimately, to understand how these variables may lead to psychopathology onset, a systems-level approach is likely to be essential, given the extremely large number of variables involved in various combinatorial fashions, the fact that the interactions of these variables are likely to be nonlinear, and the complexity of defining how these variables derail the trajectories of brain development. The emerging field of prediction modeling, which applies concepts such as dynamic systems theory, network theory, catastrophe theory, as well as instability mechanisms may hold the promise of determining what and how specific variables may influence and trigger the onset of specific psychopathology (Nelson et al. 2017; Rosenberg et al. 2018). Thus, effective early intervention and prevention strategies requires the development of strategies that can modify or ideally normalize the pathogenetic effects of these variables at specific point in time during brain maturation.

Acknowledgments

The authors' laboratory is supported by the National Institutes of Health.

8

Biological Mechanisms Underlying Risk for Emerging Psychopathology in Youth

Matcheri S. Keshavan and Shreya V. Nallur

Abstract

For many years it was believed that the fundamental properties of the brain were sculpted mainly *in utero* and in the early postnatal years, but data from a range of disciplines have forced a reassessment of this notion. The transition from childhood to adulthood, especially the critical period of adolescence, involves a profound reorganization of both architecture and functionality of large-scale networks, which is likely to constitute a vulnerability for emerging psychopathologies and opportunities for intervention.

For youth (15–24 yr) and, in particular, adolescents (10–19 yr), dramatic changes occur (physically and behaviorally) during this critical period of development. Although most teenagers successfully navigate the transition from dependence on a caregiver to being a self-sufficient member of society, adolescence is also a time of increasing incidence of several classes of psychiatric illness, including psychosis, mood disorders, and substance abuse. The pathophysiology of these disorders is increasingly understood as arising from aberrations in the maturational changes that normally occur in the adolescent brain. This chapter reviews the neurobiological changes that occur during adolescence and discuss their possible relationship to the emergence of psychopathology.

How Do Genetic and Environmental Risk Factors Interact to Produce the Expression of Mental Disorders in Youth?

The causes of schizophrenia and related psychotic disorders are complex and heterogeneous, with a multitude of risk and protective factors being suggested (Radua et al. 2018). An extensive body of literature points to genetic and environmental risk factors and their interactions (Tandon et al. 2008; van Os et al. 2008). In reviewing this large literature, it is important to consider some key caveats. First, most of what we know for establishing causality comes from epidemiological data wherein guidelines exist about how to evaluate the strength of causal relationships (Hill 1965). These include the strength of association between a putative causal factor and its effect, consistency of the observations between populations and studies, specificity of the relationship (no other explanation for the relationship), temporality (cause precedes the effect), dose effect (the greater the exposure, the higher the association), the availability of a plausible mechanism (subject to what is known), and laboratory or experimental data showing the causal effect (e.g., animal models). These strict criteria (including well-known causal associations such as between cigarette smoking and cancer) are rarely met *in toto* in medicine, and even less so for complex, multidetermined conditions such as schizophrenia. They offer, however, a framework with which to evaluate the emerging literature on etiology of this illness.

Second, one needs to make the distinction between risk indicators and risk factors. In a recent overarching study involving 55 systematic reviews and meta-analyses of 683 individual studies and 170 risk or protective factors implicated in psychotic disorders, Radua et al. (2018) concluded that only prior ultra-high risk (UHR) state and being African-Caribbean in England emerged as convincing risk factors. However, premorbid antecedents such as the UHR state (a risk indicator) are not the same as actual risk factors (e.g., genetic factors, trauma, or substance abuse) which cause these antecedents in the first place.

Third, causal factors rarely work in isolation. For example, while ethnic minority status is likely to represent a true risk factor, several factors (e.g., social defeat, social isolation, substance abuse, and discrimination in health care) may all contribute interactively. Finally, a distinction needs to be made between cause (etiology) and mechanism (pathophysiology). Thus, while discussing causal factors, we do not delve into pathways of pathogenesis (e.g., inflammation, oxidative stress, alterations in brain circuitries, or neurochemistry).

Genetic Factors

Family studies have shown that biological relatives of schizophrenia patients are at higher risk for the disorder than the general population, proportional to the proximity of the relationship and number of affected relatives. While a familial relationship alone is not sufficient to establish the genetic contributions to these disorders, it incontrovertibly plays a major role in modulating risk for schizophrenia, often termed "vertical" transmission. Twin studies allow estimation of the etiologic variance contributed by shared genetic factors and environmental factors. Concordance of schizophrenia in monozygotic (MZ) twins (who share 100% of the genes) is about 40–50% whereas in dizygotic (DZ) twins the rate is around 15%. This suggests that even when genes are fully or largely shared, environmental factors play a major role. Schizophrenia is highly heritable: a meta-analysis of 12 twin studies showed, for example, an MZ/DZ ratio of 0.92/0.52, and heritability of 81% (Sullivan et al. 2003). Shared environmental effects were also significant, but smaller. Together, these findings, along with current estimates that less than one-third of schizophrenia risk arises from the sum of risks contributed by known gene variants, have led to a search for "missing heritability." Clearly, there is a large void in understanding the basic etiological processes of schizophrenia and related psychotic disorders.

It is worth noting that MZ twins also share their environment more than DZ twins. Adoption studies address this by examining children of schizophrenia probands who were adopted at birth by families with no history of schizophrenia, compared to children of nonschizophrenia probands who were adopted away at birth. Several adoption studies have shown that children of parents with schizophrenia have substantially increased risk for the disorder, as shown by significantly more schizophrenia in the adopted-away offspring of schizophrenia probands.

An important milestone in psychiatric genetics is the concept of endophenotypes. As proposed by Gottesman and colleagues (Gottesman and Gould 2003; Gould and Gottesman 2006; Hasler et al. 2006; Lenzenweger 2013), endophenotypes are stable, heritable, quantitative trait-like abnormalities that co-occur with psychiatric illnesses at higher frequencies in first-degree biological relatives than they do in the general population. Gottesman and Gould also proposed that the identification of endophenotypes would aid the search for underlying susceptibility genes for the disorder in question. Several endophenotypes have been proposed over the last two decades (Braff et al. 2008), including cognitive deficits and brain volume abnormalities (Prasad and Keshavan 2007; Stone and Seidman 2016).

Traditional approaches for identifying implicated genes have included linkage analysis and association studies. *Linkage analysis* seeks to investigate the loci *where* the risk genes may be located on *regions* of chromosomes that tend to travel together within the families due to recombination events during meiosis I of the germ cells. Linkage analysis is performed on affected sibling pairs, other relatives, small nuclear families, or larger pedigrees (Glatt et al. 2007). Several chromosomal regions such as 1, 2q, 5q, 3q, 4q, 5q, 6p, 6q, 8p, 10p, 13q, 15q, and 22q (p refers to the short arm, and q refers to the long arm of chromosomes) have been linked to schizophrenia risk (Levinson 2003; Tsuang et al. 2011). In contrast to linkage studies, *genetic association studies* inform about *what* genetic variations may underlie risk for neuropsychiatric disorders. *Functional candidate genes* may be selected based on *a priori* knowledge of a gene's biological function that may impact the trait or disease in question. An example is the gene which codes for the dopamine receptors (*DRD3*). Genome wide association studies (GWAS) employ a case-control design which tests tagged single nucleotide polymorphisms (SNPs) from all regions of the human genome for association with a disorder. It involves comparing the number of common variants (i.e., typically variants that occur in $\geq 5\%$ of the population) among those with versus those without the disorder, and making the appropriate adjustment for the large number of statistical tests performed. GWAS studies have strongly pointed to the human leukocyte antigen (HLA) locus, suggesting dysregulation of the immune system as a possible factor in schizophrenia etiology. *DNA sequencing* refers to determining the precise order of nucleotides in the genome or in a particular gene of interest. Whole genome sequencing attempts to sequence the entire genome, whereas exome sequencing focuses on protein-coding sequences. DNA sequencing studies have identified several genes that affect immune mechanisms, synaptic function, voltage-gated calcium ion channels, and synaptic plasticity, essential to learning and memory (Schizophrenia Working Group of the Psychiatric Genomics Consortium 2014).

Environmental Risk Factors

As noted earlier, genetic factors do not explain all of the variance associated with the onset of schizophrenia. Even among MZ twins, who share 100% of the genes, the risk for schizophrenia is about 40–50%. This suggests that a sizable portion of the etiological variance is not explained by genetic factors, and that schizophrenia is the result of an interaction between multiple genetic and environmental factors. There are several challenges in examining environmental factors. The number of known associated environmental factors has been increasing, thus widening the analytical space; environmental factors may also interact with each other which further complicates the analyses. A series of environmental factors associated with schizophrenia are given in Table 8.1.

Table 8.1 Environmental factors that are implicated in the risk for schizophrenia. Herpes simplex virus, type 2 (HSV2), catechol *O*-methyl transferase (COMT), alpha serine/threonine-protein kinase gene (AKT1).

Environmental Factors	Associated Risk	Caveats	Key References
Seasonality of birth	Winter birth (ca. 5–8%)	Highly replicated finding with unclear mechanisms	Torrey et al. (1997)
Perinatal complications	Hypoxia	Perinatal complications interact with each other, but are not always present	Geddes and Lawrie (1995)
Maternal infections	First and second trimester infections	Prenatal exposure to influenza, toxoplasmosis, and HSV-2 increase risk	Brown (2006)
Postnatal infection	Serious infections that require hospitalization	May increase risk independently as well as through interaction with autoimmune disorders	Benros et al. (2011)
Substance use	Cannabis	Adolescent exposure is associated with risk for schizophrenia; interaction with *COMT* and *AKT1* variants are reported	Semple et al. (2005)

Table 8.1 (continued)

Environmental Factors	Associated Risk	Caveats	Key References
Nutrition	Malnutrition (1st and 2nd trimester); reduced Vitamin D, iron, and folate levels; increased homocysteine	Dutch and Chinese famine studies support the association between nutritional deficiencies and schizophrenia risk	Valipour et al. (2014)
Autoimmune disorders	Increases risk and interacts with serious postnatal infection	May be mediated through inflammation; autoantibodies to neuronal cell surface proteins may also lead to schizophrenia symptoms	Benros et al. (2011)
Childhood trauma	Trauma varieties before age 16 yr	Moderate evidence; more studies needed	Brown (2011)
Place of birth and residence	Urban birth associated with dose-dependent risk	Consistently replicated but reasons uncertain; urbanicity effects may be mediated, e.g., by exposure to infections, drugs, stress, and trauma	Pedersen and Mortensen (2001)
Socioeconomic status	Lower status associated with higher risk	Recent studies appear to show higher risk in relation to low social status at birth	Wicks et al. (2005)
Stress	Repeated, severe stress	Prenatal stress may constitute especially high risk	Morgan and Fisher (2007)
Social group	Ethnic minorities have elevated risk	Unclear; migration status may contribute	Cantor-Graae and Selten (2005)
Immigration	Recent immigrants have elevated risk	Observed even in the second generation	Radua et al. (2018)
Social support	Inadequate support increases risk	Poor social support may interact with stress	Veling et al. (2008)
Paternal age	Dose-dependent increase relative to advanced paternal age	Highly replicated association with risk	Miller et al. (2011)

Epigenetics and Gene–Environment Interactions

Challenging traditional inheritance paradigms, epigenetics involves several mechanisms that provide regulatory information to a genome without altering its primary nucleotide sequence, thus resulting in heritable gene expression changes and nonheritable, long-term transcriptional alterations (Allis et al. 2007). Epigenetics consists of interacting molecular mechanisms—including (a) DNA methylation, (b) histone modifications, and (c) noncoding RNA (ncRNA)-mediated regulation of gene expression through which dynamic changes to promoters, distal regulatory regions, imprinting, and X-chromosome inactivation occur during development or cellular differentiation (Allis et al. 2007; Avner and Heard 2001; Bourc'his and Bestor 2004; Colantuoni et al. 2011; Kouzarides and Berger 2007; Meissner et al. 2008; Numata et al. 2012; Tadokoro et al. 2007). Several epigenetic abnormalities have been reported in schizophrenia and related neurodevelopmental disorders, leading to altered gene expression during development and adulthood. Environmental factors that lead to epigenetic modifications may either reduce or exacerbate the expression of molecular and behavioral phenotypes associated with schizophrenia and related disorders.

How Can We "Connect the Dots" between Genes and Pathophysiology That Emerge in Early Adolescence and Adulthood

Schizophrenia is currently viewed as a disorder of disrupted connectivity across diverse neural circuitries, resulting from diverse pathophysiological processes. Currently, it is, however, unclear which of these processes is primary to the cause of the illness, and which ones are downstream consequences of a cascading pathogenic process that may begin early in development. While it is possible that all these processes may converge onto a final pathophysiological end result, which we call "schizophrenia," it is more likely that different subgroups of the illness may have distinct pathophysiological processes, and perhaps distinct causes. This latter view is supported by the enormous genetic heterogeneity observed in psychotic disorders.

The large phenotypic heterogeneity of schizophrenia (Tsuang 1975) makes a single causative gene, or a few genes of major effect, highly unlikely. More likely scenarios include a large number of common genetic variations of small effect (polygenic inheritance), rare genes of large effect, and copy number variations (CNVs) (Rees et al. 2015).

A large-scale GWAS study showed 108 schizophrenia-associated genetic loci involving 341 protein-coding genes reaching genome-wide significance (Schizophrenia Working Group of the Psychiatric Genomics Consortium 2014). Among these genetic loci were genes related to previously implicated theories of schizophrenia pathophysiology: several glutamatergic genes and one dopaminergic gene (DRD2). More recent GWAS studies and related extensions have confirmed previously implicated genes, identified new neurofunctional targets, and provided novel biological insights into the pathophysiology of schizophrenia. In addition, another large GWAS study of 11,260 cases and 24,542 controls identified 145 loci: 50 were novel and 33 were determined to contain candidate causal genes (Pardinas et al. 2018). These clustered into six independent gene sets associated with schizophrenia, which included targets of the fragile

X mental retardation protein (FMRP), abnormal behavior, abnormal nervous system electrophysiology, voltage-gated calcium channel complexes, abnormal long-term potentiation, and the 5-HT2C receptor complex (Pardinas et al. 2018). Table 8.2 highlights a few of the more novel or consistent targets from these and other GWAS studies and directs readers to sources for more detailed discussions.

GWAS data can also be combined with other genomics approaches to yield insights into the underlying biological mechanisms of schizophrenia. For example, by combining GWAS data with expression quantitative trait loci (eQTL) analyses, Dobbyn et al. (2018) identified a number of candidate genes

Table 8.2 Disease and representative animal models for schizophrenia. THC: delta9-tetrahydrocannabinol; NMDA: N-methyl D-aspartate; DISC1: disrupted in schizophrenia.

Disease Model	Animal Model Example	Key Reference
Disease Expression Models		
• Impaired information processing	Altered sensory gating	Geyer and Braff (1987)
	Aberrant salience	Gray (1995)
Pathophysiology Models		
• GABA		Berretta et al. (2001)
• Dopamine	Stimulant-induced sensitization	Borison and Diamond (1978)
• Altered glutamatergic neurotransmission	Abnormal prepulse inhibition and neural oscillations with NMDA antagonists	Ehrlichman et al. (2009), Geyer et al. (2001), Javitt et al. (1995)
Etiology Models		
• Genetic	DISC1 mutant mice with working memory deficits; 22q deletions in mice	Koike et al. (2006), Paylor et al. (2001)
• Infection/ inflammation	Maternal immune activation model	Nyffeler et al. (2006)
• Peri/neonatal lesions	Methylazoxymethanol acetate; neonatal ventral hippocampal lesions	Lavin et al. (2005), Lipska et al. (1992)
• Nutrition	Dietary omega-3 fatty acid deficiency effects on adolescent behavior and dopamine availability	Bondi et al. (2014)
• Cannabis	THC-induced sensitization of amphetamine motor effects in mice	Gorriti et al. (1999)
• Social stress	Social defeat effects on behavior in Disc1 mutant mice	Haque et al. (2012)

for which genetic variation for expression colocalizes with genetic variation for schizophrenia risk, including *IREB2* and *STAT6* among others. This suggests that the implicated genes may play a causal role in schizophrenia. Gusev et al. (2018) integrated schizophrenia GWAS data with expression data from brain, blood, and adipose tissues in a transcriptome-wide association study (TWAS) to identify multiple novel gene targets implicated in schizophrenia, such as *MAPK3*. They found that total brain expression of *MAPK3* was associated with schizophrenia. Since *MAPK3* induced neurodevelopmental changes in zebra fish (Pardinas et al. 2018), this makes it an attractive target for further investigation. In another fascinating study using a combination of GWAS analyses and single-cell RNA sequencing, Skene et al. (2018) found that the common genetic findings for schizophrenia mapped most consistently "to just 4 of 24 main brain cell types: medium spiny neurons, pyramidal cells in hippocampal CA1, pyramidal cells in the somatosensory cortex, and cortical interneurons," suggesting that these discrete cell types are central to the etiology of schizophrenia.

Other recent developments suggest that several *de novo* mutations may also contribute to schizophrenia risk. *De novo* mutations can arise from mutations occurring in the germ cell for the first time in one of the parents. Alternatively, such mutations can occur in the fertilized egg during embryogenesis. It is too early to comment on what proportion of schizophrenia patients carry *de novo* mutations compared to the mutations transmitted by the parents. Overall, such emerging data could partly address "missing heritability."

One series of observations has generated particular attention, connecting the dots with previous theories and observations. First, based on the typical onset of schizophrenia during adolescence, Feinberg (1982) initially suggested aberrant peri-adolescent pruning of synapses (too much pruning, too little pruning, or pruning of the wrong synapses) to underlie the pathogenesis of schizophrenia. We (Keshavan et al. 1994) subsequently suggested an exaggerated pruning of synapses in this illness. While there is no direct evidence of excessive pruning, there are several compelling observations which indirectly support this view, such as decreased dendritic spine density in postmortem brains of schizophrenia patients (Glantz and Lewis 2000) compared to healthy subjects and individuals with major depressive disorder. As mentioned earlier, GWAS studies have replicated the association of the HLA region in relation to risk for schizophrenia. Since the HLA region is highly complex and gene dense, further studies by Sekar et al. (2016) showed that a CNV within the HLA region accounted for a portion of the risk for schizophrenia (Sekar et al. 2016). Interestingly, Beth Stevens and colleagues demonstrated that complement proteins, known components of the innate immune system, were repurposed for another role; namely, tagging the synapses for phagocytosis (Stephan et al. 2012) and, hence, in synaptic pruning processes during adolescence (Sekar et al. 2016). *Complement genes C4A* and C4B that share 99% sequence homology are part of this gene location, and individuals with higher copy numbers of the *C4A* long form (*C4AL*) showed a stronger association with schizophrenia. They also showed that both *C4A* and *C4B* mRNA levels were elevated in five selected regions of the brains of schizophrenia patients compared to healthy controls; approximately 40% higher expression was reported. In addition, they showed that *C4* knockout mice (i.e., without *C4* activity) had decreased synaptic pruning during brain development. A recent study using phosphorus magnetic resonance spectroscopy on schizophrenia patients and controls revealed that increasing *C4A* copy numbers was associated with greater neuropil contraction, suggesting a gene dosage effect on the possibility of increased synaptic pruning (Prasad et al. 2018). Taken together, these observations point to the possibility of identifying subgroups of psychotic disorders where a known set of risk genes work via a known pathophysiological mechanism to produce an observable illness phenotype.

A continuing challenge in understanding the causes of psychotic disorders is that many biological findings (Tamminga et al. 2014) and the implicated susceptibility genes overlap between psychotic disorders as well as between psychotic, affective, and developmental disorders (Cross-Disorder Group of the Psychiatric Genomics Consortium 2013). For this reason, the Research Domain Criteria (RDoC) approaches outlined earlier are needed to advance the field, as they permit examination across multiple disorders and can capture the continuous variation between health and disease. Recent studies such as the Bipolar and Schizophrenia Network for Intermediate Phenotypes (B-SNIP) are beginning to show that it is possible to identify biological subtypes that cut across DSM psychotic disorders; this may lead to better validation by external validators such as neuroimaging data (Pearlson et al. 2016). Transdiagnostic overlaps are seen in gene expression as well. Using transcriptomic profiling of molecular brain-based phenotypes across autism, schizophrenia, bipolar disorder, depression, and alcoholism, compared with matched controls, Gandal et al. (2018) showed shared polygenic overlap underlying a substantial proportion of cross disorder expression.

What Are the Core Modifications to Circuit Properties During the Transition from Childhood to Adulthood?

Alterations in neuroplasticity underlie several major psychiatric disorders, such as schizophrenia and autism. The typical onset of psychotic symptoms and cognitive decline during adolescence as well as observations of pronounced gray matter reductions around the onset of this illness have led to the hypothesis that schizophrenia may be related to an exaggeration of the normative synaptic pruning processes around adolescence. This view, originally proposed by Irwin Feinberg (Feinberg 1982; Keshavan et al. 1994), has received subsequent support through observations of dendritic loss and synapse reductions in postmortem studies (Glantz and Lewis 2000). Reduced synaptic redundancy may also be expected to lead to diminished brain plasticity, which can account for the cognitive deficits, negative symptoms, and functional disability central to this illness.

Evidence to support reduced cortical plasticity in schizophrenia comes from novel neuroimaging experiments that incorporate brain stimulation and electroencephalography. Transcranial magnetic stimulation (TMS) has been used to study *in vivo* cortical plasticity in schizophrenia. This method uses focal magnetic fields to penetrate the cranium. The resultant electric currents then depolarize the underlying cortex, thus inducing action potentials in targeted brain regions. The output of cortical activation (in this case motor cortex) is measured using electromyographic recordings of hand muscle contractions. The most common method has been to compare motor-evoked potentials (MEP) and motor thresholds (MT) before and after repetitive brain stimulation with repetitive TMS (rTMS) or transcranial direct current stimulation (tDCS), which uses direct currents to shift the resting membrane potentials of underlying neurons. These techniques use synaptic plasticity-inducing protocols that result in cortical excitability changes mirroring LTP (high-frequency rTMS and anodal tDCS) or LTD (low-frequency rTMS and cathodal tDCS).

Compared to healthy controls, LTD-like plasticity is reduced in schizophrenia, as evidenced by lack of expected low-frequency rTMS-induced changes in MEP amplitude. Schizophrenia patients also show lesser facilitation of visual- and auditory-evoked potentials in schizophrenia patients as compared to healthy controls. Evidence to support reduced cortical plasticity in schizophrenia also comes from novel neuroimaging experiments that incorporate brain stimulation and electroencephalography. Deficient cortical plasticity may link these deficits to impairments in cognitive functions, like learning and memory (Frantseva et al. 2008; Wamsley et al. 2012). Aberrant hyperplasticity may also underlie psychotic symptoms (Keshavan et al. 2015).

Genes, Environment, and Impaired Plasticity in Schizophrenia

Schizophrenia is highly heritable. In recent years, several genetic loci with small to moderate effects have been identified in GWAS. Interestingly, not only do these genes regulate glutamatergic, GABAergic, and dopaminergic transmission, they also regulate several aspects of brain development and plasticity (discussed above). One novel line of work has used human-induced pluripotent stem cells to examine alterations in neurogenesis in schizophrenia. In this method, fibroblasts are obtained from individuals and reprogrammed into pluripotent stem cells. In one such study in patients with schizophrenia, these neurons displayed a significant decrease in the number of neurites and neuronal connectivity (Brennand et al. 2011).

Environmental factors may mediate the dendritic spine reductions observed in schizophrenia. Chronic stress and prenatal stress have been correlated with reduced dendritic arborization in animal models (Markham et al. 2013), while environmental enrichment and learning are associated with increased dendritic arborization (O'Malley et al. 2000). In summary, plasticity in schizophrenia may be abnormal due to genetically mediated changes in NMDA receptor function, GABA-mediated inhibition, and neurogenesis. These abnormalities eventually lead to observable neuropathological abnormalities in dendritic spine density and complexity. Epigenetic factors may also mediate the impact of environmental factors on plasticity processes via noncoding RNAs (Spadaro and Bredy 2012).

How Might Animal Models Guide Our Understanding of Psychopathology and the Development of Interventions?

Animal models of schizophrenia initially focused on the dopaminergic theory of this illness based on observations that all antipsychotics work by blocking dopamine receptors. Amphetamine-induced stereotypic behaviors provide one example. Dopamine-blocking antipsychotics consistently block this behavior, and this effect directly correlates with the antipsychotic potency of the drugs in clinical settings. While they were helpful in screening new compounds for antipsychotic efficacy, most of these models, however, lacked face, construct, and predictive validity. To be valid, an animal model needs to reveal the complex presentations of the illness (face validity), resemble the neurobiological observations seen in the disease (construct validity), and replicate causal relationships between the risk factors observed in the human condition and the phenotypic manifestations (predictive validity). Few extant animals do this.

As knowledge has increased on the physiology of psychotic disorders involving brain development, glutamate and the genetic factors, so too have animal models focused on these new insights. Etiological models have been designed based on known susceptibility genes and environmental risk factors for the illness (e.g., as obstetric complications, malnutrition, inflammation, and intrauterine exposure to alcohol); see Table 8.2 for information regarding well-known animal models of schizophrenia. Each animal model recapitulates one or another proposed disease model of the illness, regardless whether it is based on known aspects of clinical expression, pathophysiology, or presumed etiology. None of the models, however, recapitulates all aspects of this heterogeneous disease entity.

What Are the Implications of Causal Understanding for the Development of Biomarkers During this Period? How Can This Inform the Development of Interventions?

What we know about the etiology of schizophrenia may already be yielding better approaches to diagnosis, treatment, and prediction. Using a combination of risk markers and indicators in the clinical or familial high risk for schizophrenia, it is possible to predict conversion to psychotic disorders with a moderately high level of specificity (Carrión et al. 2016; Padmanabhan et al. 2017). A small minority of schizophrenia patients have rare large effect gene mutations or CNVs; this points to the value of genetic counseling (Gershon and Alliey-Rodriguez 2013). Several studies now suggest the value of pharmacogenetic prediction of side effects (e.g., agranulocytosis with clozapine) and the efficacy of antipsychotics, which may be increasingly used in clinical practice (Zai et al. 2018).

Understanding causes will clearly help in developing innovative therapeutic targets and potentially better diagnosis and treatments for complex illnesses like schizophrenia. Using large-scale GWAS datasets from the Psychiatric Genomics Consortium, potential "druggable" genes have been identified that encode proteins which can serve as targets of currently approved medications elsewhere in medicine (e.g., glaucoma, epilepsy, and hypertension) (Lencz and Malhotra 2015). Some of the 20 genes identified are known to be implicated in neuropsychiatric disorders, such as *DRD2* (dopamine), *CACNAC1c* (calcium channels), *GRIN2A* (glutamate receptors), and *HCN1* (voltage-gated potassium channels). GWAS studies also allow the characterization of disease gene networks to elucidate drug-disease relationships. Kauppi et al. (2018) recently examined protein interactomes to map antipsychotic drug targets to gene networks related to schizophrenia. Antipsychotic drug targets overlapped with the core disease gene network modules, comprising several pathways not limited to dopamine. Other risk genes not connected to antipsychotics may be targets for novel compounds that address unmet treatment goals, such as cognitive and negative symptoms.

Continuing challenges in this field include the lack of specific or satisfactory treatments, and the paucity of actionable biomarkers or laboratory tests for early detection, outcome prediction, prevention, and differential treatment selection. We still do not understand much of the heritability of psychotic disorders; known liability genes have relatively small effect sizes, accounting only for a small proportion of the genetic risk. Most of the implicated risk genes are noncoding genes (i.e., intergenic or intronic), whose functional significance remains unclear. A large part of the "missing heritability" in schizophrenia may be caused by unknown gene–gene interactions (epistasis). The lengthy drug development process and diminishing investment by industry in psychopharmacological research are factors that contribute to delays in treatment development (Keshavan et al. 2017).

Several recent initiatives offer promise. Progress toward bridging the "missing heritability" will benefit from the PsychENCODE initiative by NIMH (Akbarian et al. 2015). This initiative seeks to characterize the function of noncoding genomic elements in cell- and tissue-specific samples in the brain in health and neuropsychiatric illness. New bioinformatics and analytical tools are helping to clarify the interactions between genomic data with environmental, proteomic, epigenomic, and interactomic data to better understand disease mechanisms. These insights will help identify better therapeutic targets than single gene products (Gebicke-Haerter 2016). Finally, induced pluripotent stem cells from patient populations can yield cell-based *in vitro* phenotypes to model human illness and generate novel biomarkers for diagnosis and treatment development (Haggarty et al. 2016).

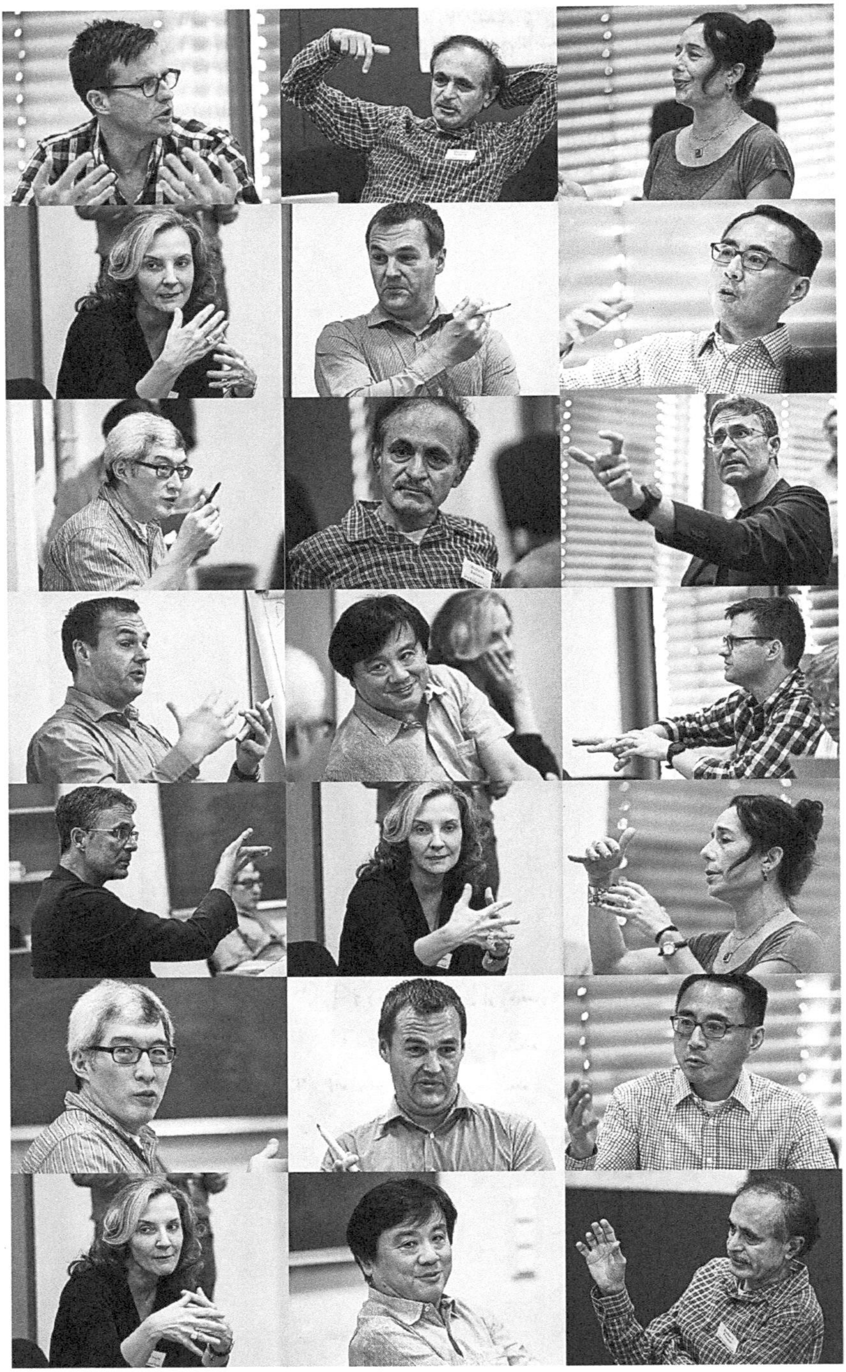

9

The Development of Brain Circuits during Youth

A Framework for Understanding Emerging Mental Disorders and Early Intervention

Christopher G. Davey, Matcheri S. Keshavan, Sophia Frangou, Francis Lee, Beatriz Luna, Andreas Meyer-Lindenberg, Akira Sawa, Peter J. Uhlhaas, and T. Wilson Woo

Abstract

Given the disease burden of mental health in youth, the development of age-appropriate treatments and effective prevention strategies needs to be prioritized. This, however, requires a better understanding of how and why mental disorders emerge. The clustering of the onset of mental disorders in youth suggests that there may be identifiable underlying brain circuit changes during this period, and that examination of normal and abnormal circuit development can improve our understanding of emerging mental disorders. This chapter synthesizes evidence related to multiscale changes in large-scale networks that occur during youth and highlights their relevance to emerging psychopathology. The impact of environmental risk factors is explored and strategies for future research proposed.

Introduction

Three-quarters of all mental disorders emerge before the age of 24 yr (Kessler et al. 2005, 2015; Paus et al. 2008). They lead to more years lost to disability in youth than any other group of illnesses—more than twice as many as the next

Group photos (top left to bottom right) Chris Davey, Matcheri Keshavan, Beatriz Luna, Sophia Frangou, Peter Uhlhaas, Wilson Woo, Francis Lee, Matcheri Keshavan, Andreas Meyer-Lindenberg, Peter Uhlhaas, Akira Sawa, Chris Davey, Andreas Meyer-Lindenberg, Sophia Frangou, Beatriz Luna, Francis Lee, Peter Uhlhaas, Wilson Woo, Sophia Frangou, Akira Sawa, Matcheri Keshavan

two leading causes combined (unintentional injuries and infectious diseases) (Gore et al. 2011). There is evidence that the burden might be increasing, driven by increased rates of affective disorders in young women (Collishaw 2015).

We need to better understand the underlying causes of emerging mental disorders during youth so that we can develop age-appropriate treatments and effective prevention strategies. We refer to "youth" as a period that encompasses development from puberty to about the age of 25 years, extending beyond what has traditionally been referred to as "adolescence" on the basis of evidence of continuous brain development over the extended period (Gogtay et al. 2004; Lebel and Beaulieu 2011). Here, we use the terms interchangeably to refer to the same period. The major disorders that emerge in youth are schizophrenia (and other psychotic spectrum disorders), bipolar disorder, depression, and substance use disorders (Kessler et al. 2005, 2007). We will also include anxiety disorders in our discussion: while they begin to emerge in childhood, many anxiety disorders do not develop until adolescence, and they are risk factors for, and frequently comorbid with, other youth-onset disorders (Lewinsohn et al. 1997).

The clustering of the onset of mental disorders in youth suggests that there may be identifiable underlying brain circuit changes during this period, and that examination of normal and abnormal circuit development can improve our understanding of emerging mental disorders. Importantly, this period is marked by heightened plasticity, and the development of brain circuits that support important cognitive processes; thus, it affords an opportunity for early intervention that can potentially change developmental trajectories (Larsen and Luna 2018). A deeper understanding of the relationship between brain development and psychopathology can lead to the identification of developmentally targeted treatments. Since the large majority of treatments for mental disorders have been developed in adult patients, it is often unclear how effective they are for emerging mental disorders in youth.

In this chapter we synthesize the evidence related to the multiscale changes in large-scale networks that occur during youth with the goal of highlighting their relevance to emerging psychopathology. We explore how these interact with environmental risk factors, and propose key strategies for future research that can inform early intervention efforts.

Plasticity and Brain Organization

Molecular and Cellular Plasticity

Brain development is influenced by multiple molecular and cellular processes, which, if impaired, can disrupt maturation and confer increased risk of mental illness. Histological and animal models provide evidence for maturational processes specific to the adolescent period, which show critical period plasticity in association cortices and, in particular, in the prefrontal cortex (PFC). One of the most significant developmental changes that occurs during youth is the pruning of synaptic connections that have not been strengthened by environmental inputs or by internal experiences (Bourgeois et al. 1994; Huttenlocher 2002; Petanjek et al. 2011). Long-term potentiation and depression, and their influence on excitatory-inhibitory (E-I) balance, are key features of the process.

The E-I balance in youth is influenced by changes in the relative dominance of GABAergic compared to glutamatergic neurotransmission, associated with the maturation of fast-spiking parvalbumin (PV) interneurons (Larsen and Luna 2018). These neurons are particularly enriched in prefrontal regions and act to regulate perisomatic inhibition levels (Freund 2003; Sohal et al. 2009; Soltesz et al. 2005; Tukker et al. 2007). PV interneurons are important for the generation of high-frequency oscillations that support the development in youth of higher cognitive processes such as working memory (Sohal et al. 2009; Wang and Buzsáki 1996).

From puberty, there is an increase in inhibitory tone mediated by an increase in alpha-1and gamma-2 subunits of the GABA receptor in layer 3, coupled with a decrease in alpha-2 and -5 subunits in the same layer (Cruz et al. 2003; Datta et al. 2015; Duncan et al. 2010; Hashimoto et al. 2009). Subunits of glutamate receptors are largely unchanged (Datta et al. 2015). The increased inhibitory tone affects E-I balance and changes the way neuronal activity is sculpted via the effects of PV interneurons on high-frequency oscillatory brain activity.

Recent research has shown that glial cells, such as astrocytes and microglia, also have important roles in the regulation of E-I balance. Glial cells contribute to oxidation–reduction (redox) homeostasis (Ogundele et al. 2014) and the mediation of inflammatory responses (Colombo and Farina 2016). These processes are particularly relevant to neurons, especially the highly energy-dependent PV interneurons (Steullet et al. 2016). In addition, NMDA signaling and receptor concentration as well as increasing levels of brain-derived neurotrophic factor (BDNF) precipitate neuronal plasticity, especially experience-dependent plasticity (Malenka and Bear 2004).

Large-Scale Plasticity

Structural magnetic resonance imaging studies have been consistent in describing anatomical changes during youth. Gray matter (GM) development follows an inverted U-shaped developmental trajectory, increasing in volume during childhood, reaching a peak in adolescence, and declining steadily thereafter (Giedd et al. 1996a; Lenroot et al. 2007). By contrast, white matter (WM) volume increases linearly from childhood to the middle of the third decade, with boys showing a steeper rate of increase during adolescence (Giedd et al. 1996a; Lenroot et al. 2007). Total cerebral volume and the GM volumes of the frontal and parietal lobes seem to attain their peak at age 11 yr in girls and 12–14 yr in boys (Giedd et al. 1996b; Gogtay et al. 2004; Lenroot et al. 2007; Raznahan et al. 2014). Diffusion tensor imaging (DTI) studies show significant developmental enhancements in WM integrity during youth development, confirming histological studies of increased myelination in frontal, temporal, and parietal cortical regions as well as in striatum and hippocampal-cingulate relays (Benes 1989; Yakovlev and Lecours 1967). Among the subcortical brain tracts, the uncinate fasciculus and cingulum show particularly protracted maturation into young adulthood (Lebel et al. 2012; Simmonds et al. 2014). In contrast to this pattern of increased integrity, there is also evidence for normative decreases in WM integrity in circuits relevant to psychopathology, including WM connections from the PFC to basal ganglia (Larsen et al. 2018) and to amygdala (Jalbrzikowski et al. 2017).

Gonadal Hormones and Plasticity

Puberty marks the beginning of adolescence and is a major driver of plasticity. Peaks in GM and WM volume correspond to the sexually dimorphic ages of gonadarche onset and suggest possible interactions between sex hormones and brain development, although correlations do not necessarily imply causal relationships (Giedd et al. 1996a, 1999). Limbic and primary sensory cortices increase in thickness with increased testosterone in boys, whereas higher testosterone levels appear to accelerate frontal cortical thinning; the latter effect is more pronounced in girls than in boys (Bramen et al. 2012).

Early pubertal changes in subcortical regions include increases in amygdala volume in males and increases in striatal and hippocampal volume in females (Lenroot et al. 2007; Neufang et al. 2009). Positive associations have been observed between circulating estrogen levels and parahippocampal GM volumes, as well as between testosterone levels and diencephalic brain structures (Neufang et al. 2009). Pubertal timing is a factor for the onset of mental illness: early life stresses can precipitate premature puberty (Braithwaite et al. 2009; Sun et al. 2017), and early puberty is a risk factor for later mental disorders (Graber et al. 2004; Tremblay and Frigon 2005).

Developmental Changes in Specific Brain Circuits

Above, our discussion focused on molecular and global changes in brain reorganization during youth. Here we examine developmental changes in specific brain circuits, an approach that is compatible with frameworks that seek to understand the relationship between circuit function and psychopathology, such as the Research Domain Criteria (RDoC) (Casey et al. 2014; Insel et al. 2010). Mental disorders are not likely, however, to be defined by abnormalities of particular circuits in isolation; instead, abnormalities in one circuit will affect another. In the complex interactions that result, symptoms of mental illness emerge.

Fronto-Amygdala Circuit

Development of fronto-amygdala circuitry in youth plays a significant role in fear-related disorders (Baker et al. 2014), as well as in depression (Carballedo et al. 2011), schizophrenia (Liu et al. 2014b), and bipolar disorder (Anticevic et al. 2013).

In the infant-juvenile period, amygdala projections to PFC precede the development of reciprocal connectivity from the PFC to the amygdala. In rodents, significant PFC projections to the basolateral amygdala (BLA) are not seen until postnatal days 10 to 15, which is delayed relative to PFC projections to the thalamus and striatum (Arruda-Carvalho et al. 2017; Bouwmeester et al. 2002). Around the time of adolescence, there is another surge in BLA connectivity to the PFC—selectively to the prelimbic PFC—that leads to a transient increase in PFC dendritic spine formation (Pattwell et al. 2016).

Parallel behavioral studies have linked development changes of this circuit to attenuated extinction learning during adolescence. Rodent studies suggest that a lack of synaptic plasticity in prefrontal regions during adolescence is associated with blunted regulation of fear extinction (Pattwell et al. 2012). The selective surge in BLA–PFC connectivity during adolescence (Pattwell et al. 2016) could support a cyclic loop of BLA–PFC and PFC–BLA activity that correlates with resistance to cued fear extinction at this age.

In humans, PFC–amygdala functional connectivity exhibits specialization during adolescent development. This involves a reduction in structural and functional connectivity between PFC and amygdala, with differences in the timing of these processes associated with anxiety and depressive symptoms (Jalbrzikowski et al. 2017). Based on functional MRI studies, immature connections between amygdala and medial PFC in childhood reach adult-like patterns in adolescence (Gee et al. 2013). This developmental switch represents a potential neurobiological basis for the improvements in emotion regulation observed across development.

Frontostriatal Circuit

The development of frontostriatal circuits plays a role in adolescent peaks in sensation seeking (Chambers et al. 2003; Spear 2000) and improved cognitive control (Luna et al. 2015). Aberrant function is implicated in schizophrenia (Eisenberg and Berman 2010), depression (Forbes and Dahl 2011), and substance use disorders (Casey and Jones 2010).

Frontostriatal circuits are composed of distinct efferent cortical connections to the striatum, proceeding to the thalamus, and then projecting back to PFC (Alexander et al. 1986). The frontostriatal circuit most relevant to psychopathology is the reward circuit, composed of connections from ventral striatum to orbitofrontal cortex and amygdala (Alexander et al. 1986; Choi et al. 2012; Fudge et al. 2004; Haber and Knutson 2010).

The striatum is the main target of dopaminergic projections from the ventral tegmental area (VTA), which then project to the PFC. Dopaminergic innervation of the PFC is one of the drivers of PFC maturation. The density of dopaminergic innervation of supragranular layers progressively increases and then plateaus before decreasing to adult levels by early adulthood (Rosenberg and Lewis 1995). Dopaminergic activity accelerates the development of PV interneurons (Porter et al. 1999), and dopamine shows an increased ability to excite PV interneurons during puberty (Tseng and O'Donnell 2007). This facilitates inhibitory circuit function and decreases the E-I balance (O'Donnell 2010), playing a role in triggering critical period dynamics (Takesian and Hensch 2013; Toyoizumi et al. 2013). In rodent models, adolescent social stresses can disturb this dopaminergic maturation, causing disordered behaviors (Niwa et al. 2013).

Ventral striatal regions show hyperactivity in the presence of impending rewards during youth, which moderates with the emergence of adulthood (Galvan et al. 2005; Geier et al. 2010; Luna et al. 2013; Van Leijenhorst et al. 2010). Related to this, functional connectivity between VTA and ventral striatum during reward states is greater in adolescents than in adults, although there is no difference in resting state connectivity (Murty et al. 2018).

Functional connectivity between PFC and striatum declines during youth (Dosenbach et al. 2010; Porter et al. 2015; Supekar et al. 2009). Consistent with this, the recruitment of prefrontal systems in the service of cognitive control decreases as executive function improves through childhood, showing more stability in adolescence (Ordaz et al. 2013; Simmonds et al. 2017), but not stabilizing completely until adulthood (Montez et al. 2017). There is also evidence that striatal systems exert less influence on prefrontal systems. While WM fiber integrity from cognitive networks that feed into convergence zones in the basal ganglia to determine action have been shown to be stable through adolescence, fibers that come from limbic regions decrease, resulting in greater relative input from cortical regions (Larsen et al. 2018). These findings suggest that executive frontal processing is available by adolescence, but striatal reward processing decreases. This specialization indicates that during adolescence there is access to prefrontal executive control, but behavior is driven by reward systems (Luna et al. 2015), which is relevant to the peak incidence of substance use disorders during the period.

Hippocampal-Prefrontal Circuit

The projection of neurons from the hippocampus (HPC) to the PFC has an important role in cognitive and affective processes. Dysfunction of the HPC-PFC circuit is particularly implicated in schizophrenia, depression, and anxiety disorders (Godsil et al. 2013).

Accumulating genetic and connectivity evidence suggests that the HPC is best understood along an anterior-posterior gradient. The anterior HPC is more closely linked to subcortical structures such as the amygdala and the hypothalamic-pituitary-adrenal axis, whereas the posterior HPC has reciprocal connections primarily with the PFC (Bannerman et al. 2014). Consistent with this connectivity pattern, the anterior HPC is more involved in contextually dependent emotional processing, including fear extinction and stress responsivity (Bannerman et al. 2003, 2004, 2014; McHugh et al. 2011), whereas the posterior HPC is primarily involved in cognitive processing, particularly episodic memory and spatial learning (Bannerman et al. 2014; Kim and Fanselow 1992; McHugh et al. 2011; Moser et al. 1993; Moser and Moser 1998).

While PFC shows protracted development (Gogtay et al. 2004), the HPC may have an even later timetable for maturation, with synaptogenesis peaking at approximately 10 years of age in PFC, compared to 13 years of age in the HPC (Ghetti and Bunge 2012; Petanjek et al. 2011). In particular, the anterior HPC has been found to show volumetric increases into early adolescence before volumes decrease (Abrahám et al. 2010; Daugherty et al. 2016; DeMaster et al. 2014; Gogtay et al. 2006; Lee et al. 2014b; Tamnes et al. 2014). The relatively extended period of volume increase is also a consequence of ongoing myelination (Benes 1989, 1994).

The HPC-PFC circuit does not fully myelinate until puberty in rodents, monkeys (Benes 1989), and humans (Simmonds et al. 2014). This might explain the delayed emergence of prefrontal abnormalities subsequent to hippocampal damage, such as in the neonatal ventral hippocampal lesion (NVHL) model of schizophrenia (Lipska et al. 1993). In humans, DTI studies have shown that WM integrity of the uncinate fasciculus, which provides major connections between PFC and HPC, continues to increase through young adulthood (Lebel et al. 2012; Simmonds et al. 2014). Activation of this part of the circuitry via contextual elements has been shown to ameliorate observations of diminished cued and contextual fear extinction observed during adolescence (Pattwell et al. 2016). Importantly, increased dopamine activity during the pubertal period has been shown in rodent models to enhance circuit integration across the HPC and PFC (Tseng and O'Donnell 2005, 2007). These findings indicate that developmentally informed treatments which engage this developing HPC-PFC circuit (e.g., contextually based extinction learning) might help to prevent the emergence of anxiety disorders following stressful or traumatic events.

Developmental Integration and Specialization

Distributed Functional Brain Networks

It is well established that the brain is organized into distributed functional networks that support multiple mental operations (Doucet et al. 2011; Power et al. 2011). The most replicable networks include the default mode network (Raichle et al. 2001), the central executive network (Corbetta and Shulman

2002), and the salience network (Seeley et al. 2007), all of which support diverse and mostly internally guided processes. Other networks, particularly the auditory, visual, and sensorimotor networks, are known to support more specialized and mostly externally driven functions. Despite the robust and reproducible description of these brain networks in adults, there is less information about their maturation during adolescence.

While initial studies suggested possible changes in local to distributed function during development (Fair et al. 2009; Gu et al. 2015; Supekar et al. 2009), these studies were found to be undermined by greater motion in younger subjects (Power et al. 2012). Recent studies have demonstrated that the organization of networks is established by childhood (Fair et al. 2013; Marek et al. 2015), with changes in network integration, particularly involving cognitive networks, increasing into adulthood (Marek et al. 2015). Similarly, hub architecture (i.e., the organization of critical regions that provides high-level integration) is in place by childhood, while cortico-subcortical connections strengthen into adolescence (Hwang et al. 2013). This foundational network organization establishes divergent specialized information streams that are core to cognition and behavior (Grayson and Fair 2017). The anatomical extent of network modules, however, may become more variable into adulthood, suggesting that there is ongoing specialization (Gu et al. 2015).

A hallmark of youth is a change in the way we understand ourselves and others; this is underpinned by developmental changes in the "social brain," a widely distributed network that supports social cognition (Blakemore 2008). Task fMRI has established a social brain network that incorporates medial PFC, superior temporal sulcus, inferior parietal lobule, amygdala, anterior cingulate cortex, and anterior insula (Blakemore 2008; Mars et al. 2012). Social processes are strongly bound to affective processes, and the integration of cortical regions with subcortically based circuits is core to adolescent development (Simmonds et al. 2014; Spear 2000). The social brain becomes more influenced by motivational drives, particularly in relation to sex, drug use, and other peer-influenced behaviors (Davey et al. 2008). These are moderated by the maturation of top-down cortical influences, with improvements in the regulation of affective processes as this circuitry diminishes its influence over established cognitive systems through adolescence (Steinberg 2005).

Developmental Specialization of Brain Function

Taken together, developmental changes in circuitry and network dynamics during adolescence indicate a process of specialization as adult trajectories become established. PFC connectivity with critical regions that support affect (particularly the fronto-amygdala and frontostriatal circuits) demonstrate a transition from heightened affective influence on prefrontal systems during adolescence, which decreases with the emergence of adulthood. This allows cognitive systems to provide better control and hippocampal systems to establish contextual flexibility. In particular, adolescence is a time when network organization becomes more firmly established and PFC systems are available at adult levels. This supports the ability of young people to make complex decisions, but in the context of affective influences that drive adaptive information-seeking abilities needed for specialization (Larsen and Luna 2018).

The process of specialization in adolescence proceeds in a "use it or lose it" manner, as brain processes identify the systems that have been in high use and that are therefore relatively strengthened. In this light, psychiatric disorders can be viewed as resulting from processes that integrate genetic predispositions with experience-dependent use. If the disadvantageous function influenced by genetic predisposition has been the developmental norm for a young person, the brain will fortify this norm and an adult trajectory of psychiatric illness can ensue.

Alternatively, the process of specialization itself can become impaired, as happens in schizophrenia. There is evidence of aberrant maturation of perineuronal nets in schizophrenia, which prolongs the development of neural sculpting to the detriment of PFC functioning (Enwright et al. 2016). These impairments are likely to impact established network and circuit processing, further undermining normative trajectories. For example, the modularity of networks has been found to be reduced in schizophrenia, which might lead to aberrant activity of self-oriented task-negative circuits and the development of psychotic symptoms (Collin and Keshavan 2018).

Environmental Risk Factors for Abnormal Adolescent Brain Development

Adolescent brain reorganization can be influenced by environmental exposures that are present earlier in development (e.g., perinatal complications) as well as risk factors that occur during adolescence (e.g., substance abuse, psychosocial stress). It is understood that these exposures interact with genetic predisposition and epigenetic influences to increase the risk of psychopathology (Figure 9.1).

Early Risk Factors

Early risk factors include intrauterine exposures and those experienced during childhood. Maternal infection is an important risk factor for psychopathology, as it can elicit immune disturbances in the fetus, influencing the initial priming of long-lasting microglia (Bilbo and Schwarz 2009). The affected microglia show aberrant responses to stressors postnatally, including in their regulation of synaptic maintenance processes (such as pruning), thereby influencing E-I balance (Mottahedin et al. 2017). Childhood adversity (e.g., maltreatment, abuse) is a particularly potent distal risk factor for adolescent and adult

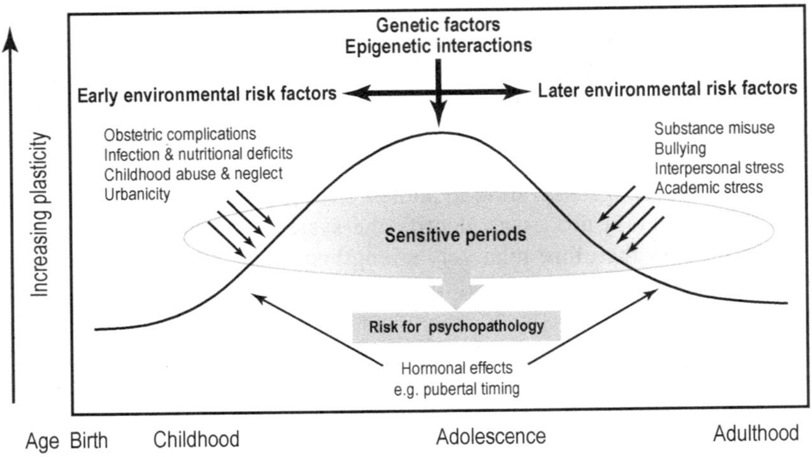

Figure 9.1 Brain reorganization is influenced by environmental exposures, present early in development, and risk factors that occur during adolescence. These exposures interact with genetic and epigenetic factors to increase the risk of psychopathology.

psychopathology. The effects of adversity might partly be mediated through functional and structural changes in the HPC (Dannlowski et al. 2012).

Late Risk Factors

Late risk factors act on brain development after the onset of puberty and can interact with early risk factors to amplify risk further. Cannabis use, which emerges as a significant environmental exposure during adolescence, provides a good example of a late risk factor. The particular culprit is tetrahydrocannabinol (THC), the major physiologically active component in cannabis preparations. Previous work indicates that THC can dysregulate the E-I balance of cortical circuits by affecting cannabinoid 1 receptors (CB1R) (Robbe et al. 2006), which are highly expressed on GABAergic interneurons and astrocytes, thus leading to disruption of neural oscillations (Renard et al. 2017; Skosnik et al. 2012). Importantly, the expression of CB1Rs in the PFC increases until adulthood, thus contributing to developmental modifications in network inhibition (Eggan et al. 2010a). The influence of THC on these processes constitutes a potential candidate mechanism for the generation of cannabis-induced cognitive deficits and possibly for the development of psychosis. This is supported by recent evidence that THC exposure during adolescence is associated with poor visuospatial working memory (Verrico et al. 2014) and highlights the importance of developmental timing for the effects of risk factors on circuits.

It is important to note that human studies have predominantly been retrospective. This makes it difficult to assess whether working memory impairments precede use and might, in fact, be a risk factor for it. A recent study found that working memory impairments and associated aberrations in frontoparietal activation in early adolescence were risk factors for later cannabis use (Tervo-Clemmens et al. 2018). Adolescence is a period when rates of experimentation with cannabis are high, which mostly does not result in mental illness. Those who do develop mental disorders are likely to have other risk factors that make them more sensitive to the effects of cannabis. The interactions between brain developmental processes and environmental exposures are complex.

Treatment Implications

We argue that understanding circuit modifications during youth can provide a neuroscientifically informed platform for refining or developing interventions for emergent psychopathology. Specifically, the efficacy of treatments might be increased if they map selectively to the specific relevant brain circuits at the appropriate developmental period. In particular, an understanding of heightened plasticity during critical period specialization can identify the period where interventions may be most effective. A neuroscience-informed platform for early intervention needs to consider

1. the developmental timing of brain circuits relevant to psychopathology,
2. the selection and development of appropriate therapies (neurobiological, pharmacological, and psychological) to target these circuits, and
3. the testing of the efficacy and side effects of treatments in relation to the developmental stage of the brain circuits.

One example of such an approach comes from a study of developmental timing of alterations in fear circuits (Pattwell et al. 2011). Diminished cue-based fear extinction during peri-adolescence, compared to earlier and later periods, significantly reduced the effectiveness of treatments for anxiety disorders that relied on extinction mechanisms during this period. Conversely, context-based extinction learning was specifically *enhanced* during peri-adolescence (Pattwell et al. 2016). These data suggest that treatment response to standard cue exposure-based cognitive behavioral therapy varies nonlinearly with age, with the poorest response in adolescents (Drysdale et al. 2014). This highlights the importance of optimizing treatment strategies based on age as well as the potential importance of developing contextual extinction-based therapies and related preventive interventions for youth.

Evidence from preclinical research indicates that early circuit impairments can be reversed during youth. A study that examined oxidative stress in NVHL rats, an established neurodevelopmental model of schizophrenia, provides a pertinent example (Cabungcal et al. 2014). The administration of the antioxidant N-acetyl cysteine to juvenile and adolescent rats prevented the expected reduction of prefrontal PV interneuron activity as well as anticipated electrophysiological and behavioral deficits. This suggests that presymptomatic oxidative stress yields abnormal adult brain function in a developmentally compromised brain and highlights redox modulation as a potential target for early intervention (Do et al. 2015). Redox imbalance is reproducibly reported in patients with psychosis from early disease stages, and the use of safe antioxidants such as sulforaphane might be potential therapies (Shiina et al. 2015).

Similarly, intervening to correct E-I imbalances in adolescence using cognitive approaches might ameliorate the emergence of aberrant behaviors. For example, in NVHL rats, adolescent cognitive training was shown to prevent adult cognitive control impairment (Lee et al. 2012). The findings suggest that cognitive training during the adolescent period might (a) tune compromised neural circuits to develop in the service of adult cognition and (b) attenuate schizophrenia-related cognitive impairments that manifest in adulthood.

Strategic Research Priorities for Early Intervention

In the preceding sections we proposed that the unfolding of psychopathology across stages of mental disorders might parallel the development of relevant brain circuits. While our knowledge of brain development during youth has significantly expanded in recent years, highly significant knowledge gaps still exist. Addressing these gaps will be necessary if we are to develop a developmentally sensitive, neuroscience-informed, circuit-based framework for implementing effective interventions during youth. These gaps can be addressed by attending to the following strategic priorities.

Resolving Conceptual Frameworks for Youth Mental Health

Adolescence is described as a "sensitive period," implying that there are unique developmental events that occur during this period, and that alterations in the normal developmental trajectory will lead to vulnerabilities to mental illnesses. However, there are alternative views. It might be that the accumulation of risks, which are causally linked, better explains the emergence of mental illnesses. Models that integrate sensitive periods with risk models might provide insights that more directly inform treatment strategies by identifying systems underlying risk and the peak timing for intervention.

Critical period and *sensitive period models* assume that there are stages in human development during which the influence of external agents have particularly potent effects on subsequent development and vulnerability to illness. Implicit in the critical period model is the notion that the influence of external agents, when they occur during youth, alter the function or structure of biological tissues or systems through processes of "biological programming" (Kuh et al. 2003; Papachristou et al. 2013). Conversely, the influence of the same agents during other developmental stages will be minimal or absent.

Less strictly defined than critical periods, sensitive periods refer to stages in development when the influence of external agents may have strong effects on disease risk, but which can be modified by subsequent experiences or exposures (Kuh et al. 2003; Papachristou et al. 2013). Understanding the molecular mechanisms underlying periods of heightened plasticity can help us identify circuits that might be particularly susceptible at particular points in time (Larsen and Luna 2018).

Different insights can also be gained by considering the *accumulation of risk model*, which emphasizes that exposures or insults act in a cumulative fashion to increase gradually the risk of disease or mortality. The model postulates that cumulative differential lifetime exposure is the main explanation for observed individual differences in disease risk (Kuh et al. 2003; Papachristou et al. 2013). An extension of this is the *chain of risk model*, which proposes that factors may be linked in chains (or cascades), whereby each exposure leads to further adverse exposures or experiences. Each link in the chain may have an independent effect on disease risk, otherwise disease onset may be predicated only by the final link (Kuh et al. 2003; Papachristou et al. 2013). Support for these models can be determined by modeling and testing pathways to show how risk factors relate to adolescent development, by assessing the cumulative effects of prolonged exposure or clustering of factors, and by identifying chains of risk that have not yet been fully described.

Building Global Data Repositories to Determine Normative Centile Curves

While our knowledge of circuit development has advanced, the field lacks robust evidence for the age-related trajectories of brain, cognitive, and behavioral phenotypes. In most fields of medicine, age-related trajectories derived from healthy individuals are used as references to identify deviations from the expected range, which are then used to trigger further investigations or interventions. An important example is the age trajectory of body mass index, which has been instrumental in informing public health policies relating to cardiometabolic health (Johnson et al. 2015). To move forward, the field requires international initiatives to pool data, already acquired in population-based adolescent samples, and enable us to derive age-related trajectories of key phenotypes. That is, there is a wealth of "big data" available that provides the power, individual variability, and unique contextual and genetic information to advance our understanding significantly. We also need to harmonize brain, cognitive, and behavioral phenotypes to minimize interstudy differences in terminology and methodology. This would benefit from prospective large-scale longitudinal studies that can clarify factors associated with risk and resilience to mental health outcomes (Feldstein Ewing et al. 2018; Frangou 2011).

Detailed Mapping of Brain Circuits to Psychopathology and Cognition

Above, we highlighted several brain circuits that show age-related changes in activity and connectivity during youth. This circuit-based approach has been promoted by the RDoC initiative (Insel et al. 2010), where the focus is on shared dimensions of impairment that may be particularly relevant to understanding developmental specialization of trajectories. This is particularly valuable given that it is often difficult to diagnose psychiatric illness early in development, when adult brain and cognitive trajectories have not yet been established. With the possible exception of the fronto-amygdala circuit, our knowledge of the age-related trajectories of these circuits lacks detail. Although there is a degree of face validity in linking different circuits to cognitive and behavioral phenotypes, a principled and comprehensive characterization of the link between adolescent changes in these circuits with psychopathology is still missing. This area of research is best addressed by integrating animal and human studies. Human studies could highlight phenotypes of key relevance to adolescent psychopathology and systems-level brain processing, which could then be examined in preclinical designs that allow for more detailed mechanistic dissection of the neural underpinning of these phenotypes and effects of treatments.

Multivariate Models of Risk, Disease, and Resilience in Youth

Previous research has identified multiple risk factors for adolescent psychopathology, including polygenic instruments of genetic risk, polyenvironmental risk (comprising biological factors, such as obstetric trauma and infections, and nonbiological exposures, such as psychosocial trauma as well as social and family adversity), and epigenetic markers linking exposures to molecular changes. It is widely accepted that adolescent mental health problems arise from complex interactions between these factors. However, examination of these interacting "omic" influences requires advanced multivariate modeling, large samples, and significant computing power to handle simultaneously high-dimensional data sets. This is an emerging field with multiple groups endeavoring to define optimal statistical algorithms and test their external validity (e.g., Nymberg et al. 2013; Xia et al. 2018).

Clarifying the Role of Sex and Pubertal Changes for Youth Mental Health

We have outlined what is known about the molecular factors that are involved in the initiation of puberty. With the onset of puberty, significant changes in brain circuits begin, including the sexual dimorphism of brain regions. It is also from puberty that most serious mental illnesses start to emerge and become diagnosable. Significant gaps in our knowledge remain, however, about how pubertal processes exert their influence on brain development. Few studies have examined the association between gonadal steroid levels and measures of brain processes, such as white matter integrity, brain function (including resting-state fMRI), and neurochemistry (MRS) in adolescence. Similarly, the relationship between gonadal steroid levels and functional brain changes are limited to a small number of tasks (e.g., Braams et al. 2015; Fareri et al. 2015). Even fewer studies have focused on the association between gonadal hormones and adolescent changes in the intrinsic architecture of the brain functional connectome.

Integrative Systems Neuroscience of Large-Scale Network Development

While considerable evidence has been obtained for neuroanatomical development in youth, there remains a substantial knowledge gap in understanding the relationship to fundamental systems neuroscience parameters, important for large-scale brain activity. These include systematic studies into maturation of neural oscillations as well as circuit motifs that are involved in the sculpting of neuronal dynamics, such as E-I balance parameters. In addition, there remains only circumscribed evidence for neurotransmitter systems changes during youth, despite evidence for late-occurring changes in dopamine-NMDA receptor interactions, for example (Tseng and O'Donnell 2005). Extending these data and establishing links with large-scale network measures (EEG, MEG, fMRI) will be critical for understanding more fully the emergence of psychiatric disorders and their relationship to ongoing brain maturation during youth.

Conclusion

We propose that the sequential unfolding of psychopathology across stages of mental disorders parallels the hierarchical development of brain circuitries, and that emerging psychopathology is related to different risk factors to which the brain is exposed during sensitive periods of circuit development (Table 9.1). Importantly, we hold that unique opportunities exist to provide a developmental lens of the precursors of mental illness by understanding development—and in particular adolescent development—as a period when adult trajectories become established that can lead to lifelong psychiatric diagnoses. While there are many gaps in our knowledge of these brain–behavior relationships, they offer a framework for further research. Fine-grained studies of developmental neurobiology and their psychopathologic correlates are needed, using state-of-the-art tools from cognitive and affective neuroscience, imaging, and molecular biomarker research. From this, we hope that new treatment approaches

Table 9.1 Brain development processes and their relevance to emerging psychopathology: prefrontal cortex (PFC), posttraumatic stress disorder (PTSD), ventral tegmental area (VTA).

	Behavior/Cognition	Developmental Modifications	Relevance for Emerging Psychopathology
Fronto-Amygdala Circuit	Fear extinction, anxiety	Early amygdala influence on medial PFC, reverses direction	Anxiety, depression, bipolar disorder, schizophrenia
Frontostriatal Circuit	Sensation seeking, reward processing, cognitive control	Increased dopamine projections from VTA to PFC, reduced PFC-striatal connectivity	Substance use disorders, schizophrenia, bipolar disorder, depression
HPC-PFC Circuit	Memory, contextual encoding, learning	Increasing hippocampal (CA1) innervation of PFC	Schizophrenia, anxiety (including PTSD), depression
Distributed Brain Networks	Mentalizing, cognitive control	Network integration and specialization, increasing top-down cortical control	Schizophrenia, depression, substance use disorders

can be developed to address circuit abnormalities, which might ameliorate the experience of youth-onset mental ill-health into adulthood.

Developing and Implementing Prevention and Early Intervention

10

Novel Modalities for Assessment and Intervention in Youth Mental Health

Digital Interventions and Omega-3 Fatty Acids

Mario Alvarez-Jimenez, G. Paul Amminger, Maximus Berger, John Gleeson, and Andrew M. Chanen

Abstract

Extant interventions and services for young people with mental ill-health and their families have significant limitations, including poor access to services, relapse prevention, social recovery, research translation, and family support as well as limited effectiveness and significant adverse events of pharmacological interventions. Based on research literature and the authors' work in the field, this chapter reviews three avenues for progress: novel digital, family, and transdiagnostic biomarker-guided interventions.

Main findings and conclusions: Despite their potential and consistent evidence supporting their effectiveness, digital interventions have not been integrated into youth mental health services. Integration of digital interventions into mainstream services is likely to create a new paradigm, driven by ongoing innovation and rapid evaluation and clinical implementation. Family interventions need to move away from a narrow focus on psychotic disorders, patient symptoms, and relapse to include overlooked populations, transdiagnostic processes, family burden, and the mental and physical health of families. Finally, transdiagnostic prevention and treatment of severe psychiatric disorders is a promising avenue for reducing the burden, mortality gap, and adverse effects of current medications. Supplementation of n3PUFA via fish oil is proposed as a prototype of a transdiagnostic, benign, biomarker-guided intervention.

Key Limitations of Current Interventions and Mental Health Services for Youth

The past 25 years has seen significant progress in interventions and models of care designed to improve the clinical symptoms of young people with mental ill-health and to support their families. Early intervention is now seen as the most promising and evidence-based approach to improve the long-term outcomes of mental disorders (McGorry et al. 2008a). Specialist early intervention services for psychosis originated in the early 1990s, with a focus on reducing treatment delays, providing youth-friendly, phase-specific support, and preventing the development of long-term functional and social disability (McGorry et al. 2008a). Over the past two decades, several randomized control trials (RCTs) conducted across countries and mental health systems have demonstrated that these services improve psychotic symptoms, reduce relapse rates, foster patient satisfaction, and result in tangible economic benefits (Alvarez-Jimenez et al. 2011; Bird et al. 2010; Craig et al. 2004; Melle et al. 2004; Petersen et al. 2005). The success of the reforms supporting early intervention for psychosis has led to the extension of this model to other mental health conditions, including the development of youth mental health services for both subthreshold clinical conditions as well as severe mental health disorders, such as borderline personality disorder or complex depression (Chanen and McCutcheon 2013; Rice et al. 2017). Despite these advances, current youth mental health interventions and services have major limitations:

- *Relapse prevention failure*: Youth mental health services are not equipped to effectively prevent relapse. The result is that up to 80% of young people with depression or psychosis will suffer repeated recurrences after initial treatment response, thereby increasing the risk of long-term disability (Alvarez-Jimenez et al. 2012; Kennard et al. 2006).
- *Social recovery failure*: Existing interventions have limited impact on key domains of social recovery, such as social connectedness, employment, or well-being (Horan et al. 2006). Not only are these deficits the most disabling and costly aspect of mental illness, achieving social recovery is the most valued goal for young people and their families.
- *Innovation failure*: The variety of evidence-based treatments available to young people has remained largely unchanged over the past four decades, and has been limited to psychotherapies or psychotropic medications. No specific guidelines on the indications for psychological treatment versus medication have been provided for most psychiatric disorders. While public views tend to favor the psychotherapies as first-line interventions, one problem with this approach is workforce capacity constraints, leading to failure of access to services.
- *Access failure*: Seven out of ten young people and the majority of their families do not have access to evidence-based interventions (Reavley et al. 2010). Even when they receive treatment, many discontinue

treatment too soon, and they have no access to personalized support when they need it.

- *Research translation failure*: Research translation is painfully slow, with up to 17 years of delay between treatment innovations and their dissemination across mental health services (Mohr et al. 2018).

Digital Interventions and Youth Mental Health Reform: Can Technology Drive the Next Transformation in the Field?

The Promise and Unmet Expectations of the First Generation of Digital Interventions

One avenue to address the limitations of current interventions and youth mental health services is to harness digital technologies to increase their accessibility, attractiveness, cost-effectiveness, and impact. Digital mental health interventions include devices and programs that harness digital technology to foster improved mental health outcomes (Michie et al. 2017). This can include computer-based interventions (with or without online access), online-based interventions (e.g., self-guided online programs, online interventions including therapist support), mental health mobile applications (e.g., interventions delivered by mobile applications, such as ecological momentary interventions), or virtual reality-based interventions. The most widely researched type of digital mental health interventions are online-based interventions. Indeed, there is strong evidence for the effectiveness of online interventions in both adults and young people, particularly for high prevalence mental health disorders such as depression and anxiety disorders, from over 100 clinical trials (Richards and Richardson 2012). Encouraged by this evidence, mental health-care systems have attempted to integrate digital technologies, as in the Australian national E-mental health strategy, which recommends integrating online support with youth mental health services (Australian Government Department of Health and Ageing 2012). Yet, around the world, integration of digitally enabled support with current models of care has not been implemented, leading to fragmentation of online support and youth mental health services. Despite being evidence-based, online interventions are rarely taken up by young people or clinicians in the real world (Mohr et al. 2018). Concurrently, there has been an explosion of mobile applications claiming to improve well-being and to reduce depression or anxiety, yet very few have quality evidence to support their safety or effectiveness. Consequently, while young people have more ready access to potential supports than ever before, they have no means to determine their quality. Conversely, when they do access mental health services and face-to-face interventions, these are not complemented by personalized and engaging digitally based support to enhance their generalizability and impact.

Further limitations that have significantly hampered the promise and impact of existing online supports include very high attrition rates, especially among online interventions without human support, usually after only one or two sessions, thereby limiting their ability to address relapse prevention (Gilbody et al. 2015). Also, online support has primarily focused on clinical symptoms, with little attention paid to social, educational, employment, and other functional outcomes. Finally, online interventions have typically targeted mild to moderately high-prevalence disorders; very few have addressed severe mental health conditions (e.g., psychosis, bipolar disorder, or borderline personality disorder).

Drawing on our work on online interventions in youth mental health, we propose that for digital interventions to be able to deliver on their promise to revolutionize mental health services, the new generation of technology-driven interventions needs to harness contemporary methodologies and technologies to promote sustained engagement, so that long-term outcomes, such as relapse prevention, can be addressed. Such interventions will need to draw upon novel as well as robust psychological models that focus on well-being and social functioning. Moreover, they will need to be designed from the outset to be integrated with real-world mental health services and settings, at all stages of treatment, and they will need to integrate a new blend of multidisciplinary expertise, including that of young people and families.

Toward Long-Term Engagement: The Science of Developing Online Interventions in Youth Mental Health

Commercial online social media platforms such as Facebook, Instagram, and Snapchat have a well-demonstrated capacity to engage young users, even to the point of becoming addictive. Driven by the "attention economy," whereby harvesting attention has become their key metric of business success, these platforms run thousands of tests with their users and take advantage of known social and cognitive biases to devise (disguised) strategies that capture users' attention. The results of this approach are remarkable: 50% of 18- to 24-year-olds go on Facebook when they wake up, 90% of young people use online social media daily, and young people under the age of 25 use Snapchat 20 times for over 30 minutes every day (Hadad 2015; Rideout 2015; Smith 2016). Unfortunately, accumulating evidence shows that using online social media platforms can have detrimental effects upon youth. These include high rates (around 23%) of cyberbullying (which is strongly associated with depression and is often suffered in silence), increased anxiety, negative body image and, paradoxically, an increased perceived social isolation among those feeling lonely (Rideout 2015). Purely harvesting attention, as it turns out, can have severe adverse consequences for young people. On the other hand, most evidence-based online interventions have been designed to replicate traditional, effective, face-to-face therapeutic principles (e.g., cognitive behavioral therapy), with little attention to design choices aimed at promoting sustained engagement. The result is that these interventions have traditionally been plagued by disappointing engagement rates over the longer term.

Building on the useful knowledge that digital interventions can deliver effective psychological support, we need to advance the science of developing digital interventions in youth mental health. The design and development process of new digital interventions is critical to ensure quality interventions that are safe, engaging, and effective. The field needs to fully embrace and adapt best practices in software design as well as persuasive methods and strategies. As scientists and clinicians, we need to promote the "well-being economy" as an alternative model, where supporting meaningful and lasting benefits is the end goal. As such, the new generation of technology-based interventions needs to harness the appeal and therapeutic potential of online social media technologies, while engineering digital interventions that enable meaningful and positive relationships and foster well-being in an ethical, safe, and transparent manner. Advancing the well-being economy will require a new blend of multidisciplinary expertise, including clinical psychologists, creative writers, software developers, artists, experts in human computer interaction, game developers, and experts in machine learning who work in partnership with end users.

Developing New Methodologies to Evaluate the Effects of Digital Interventions

Rapid development of online technologies has outpaced the timeline of conventional RCTs. This is, however, not the case for RCTs that evaluate mobile health interventions (which can recruit from a global pool of potential participants, thereby conducting fast and efficient RCTs) in high prevalence conditions, such as depression and anxiety. This limitation applies to studies conducted in traditional clinical services that recruit specific populations (e.g., young people with psychosis or at clinical risk of developing psychosis) (Alvarez-Jimenez et al. 2018) with prolonged follow-up periods (e.g., 18 months or longer). In the latter case, studies can take up to five years to be completed (Alvarez-Jimenez et al. 2019). This results in evaluations of interventions that are obsolete by the time trial results become available, preventing real-world implementation.

Novel research frameworks put forward solutions to this issue, balancing the need for ongoing technological improvements while maintaining the internal validity of the interventions being tested (Mohr et al. 2015). In this way, the core elements and theoretical principles of a technology-based intervention can be operationalized and remain consistent during the evaluation process, while allowing for ongoing quality improvements in functionality, thereby maintaining technological currency (Mohr et al. 2015). That said, rigorous methodologies need to be developed and applied to reliably measure the intervention principles and their consistent implementation throughout the trial.

An additional alternative to conducting traditional, slow, and expensive clinical trials of digital interventions in the context of clinical services (which lack a direct pathway to clinical implementation) is to make youth mental health services digitally enabled by integrating digital interventions designed to enhance their impact. By providing technology-enabled support to all young people using these services—potentially hundreds of thousands—we could then conduct rigorous, fast, and efficient RCTs of progressive updates, releases, and new digital tools delivered as part of the service. Crucially, the results of these RCTs can be readily implemented in the clinical service by making the new intervention available to all service users (vs. the up to 17-year delay in current research translation).

Integrating Digital Interventions and Assessments into Youth Mental Health Services

Rather than evaluating digital interventions where real-world implementation and integration is an "after the fact" procedure, digital interventions need to be designed from the outset to be integrated within youth mental health services. This implementation needs to occur at all stages of treatment, including help-seeking, blended face-to-face online support, as well as digital interventions to prevent relapse and maintain the hard-won gains of face-to-face interventions. To create effective interventions that address critical issues for young people and their families and clinical services, all relevant stakeholders, including clinicians, end users, and administrators, need to be part of the design process. Importantly, new business models need to be developed that account for the need for ongoing evaluation and regular technological improvements, while also meeting the expectations of young people that they receive modern, constantly evolving, and effective support.

The integration of digital interventions and assessments into current models of care offers fascinating new possibilities. Rather than being an "add-on" or even a replacement for effective face-to-face interventions, digital technologies can be used to create a new model of synergistic care that breaks down the perceived online/offline divide. For example, at Orygen, we have developed a new blended model of care entitled Moderated Online Social Therapy + (MOST+) through which young people can access support from other young people at all times, day or night, as well as peer supporters and moderators between sessions. In addition, MOST+ includes a comprehensive array of high-quality, interactive, evidence-based interventions that can be recommended by the clinician, selected by the young person, or automatically suggested by the system, based on individual preferences and needs. The clinicians and young people are able to schedule action plans and homework based on team and geographic location. Importantly, the system can harness real-time assessment methodologies, such as ecological momentary assessments (Shiffman et al. 2008) or digital phenotyping enabled by a smartphone application (Insel 2017), to capture the changing needs and emotions of young people *in vivo*. Coupled with novel data science tools, such as artificial intelligence (D'Alfonso et al. 2017) and machine learning (Torous et al. 2018), this information can subsequently be used to identify patterns of behavior and emotions, to evaluate progress, and to tailor therapeutic interventions in real time via ecological momentary interventions (Heron and Smyth 2010; Myin-Germeys et al. 2016).

Priorities for Family Assessment and Intervention

The onset of severe mental ill-health in a young person often marks the start of a major crisis in the lives of their families. In the process of caring for their young relative, family members often suffer high levels of stress, burnout, and depression (Onwumere et al. 2011, 2018), and exposure to violence is not an uncommon result (Onwumere et al. 2014). Since mental health disorders often emerge when families expect their young person to become increasingly independent, it is not surprising that the young person experiences a sense of grief after initial diagnosis—a sense of loss or separation from family, friends, or other carers[1] (Patterson et al. 2005; Tennakoon et al. 2000).

Despite decades of robust research on the efficacy of family interventions in severe mental health disorders and clinical guidelines recommending their deployment (most notably for schizophrenia), access to effective interventions remains a lottery for most families (Bucci et al. 2016). In youth mental health, the evidence base for family intervention is less well established. Mounting evidence indicates, however, that it is effective in reducing the risk of both relapse and family/carer distress (Claxton et al. 2017).

In the context of this promising evidence and high level of unmet need, we explore key priorities for family assessment and interventions in youth mental health. Focusing on recent and potential innovations in the assessment of family needs and the delivery of family interventions to address access logjams, we identify critical targets for family interventions that have been overlooked and note specific populations of families whose needs have been largely ignored by researchers. Finally, we consider the implications of changing family structures and environments for the future of family-level assessment and interventions in youth mental health.

Innovations in Family Assessment and Intervention

The assessment of family needs can inform clinical interventions that benefit individual family members, the family system, and the individual diagnosed with the mental health disorder. Several domains of family assessment, however, require greater attention and innovation.

---

1 Here we refer collectively to people engaged in supporting young individuals (e.g., parents, siblings, friends, teachers, etc.) as "families."

Ecologically valid assessment methods have been widely utilized to assess the daily lives of patients with mental health disorders, but surprisingly little light has been shed on the everyday lives of families supporting a young person recovering from severe mental ill-health (Myin-Germeys et al. 2009). Experience sampling and emerging passive sensing methods (Cornet and Holden 2018) could provide clinically useful data regarding the problems faced by families, most notably their daily interpersonal challenges when communicating with their young person.

The physical health of families has also been largely ignored by clinicians and researchers in youth mental health. Early reports have suggested that families of early psychosis patients are frequently overweight, with high rates of hypertension, and elevated risk for type 2 diabetes (Poon et al. 2018). At the upper end of the age spectrum, it is known that the chronic stress in caring for a relative with dementia is associated with a range of physiological markers of disease, including dyscoagulation, inflammation, cell aging, and changes in immune function, compared with controls (Fonareva and Oken 2014). Embedding family health assessments in research and encouraging assessments for families in youth mental health services is worthy of consideration with the aim of prevention of disease in these populations.

Intervening with families in youth mental health offers a window of time in which intensive interventions can maintain the young person's developmental trajectory and prevent the long-term consequences of stress for family members.

There are several possible strategies to refine and extend family interventions. For example, while the targeting of "high expressed emotion" has been important for the prevention of relapse, novel models of the interactions between the family environment and patient outcomes might prove fruitful. These include the early identification of families most at risk of depression and chronic stress, as well as the association with depleted caregiving and modeling of self-efficacy for the young person. The identification of endophenotypes for mental health disorders raises the prospect of interventions for multiple family members that target transdiagnostic processes; for instance, emotional dysregulation, which is linked to personality (Gunderson et al. 2018), mood, and other disorders, is highly likely to compromise the effectiveness of the family system in solving complex interpersonal problems, especially if shared by multiple family members.

The critical issue of access to effective interventions calls for major innovations in available modes of delivery. An online model of family intervention, "moderated online social therapy," was specifically developed to integrate online therapy content with expert and peer moderation within a social networking environment, available 24 hours a day from any internet-enabled device (Gleeson et al. 2017b). An RCT is currently in progress to evaluate the effectiveness of this model for carers of youth recovering from psychosis (Gleeson et al. 2017a). A major added advantage of this model is that it can efficiently support relatively large numbers of carers who are dispersed across geographical regions, which is especially important for low-prevalence disorders, where carers are potentially at greater risk of stigma and social isolation and where experts might be in short supply. Our model also integrates a role for carer peer support workers, an element that we argue is ripe for closer empirical investigation, with good prospects for cost-effective dissemination.

Critical Targets That Have Been Overlooked

To date, family-based interventions have targeted relapse prevention and family levels of stress and burden. Although these are important targets, which we ourselves have pursued (Gleeson et al. 2010), there is an urgent need to develop and evaluate interventions that support families as they address normative parenting goals, such as how to best support a young person who is recovering from severe mental illness to maximize their personal independence, meaning in life, connectedness with others, and to establish a purposeful life. These are, in short, components of eudaemonism, which have oddly eluded the attention of researchers and clinicians alike in youth mental health (Ryff and Keyes 1995).

The issue of abuse perpetrated by family members remains an important controversy in youth mental health. Recent reviews by members of our group confirm that abuse is implicated in raising the risk for psychosis. However, significantly more work needs to be done in formulating effective approaches for working with family members, both perpetrators and victims, in these situations.

Specific Populations Ignored

There are specific populations of families that have been almost entirely overlooked by researchers and clinicians in youth mental health. Carers of youth with borderline personality disorder have been identified as the most distressed of all carers, given the interpersonal features of the disorder (Bailey and Grenyer 2014). Here, the development of a specific carer intervention would be timely in light of the emergence of an effective youth model for borderline personality disorder (Chanen et al. 2017). Orygen has developed a promising pilot intervention for this group (Pearce et al. 2017), which we plan to extend to a larger trial.

Parents of youth living with gender dysphoria are another population that faces significant stress. Support for these carers might prevent adverse outcomes in their children (Gregor et al. 2016; Hasan et al. 2017).

Other populations include First Nations families that are caring for young people with severe mental disorders, as well as families isolated in rural or remote locations. This is especially true for countries such as Australia and Canada, which have very isolated communities.

In short, the digital era offers the promise of addressing geographical and demographic obstacles to provide access for specific populations with identifiable needs.

The Broader Perspective

Contemporary models of family interventions were largely developed out of behavioral and cognitive therapy models in the 1970s and 1980s (Falloon 1988). Little consideration has been given in family research in youth mental health to the effects of secular trends in family environments. For example, in Western-developed nations, there is an expanding timeline for young adults who remain economically dependent on their parents. In addition, the age of first-time parents has been rising over the previous decades, and patterns of workforce participation have changed significantly from what they were 30 years ago, when policies like deinstitutionalization first effected a shift in the burden of care to families in the community. In addition, the structure of families has changed: family size is smaller, there are more blended families, and increasing numbers of same-sex parents are raising children.

Over the last 10–20 years, global economic changes have caused rapid cultural changes in younger generations from emerging economies. Previously, families in these societies were especially supportive and protective of relatives with severe mental health disorders, compared with Western-industrialized contexts.

These large-scale secular trends raise important questions and issues for researchers and clinicians alike in youth mental health. Since pressure on families is unlikely to reduce, researchers and clinicians will need to provide solutions to the local and global problems that continue to emerge.

Transdiagnostic Biomarker-Guided Intervention

Supplementation with Omega-3 Fatty Acids to Promote Mental Health in Youth as an Exemplar Model

Pharmaceutical interventions in youth have been limited by lack of efficacy and incidence of adverse events (Bridge et al. 2007; Hetrick et al. 2010). Given the paucity of new drug developments for psychiatry in recent years, alternative biological treatments merit investigation, in particular agents that are more benign and therefore feasible for early intervention (Amminger et al. 2017). There is also a need for pluripotent treatments that can influence core biological processes, such as monoaminergic (Sublette et al. 2004), dopaminergic (Sublette et al. 2014) and serotonergic neurotransmission (Freeman et al. 2006; Garland and Hallahan 2006), oxidative stress, and inflammation. Such treatments are potentially relevant for illness progression transdiagnostically (Berk et al. 2011). In the case of omega-3 fatty acids (n3PUFA), abnormally low levels are consistently seen across psychiatric diagnostic categories (Assies et al. 2010; Garland and Hallahan 2006; Parletta et al. 2016a, b; Reddy et al. 2004; Rice et al. 2015), providing a strong biological rationale for supplementation. Furthermore, important for both early intervention and for treatment in youth, there are minimal side effects to n3PUFA (Schlögelhofer et al. 2014). This high margin of safety coupled with an emerging broad therapeutic profile, and evidence of abnormally low levels in people with a range of mental health problems, supports the investigation of its efficacy as novel biomarker-guided therapy for young people with emerging mental health conditions across diagnostic categories.

Long-Chain n3PUFA Polyunsaturated Fatty Acids

Polyunsaturated fatty acids (PUFA) can be classified into n3 and n6 fatty acids, and have numerous and diverse functions in the human body. They are part of phospholipid molecules, the main structural building blocks of cell membranes. PUFA are bioactive molecules that play central roles in a broad range of physiological functions. For example, two particularly important PUFA, eicosapentanoic acid (EPA) and arachidonic acid, are key players in signal transduction, ion transport, and receptor sensitivity (e.g., for serotonin, dopamine, endocannabinoids), as well as precursors in the biosynthesis of the eicosanoids (prostaglandins, leukotrienes, thromboxanes), which mediate the inflammatory response (Mossaheb et al. 2012). Another key PUFA, docosahexaenoic acid (DHA), serves as a precursor for the docosanoids (resolvins, neuroprotectins), which have a neuroprotective effect. The brain is highly enriched with DHA and their derivatives, which regulate biological processes such as neurotransmission, neuroplasticity, and neuroinflammation, and thereby mood and cognitive function (Lin et al. 2017; Piomelli et al. 2007; Su et al. 2015). Moreover, n3PUFA may modulate neurotrophins (Venna et al. 2009), which might be a direct mechanism to mediate neurogenesis and antidepressant effects (Blondeau et al. 2009). Finally, elevated plasma triglyceride level is a cardiovascular risk factor (Hokanson and Austin 1996): n3PUFA have long been known to lower plasma triglyceride along with a variety of other drugs such as fibrates and statins (Patel and Budoff 2016).

n3PUFA Deficiency in Psychiatric Disorders

Low levels of n3PUFA have been consistently reported in psychiatric populations compared with healthy controls across diagnostic categories, including major depressive disorder (Assies et al. 2010), bipolar disorder, anxiety disorders (Thesing et al. 2018), borderline personality disorder (Garland et al. 2007), schizophrenia (Reddy et al. 2004), at-risk mental state for psychosis (Rice et al. 2015), autism spectrum disorders (Parletta et al. 2016a), and attention deficit hyperactivity disorder (Parletta et al. 2016a). These findings are supported by large-scale epidemiological studies. Considering that fish are the principal source of EPA and DHA, Hibbeln (1998) reported that the variation in rates for major depression across countries inversely correlated with national fish consumption. In another study, a 17-year follow-up of 256,118 Japanese people demonstrated that daily fish-eating had a positive effect in reducing the risk of death from suicide, compared with individuals having a nondaily consumption (Hirayama et al. 2004). A survey of 3204 adults in Finland found that infrequent fish consumption was associated with depressive symptoms in women, and a similar trend was noted in men (Tanskanen et al. 2001). A similar inverse relationship between fish consumption and prevalence rate has been demonstrated for bipolar affective disorder (Noaghiul and Hibbeln 2003), although the same study did not find a relationship between fish consumption and the prevalence of schizophrenia. However, there is compelling evidence supporting an association between fish consumption and subthreshold psychotic phenomena. Hedelin et al. (2010) conducted a study among 33,623 women in Sweden to evaluate the association of dietary intake of PUFA with the prevalence of positive psychotic symptoms. Among their many findings, the authors reported a risk ratio of 0.45 (95% CI 0.31–0.66) for high levels of psychotic symptoms for participants who consumed fish on three to four times per week.

Low Levels of n3PUFA Are a Risk Factor for Cardiovascular Disease

An n3 index for cardiovascular health was developed by Harris and von Schacky (2004). The n3 index is the sum of EPA and DHA in erythrocyte membranes and is expressed as a percentage of total erythrocyte fatty acids. They first established erythrocyte levels of EPA+DHA as a valid biomarker of n3PUFA status (Harris 2008). By pooling together results from prospective studies and RCTs, they identified that an n3 index <4% in erythrocyte membranes was associated with the highest risk of mortality from coronary heart disease, whereas levels >8% conferred the greatest cardioprotection. Therefore, the n3 index was proposed as a useful biomarker to estimate risk of mortality from coronary heart disease and provide targets for reducing mortality risk (von Schacky 2009). The direct roles of n3PUFA, particularly DHA (Serhan et al. 2011), in brain function and the growing evidence of their ability to improve psychiatric symptoms suggest that the n3 index might similarly provide a useful target for estimating risk of mental illness and targets for treatment.

Treatment Studies with n3PUFA in Psychiatric Disorders

Trials in Major Depressive Disorder and Anxiety Disorders

Trials evaluating efficacy of n3PUFA supplementation in major depression report conflicting findings (Bloch and Hannestad 2012; Hallahan et al. 2016; Sublette et al. 2011). Among participants with major depressive disorder, however, EPA-predominant formulations (>50% EPA) demonstrated clinical benefits, compared with placebo, whereas DHA-predominant formulations (>50% DHA) did not (Hallahan et al. 2016). Notably, the majority of trials have been conducted in adult populations, with n3PUFA as an adjunct to antidepressant medication and without selecting participants with abnormally low n3PUFA levels. Interestingly, one proof-of-concept RCT of n3PUFA in people with major depressive disorder found that participants with specific combinations of inflammatory markers were more likely to respond to EPA treatment and less likely to respond to placebo treatment (Rapaport et al. 2015). This study highlights the importance of biomarker screening to determine a participant's eligibility for trials and better treatment outcomes.

Anxiety disorders are frequently comorbid with depression. This raises the possibility that n3PUFA levels might contribute to the pathophysiology of both conditions (Ross 2009). In support of n3PUFA supplementation in people with anxiety, a study from Israel reported decreased n3PUFA levels in non-depressed patients with social anxiety disorder (Green et al. 2006). Liu et al. (2013b) found the presence and severity of comorbid anxiety in people with depression were associated with the lowest n3PUFA levels. The Netherlands Study of Depression and Anxiety showed that currently depressed patients, especially those with comorbid anxiety, had n3PUFA levels lower than those in remission or in healthy controls (Thesing et al. 2018). One RCT showed that n3PUFA supplementation lowered anxiety symptoms in medical students (Kiecolt-Glaser et al. 2011), which provides the first evidence that n3PUFA might have anxiolytic benefits.

Trials in Youth with At-Risk Mental State for Psychosis

A 12-week RCT of supplementation with n3PUFA reduced the risk of progression to psychotic disorder in 81 young people with at-risk mental state over a 12-month period, compared with a placebo (Amminger et al. 2010). A longer-term follow-up of this trial found that the brief intervention with n3PUFA was still effective. Compared with placebo, n3PUFA prevented transition to full-threshold psychotic disorder and led to sustained symptomatic and functional improvements for seven years (median) (Amminger et al. 2015). In addition to these trial results, both (negative) correlations between n3PUFA and psychopathology (Kim et al. 2016), along with a large effect size deficit for n3PUFA (compared with healthy adolescents) observed in patients with an at-risk mental state, provide a further rationale for supplementation as early intervention for incipient psychotic symptoms (Rice et al. 2015). Furthermore, a high ratio of n6 to n3PUFA, which indicates a relative deficiency of n3PUFA, is thought to have adverse health effects (Simopoulos 2011). A higher n6 to n3PUFA ratio at baseline has been found to predict mood disorders at longer-term follow-up (Berger et al. 2017).

Two large-scale studies have tried to replicate these findings. In the NEURAPRO study of 304 individuals with an at-risk mental state for psychosis (McGorry et al. 2017), 153 received n3PUFA and 151 received placebo for 6 months. No significant group difference was observed for rates of transition to psychosis. A lower than expected psychosis transition rate (11% vs. 25%) might have prevented a test of the main hypothesis; the trial also failed to show effects in favor of n3PUFA on secondary outcome measures. An important limitation of NEURAPRO (and all n3PUFA RCTs) is that the use of n3PUFA supplements unrelated to the study cannot be excluded (James et al. 2014). Therefore, secondary analyses were conducted using cell membrane-level change pre- to post-supplementation as objective measures of n3PUFA intake. Again, when analyzed as a single cohort, no association was observed between n3PUFA levels and transition to psychosis. However, increase of n3PUFA was found to be significantly related to functional and symptomatic outcome measures at 6 and 12 months (Amminger et al. 2018). In contrast to the RCT analysis, this secondary analysis, using biomarker information, showed that an increase in erythrocyte n3PUFA correlated with better clinical outcomes, thus confirming the findings of Amminger et al. (2010).

Preliminary data are available from a second, independent n3PUFA supplementation replication RCT in individuals from the North American Prodrome Longitudinal Studies (NAPLS) (Cadenhead et al. 2017). Of the 127 "clinical high-risk" patients recruited into the trial, the rate of transition to psychosis was low (10%) over 24 months of follow-up, without statistical difference between n3PUFA and placebo groups. However, the researchers noted cardiometabolic abnormalities were prevalent at baseline in this cohort of young people, and they found significant evidence that those with low n3PUFA in their diet were statistically more likely to have converted to a psychotic disorder by study end (Cadenhead et al. 2017).

Post Hoc Analysis of the NEURAPRO RCT

Therapeutic effects of n3PUFA might be stronger in subgroups characterized by certain biological or phenotypic markers (Kraemer 2016); for example, low n3 index at baseline. The post hoc analysis of the NEURAPRO RCT posed two questions:

1. Is n3PUFA supplementation specifically effective in participants characterized by low n3 index at baseline?
2. Do effects differ between participants randomized to n3PUFA or placebo?

In NEURAPRO, erythrocyte fatty acid data were collected in 285 out of 304 (94%) participants (mean age = 19.1 yr, SD = 4.6). The mean n3 index at baseline in the sample was 2.96% (SD = 1.10; median = 3%). This is 40% lower than the average n3 index (5%) in the Australian population (Swierk et al. 2011). The median n3 index of 3% places theoretically half of this cohort of young people at a substantially elevated longer-term risk of premature death from coronary heart disease (Parletta et al. 2016b; von Schacky 2009). This view and the very high rate of youth with abnormally low n3PUFA levels in NEURAPRO are consistent with the fact that people with mental health problems die at a significantly younger age (Thornicroft 2011).

To show specific efficacy of n3PUFA supplementation in people with low levels, a median split was used to group participants with low and high n3 index at baseline. Analyses tested whether change in the n3 index (an objective measure of n3PUFA intake), over the 6-month treatment period in NEURAPRO, was differentially associated with clinical improvement in groups characterized by an n3 index of <3% versus ≥3% at baseline. The Clinical Global Impression–Improvement (CGI-I) scale (Busner et al. 2009), ranging from one to seven (lower scores indicate more improvement as compared with baseline), was used. A score of one or two (i.e., very much or much improved) reflects a substantial, clinically meaningful improvement in illness severity. Figure 10.1 shows that in the <3% group, individuals with much or very much clinical improvement, when compared with individuals with less favorable outcomes, were characterized by a significantly higher increase of their n3 index (mean = 1.5, SD = 1.3 vs. mean = 0.7, SD = 1.7; mean difference = –0.8, P = 0.015); more n3PUFA intake between baseline and 6 months was associated with better clinical outcome. In the ≥3% group, this association was not observed. These findings suggest that n3PUFA supplementation should target individuals with low n3 index (<3%), who are also at risk of coronary heart disease and might benefit in terms of both mental and physical health.

To further elucidate the observed treatment effect in NEURAPRO participants with low n3 index (<3%), the same test was conducted separately in the fish oil and the placebo groups. Better clinical outcomes were consistently associated with a higher increase of the n3 index for both groups: for fish oil, the mean difference was –1.0 whereas for the placebo, the mean difference was –0.8 (Figure 10.2). This analysis suggests that treatment effects of n3PUFA in NEURAPRO occurred in both treatment arms. It also indicates the importance of utilizing biomarker information to determine the efficacy of n3PUFA supplementation versus placebo.

Clinical trial evidence suggests that n3PUFA are safe and well tolerated (Freeman et al. 2006; Schlögelhofer et al. 2014). Most commonly occurring, but clinically rarely significant, are mild gastrointestinal symptoms (e.g., a fishy aftertaste, indigestion). It has been suggested that the potential antithrombotic effect of fish oil might theoretically increase the risk for bleeding, which might be a safety concern for individual participants. However, clinical trial evidence has not supported increased bleeding with n3PUFA intake, even when combined with other agents (such as aspirin or warfarin) which might also increase bleeding (Bays 2007). Differential effects on metabolic parameters, most of which appear to be beneficial, have also been reported (Mossaheb et al. 2015).

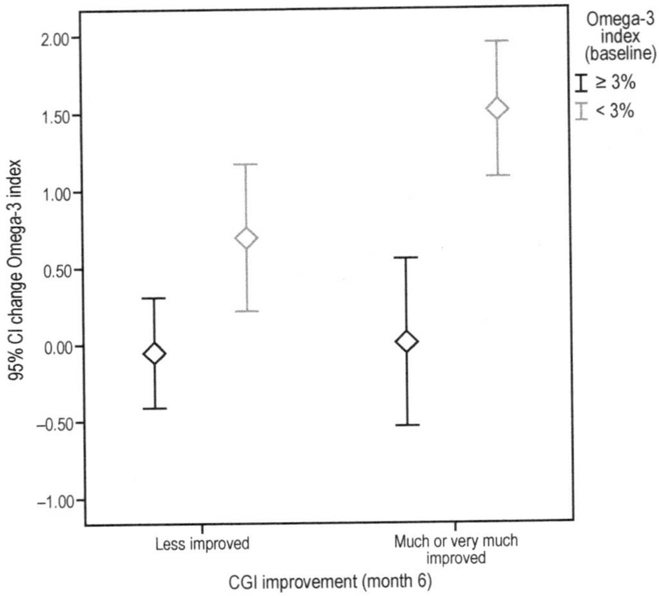

Figure 10.1 Change in omega-3 index between baseline and month 6 in participants with low or high baseline omega-3 levels by clinical improvement groups.

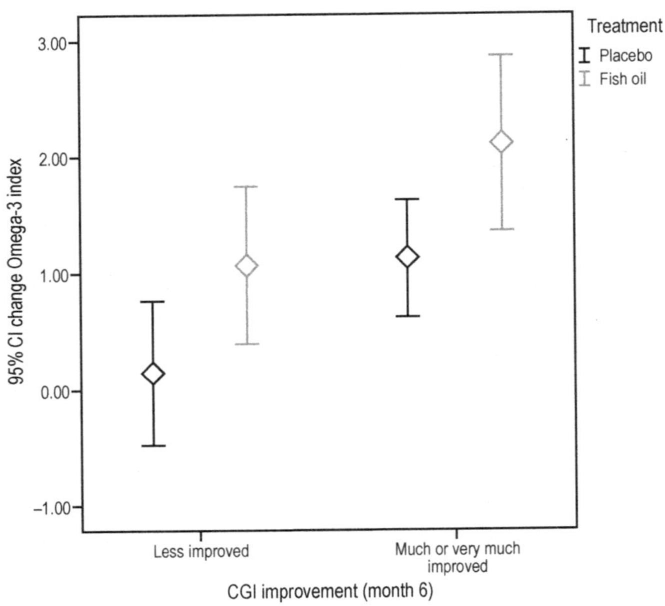

Figure 10.2 Change in omega-3 index between baseline and month 6 in participants who received fish oil or placebo by clinical improvement groups.

A recently developed capillary dried blood spot test can be used to quantify levels of n3PUFA and other relevant fatty acids in erythrocytes (e.g., n6PUFA) (Liu et al. 2014a). This has strong practical and cost advantages over conventional methods because of the need for remarkably lower blood volumes and easier shipping and storage at ambient temperatures.

Conclusions

Interventions and mental health services for youth are mired in failures of relapse prevention, social recovery, innovation, access to services, and research translation. Three avenues for progress lie in novel digital interventions, broadening the scope of family assessment and intervention, and transdiagnostic biomarker-guided intervention.

Integration of digital interventions into mainstream youth mental health services aims to create a new paradigm, fueled by fast innovation and research translation. Successful implementation has the potential to revolutionize the field through online social media and mobile technology, novel and evidence-based psychological models, and new blends of multidisciplinary expertise that will lead to new interventions designed to transform clinical practice, rather than merely translating existing face-to-face interventions into an online mode of delivery.

Digital and other technologies can also transform family intervention by providing ecologically valid family assessment. Family intervention in youth mental health needs to move away from a narrow focus on psychotic disorders, patient symptoms, and relapse and toward the inclusion of overlooked populations and transdiagnostic processes as well as family burden and the mental and physical health of families, which have the potential to yield major reductions in carer and disease burden.

Finally, transdiagnostic prevention and treatment of severe psychiatric morbidities (e.g., anxiety, psychotic, mood, and personality disorders) is a promising avenue for reducing the burden, stigmatization, and economic consequences of these disorders. A 20-year mortality gap for men, and 15 years for women, is still experienced by people with mental ill-health in high-income countries (Thornicroft 2011). Cardiovascular and metabolic risk factors are prevalent among people with mental health problems, even at a young age (Cadenhead and Mirzakhanian 2016).

Based on the existing literature and new observations presented here, n3PUFA supplementation with fish oil is proposed as a prototype for transdiagnostic biomarker-guided intervention for young people with mental health problems. This proposal introduces a new paradigm in primary health care by using easily accessible biomarker information to target an intervention with an excellent side effect profile to a group most likely to benefit for a broader range of health outcomes.

11

The "Clinical High-Risk State for Psychosis" in Youth

Global Challenges and Controversies

Lawrence H. Yang, Sarah A. Lieff, Bernalyn Ruiz, Shane D. Colombo, Drew Blasco, and PhuongThao Le

Abstract

Whereas identification of a "clinical high-risk state for psychosis" (CHR-P) marks a groundbreaking global advance in the treatment of youth with potential subthreshold psychotic symptoms, controversies regarding the CHR-P exist. This chapter explores three sets of challenges: validity of the CHR-P diagnosis, stigma and ethical concerns, and challenges in implementing CHR-P identification measures globally.

It critically analyzes the current knowledge regarding these challenges. Debates surrounding core validity of the CHR-P diagnosis include whether CHR-P is a distinct syndrome from other common mental disorders, decline of transition rates in studies over time, and the value of identifying an at-risk status when empirically validated treatments have not yet been developed. Ethical challenges include potential stigma of the CHR-P state, and the ethics of diagnosing an at-risk state that encompasses a period of adolescence and extends into youth. Challenges in implementing CHR-P interventions globally include questions of whether early mental health intervention shows sufficient economic return, and promotion of psychosis terms in cultural settings where such conceptions may be entirely novel. Addressing these controversies could facilitate adoption of the CHR-P identification into mental health-care systems globally, thus maximizing public health impact.

The Clinical High-Risk State for Psychosis: Core Concepts and Approach

A substantial proportion (80–90%) of individuals suffering from schizophrenia experience subacute (or "prodromal") symptoms prior to the onset of full psychosis (Addington and Heinssen 2012). Whereas those with a first episode of psychosis (FEP) already experience significant psychotic symptoms, individuals identified at CHR-P show subthreshold psychotic signs and need for care. Significant efforts have been made to identify, evaluate, and provide treatment in this earlier high-risk stage, so that early treatment and consistent monitoring can forestall and possibly prevent the first psychotic break and the full development of psychosis (Addington and Heinssen 2012; McGorry 1993). Roughly one-third of these cases develop FEP over a three-year follow-up (Fusar-Poli et al. 2012). CHR-P services enable interventions in the earliest stages, prior to the first episode of psychosis. Implementation of CHR-P services, such as those which have taken place in the United States, Europe, and Australia, could avert significant financial and social burdens associated with psychosis (McGlashan et al. 2010).

Initiating treatment at an earlier point can reduce the duration of untreated psychosis (DUP). Longer DUP is associated with worse outcomes, including poorer overall functioning, positive symptoms, quality of life, and response to antipsychotic treatment at six months (Niendam et al. 2009). Conversely, shortened DUP is associated with better positive and general symptom outcomes, better functioning, and a greater likelihood of being referred to outpatient treatment (Addington et al. 2015). Accordingly, early interventions in CHR-P individuals could effectively lead to a much reduced or negligible DUP, even when transition to a full psychotic disorder results.

CHR-P Identification: Operationalization

As one possibility, individuals can be identified as being on the psychosis-risk spectrum if they meet the at-risk mental state, which emphasizes psychotic-like symptoms and sharp declines in functioning (initially proposed by Yung and McGorry 1996), defined as follows:

1. The ultra-high risk state for psychosis (UHR-P), identified via the comprehensive assessment of at-risk mental state (CAARMS) criteria based on Yung and McGorry's (1996) pioneering work, provides one way of identifying the high risk for psychosis state (Yung et al. 2005).
2. Alternatively, the CHR-P state, as assessed by the SIPS/SOPS (described below), is met if an individual meets at least one of the following inclusion criteria: brief intermittent psychotic syndrome (BIPS), attenuated positive symptom syndrome (APSS), or genetic risk and decline (GRD); for definitions, see Table 11.1.

It is important to note, however, that UHR-P and CHR-P samples are similar in terms of their diagnostic makeup (i.e., BIPS, APSS, and GRD cases, symptom severity, and level of functional impairment).

As an example of how the at-risk mental state is assessed, consider the Structured Interview for Prodromal Symptoms (SIPS), which represents a

Table 11.1 Defining the three subtypes of the CHR-P syndrome (after Miller et al. 2003).

Subtype	Description
Attenuated positive symptom syndrome (APSS)	Presence of one or more positive symptoms, including but not limited to "suspiciousness/persecutory ideas," "grandiosity," or "perceptual abnormalities/hallucinations" at a prodromal rating (3–5). Symptoms developed or began to worsen over the past year and have occurred at least once per week during the previous month.
Brief intermittent psychotic syndrome (BIPS)	One or more positive symptoms experienced at a fully psychotic level. Symptoms must have started within the previous three months and occur several minutes a day at a rate of at least one time per month, up to four times per week.
Genetic risk and decline (GRD)	Includes (a) having a first-degree relative with a diagnosed psychotic disorder or meeting criteria for schizotypal personality disorder and (b) experiencing a significant decrease in functioning over the past year as measured by the GAF scale (i.e., at least a 30% drop).

significant advance in operationalizing CHR-P (Fusar-Poli et al. 2013b). SIPS includes the following measures:

- A family history questionnaire
- A scale of prodromal symptoms (SOPS)
- A schizotypal personality disorder checklist
- A global assessment of functioning (GAF) scale

All are used in combination to ascertain high-risk status using the SOPS criteria, which includes negative, positive, disorganized, and general symptoms (Miller et al. 2003). Symptoms are rated on a scale from 0–6. The 3–5 range represents mild or attenuated symptoms, with individuals experiencing prepsychotic symptoms (e.g., hearing odd noises as a perceptual abnormality) (Miller et al. 2003). In contrast to individuals who experience a full psychotic episode (i.e., who evidence total conviction in their symptoms, a rating of 6), those who experienced prodromal symptoms recognize that their symptoms may not be real (Miller et al. 2003).

As an alternative possibility, "basic symptoms" can be used to identify earlier prodromal symptoms (e.g., subjective experienced changes in self-perception, tolerance to stress, cognitive disturbances, and cognitive-perceptive disturbances). Here, to meet basic symptoms criteria, individuals must (a) exhibit ≥2 of 9 cognitive-perceptive symptoms (COPER), with a score of ≥3 in the past three months, and/or (b) demonstrate a disturbance in cognition (COGDIS), with a score of 3 over the past three months and a first occurrence at least one year ago, irrespective of earlier frequency or persistence. While the psychosis risk spectrum can include individuals who meet basic symptom criteria, basic symptom and CHR-P/UHR-P criteria, as well as CHR-P/UHR-P criteria alone, we focus on controversies associated with the psychosis risk designation using the CHR-P example.

Core Ascertainment Strategy in CHR-P

CHR-P programs mainly care for adolescents and young adults who are already showing signs and seeking help for potential mental health problems (Fusar-Poli et al. 2013b). In addition to providing comprehensive care, monitoring, and evaluation via a multidisciplinary team, CHR-P clinics engage in community outreach in an effort to increase enrollment of help-seeking individuals (Compton et al. 2008). Outreach activities include recruitment from primary schools, colleges, primary care, and other mental health services, as well as CHR-P education within the community to improve lay identification of individuals who meet CHR-P criteria (Cannon et al. 2008; McFarlane et al. 2010; McGlashan et al. 2007). The intent of ascertainment from nonmental health community sources is to identify individuals who have not yet sought tertiary mental health treatment and to improve the course of their illness while they are still in a "high-risk" state, ultimately reducing the burden of psychosis (McGorry et al. 2008a).

The Portland Identification and Early Referral (PIER) program in Portland, Maine (McFarlane et al. 2010), provides an example of a community CHR-P program. To identify CHR-P youth, PIER employed a public education campaign directed at a broad spectrum of the community (i.e., counselors at the primary and college level, clinicians in primary care, mental health, and other health-care areas). Through on-site visits as well as via a public education campaign using radio and TV ads, brochures, and customized websites (see Figure 11.1), PIER's efforts were aimed at enhancing recognition of the warning signs of early psychosis (McFarlane et al. 2010). Although there was, on average, a six-month lag

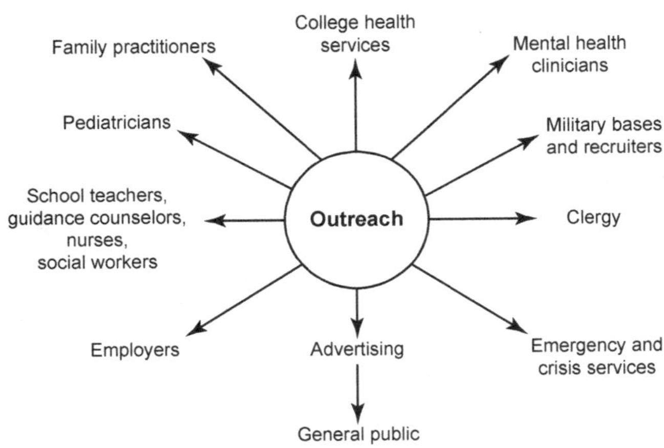

Figure 11.1 Example of community ascertainment from PIER.

between outreach efforts and referral to PIER, this community outreach program achieved its objectives: more than 50% of CHR-P referrals came from sources outside traditional mental health agencies (McFarlane et al. 2010). Further, the presence of a community CHR-P program appeared to decrease rates of first hospitalizations for psychosis in that region. A follow-up study found that there was an 8% increase in hospitalization rates related to psychosis in a control group of comparable catchment areas in which no CHR-P programs existed, compared to a 26% decrease in the catchment area for the PIER program (i.e., the experimental group) (McFarlane et al. 2014).

The Validity of CHR-P Identification: Challenges and Controversies

In this section we explore the controversies and challenges that surround the core validity of CHR-P identification. We discuss whether the CHR-P can be considered to assess a "true" syndrome with useful predictive features across populations. Conversion rates have been reportedly decreasing over time. While some studies have examined the observed declining transition rates as a potential artifact of whether participants are ascertained earlier in the course of CHR-P, others have focused on the heterogeneity between subgroups (CHR-P, UHR-P, and basic symptoms) as a source of variance. We also discuss the inconclusive state regarding the comparative effectiveness of treatment options and current controversies regarding treatment recommendations.

Declining Conversion Rates in Samples over Time

A key meta-analysis reported that the rate of symptomatic, help-seeking CHR-P youth who transition to (i.e., meet full criteria for) a psychotic disorder within three years after first identification is approximately 36% (Fusar-Poli et al. 2012). Similarly, the North American Prodrome Longitudinal Study (NAPLS) found that 35% of individuals convert to psychosis within 2.5 years of follow-up (Cannon et al. 2008). However, one controversy concerns declining conversion rates to psychosis that have been observed over time (Yung et al. 2007). Early studies identified upward of a 40% conversion rate to full psychosis over a follow-up period of two to three years after identification (Gee and Cannon 2011). In more recent studies, reported rates declined when the essentially interchangeable UHR-P state was used as the criterion: large portions of UHR-P individuals did not convert to psychosis and even remitted from a UHR-P state (Fusar-Poli et al. 2012; Nelson et al. 2013; Simon et al. 2014). One meta-analysis reported an average conversion rate of only 24% among UHR-P patients, whereas earlier publications showed significantly lower conversion rates, especially among studies with a naturalistic (i.e., nontreatment) study design (Simon et al. 2011).

With CHR-P, a similar decline in transition rates has been observed. In their study of 129 patients, separated into two periods of enrollment (2005–2009 and 2009–2013), Lim et al. (2016) found transition rates to be lower in the later-identified CHR-P sample. When the duration of prodromal positive symptoms was accounted for, however, this significant difference disappeared. This suggests that referral of youth who are earlier in their trajectory of illness to CHR-P clinics may be associated with decreasing transition rates, a trend that occurred in the more recently enrolled patients. A meta-analysis that examined eight studies (N = 773 CHR-P youth) conducted between 2002 and 2012 found that 73% of individuals identified with CHR-P did not convert during a two-year follow-up period and that an additional 46% fully remitted from baseline psychotic signs (Simon et al. 2013). Possible explanations include more effective treatments, comorbidity with other disorders, differences between earlier cohorts and more recent cohorts (e.g., higher proportion with trait risk factor), or lead time bias (the difference in time between initial CHR screening and when the onset of symptoms might occur in the absence of screening) (Simon et al. 2013). Here, CHR-P patients are diagnosed at an even earlier stage than they would have been without clinical involvement, giving the illusion that more time has elapsed in the CHR-P stage and that transition rates are declining. It may be that as programs continue to advance, in terms of being able to detect and treat CHR-P individuals at progressively earlier stages, transition rates may continue to decrease.

Another factor that may contribute to declining conversion rates to psychosis is that features of CHR-P closely overlap with that of other common psychiatric disorders. In their review of possible comorbid psychiatric conditions (e.g., isolated hallucinations, unusual bodily perceptions, hypochrondriatic fears and cenesthetic psychotic symptoms, depersonalization, obsessive-compulsive, overvalued, and delusional ideas), Simon et al. (2014) found that the vast majority (86%) of UHR-P patients reported ≥1 of these four clinical subgroups. Given the substantial overlap of these clinical symptoms with other common mental disorders, future studies should characterize the influence of comorbid clinical symptoms on transition (or nontransition) rates for psychosis.

Psychosis Risk Spectrum as Distinct Subsyndromes

Another possible explanation for why transition rates are declining is that subgroups of CHR-P, UHR-P, and individuals with basic symptoms have heterogeneous conversion rates; that is, the differing compositions of these subgroups across study samples may be a source of variance in the observed transition rates. In a meta-analysis that compared rates of those who met criteria for the UHR-P subgroup versus those meeting basic symptoms criteria of COGDIS, conversion rates were found to be similar for both criteria at two-year follow-up. This changed after two years, at which time conversion rates for COGDIS became significantly greater (Schultze-Lutter et al. 2015).

A larger meta-analysis was conducted for 33 independent studies (N = 4,227 participants) which categorized CHR-P individuals based on the presence of (a) any BIPS, APSS, and GRD, (b) APSS alone, (c) GRD alone, and (d) basic symptoms (Fusar-Poli et al. 2016). It identified a control group across studies comprised of individuals who were assessed for risk of CHR-P, but did not ultimately meet these criteria. The proportion of each subgroup having any psychotic disorder at 6, 12, 24, 36, and >48 months follow-up was then evaluated. Findings indicated that the GRD subgroup did not demonstrate a higher risk of psychosis compared with the CHR-P subgroup. The BIPS subgroup was at higher risk compared with APSS (39% vs. 19% transition rates). However, APSS demonstrated the highest proportion of CHR-P cases, comprising 85% of this meta-analytic sample. Although the BIPS subgroup demonstrated the highest conversion rates, it has been questioned whether those who meet these criteria are already psychotic (Fusar-Poli et al. 2016), which could potentially bias transition rates because those in the BIPS subcategory are more likely to transition yet they make up a relatively smaller proportion of CHR-P samples.

A more focal analysis of four distinct clinical variables—disorganized communication (from APSS), suspiciousness (from APSS), verbal memory (neuropsychological deficits), and decline in social functioning (global functioning)—was examined among 101 patients at baseline with an average three-year follow-up (Cornblatt et al. 2015). Only cases exhibiting ≥1 APSS symptoms at a moderate-to-severe level were included; cases that solely met BIPS or GRD criteria were excluded. Overall conversion rates at follow-up were 28%, and the final model had a positive predictive value of 82%. Additionally, based on data from 596 clinical high-risk participants from NAPLS-2, Cannon et al. (2016) identified predictors of conversion: unusual thought content and suspiciousness, decline in social functioning, lower performance on verbal learning and memory, slower speed of processing, and younger age at baseline. These findings, externally validated by Carrión et al. (2016) with a sample of 210 participants from the Early Detection and Intervention for the Prevention of Psychosis Program, indicate that in addition to standard prodromal criteria, domains for global functioning and neuropsychological abilities impacted psychosis conversion rates. Accordingly, identifying distinctive symptom components of CHR-P criteria offers the potential to improve predictive accuracy of conversion while also providing insight into treatment targets.

An emerging area of CHR-P research has been the characterization of social and functional outcomes for nonconverters; that is, individuals who exhibit significant decline in social functioning but have not yet transitioned to psychosis. Since nonconverters possess suboptimal functional outcomes, we need to know whether there is heterogeneity among nonconverters that might enhance our understanding of psychosis prediction. In a major NAPLS study that examined 300 CHR-P patients longitudinally, 71% (214) of CHR-P patients had not transitioned to psychosis after 2.5 years. Although there were significant declines in attenuated positive and negative symptoms for nonconverters, at least one positive symptom was present for 40% of this group at one- and two-year follow-up. When compared with their nonpsychiatric counterparts, these nonconverters had significantly poorer social and role functioning (Addington et al. 2011).

To address the issue of whether nonconverters are heterogeneous in outcome, Schlosser et al. (2012) examined 84 CHR-P participants and 58 healthy controls across a two-year period. At the two-year follow-up, 30% of their CHR-P sample had transitioned to psychosis while 20% had fully remitted; that is, they no longer exhibited prodromal symptoms at subpsychotic levels (e.g., symptomatically remitted) and demonstrated high global and social functioning (e.g., functional recovery). Of note, another 17% were symptomatically remitted but did not functionally recover; conversely, 17% did not experience symptomatic remission but functionally recovered. Those symptomatically remitted patients who did not experience a full functional recovery were more similar to healthy controls in terms of baseline and longitudinal symptoms and functioning compared with the other two groups. This can be explained by the symptomatically remitted (but functionally impaired) group also having presented initially with less severe prodromal symptoms than the other two groups; although they did not experience a full functional recovery at two-year follow-up, they did possess a more normative trajectory of psychosocial functioning over time. This suggests that the symptomatically remitted (but functionally impaired) group might more accurately represent the "false positive" cases from the perspective of risk ascertainment, whereas the functionally recovered but still symptomatic patients represent a clinical profile similar to that of their converted counterparts. Accordingly, future research should seek to follow these still symptomatic (but functionally recovered) nonconverters past the two-year follow-up period to track their continued risk for psychosis conversion.

Inconclusive Treatment Recommendations for CHR-P Status

Existing randomized controlled studies of treatment for CHR-P individuals recommend psychosocial and pharmacological interventions, in particular cognitive behavioral therapy (CBT) as effective in delaying the onset of acute psychosis (Woodberry et al. 2016). A recent review of CHR-P interventions, however, concluded that no particular treatment has demonstrated greater efficacy than any other available treatment (Woodberry et al. 2016). Partly due to overlap across different strategies, treatment recommendations are currently unable to claim whether psychosocial interventions, neuroprotective agents, or antipsychotic medications are more effective for the prevention or delay of transition to psychosis. While eight guidelines have been proposed for treating CHR-P, only two were deemed of sufficient quality, by the Canadian Treatment

Guideline developers (Addington et al. 2017), to offer treatment recommendations: the National Institute for Health and Care Excellence and the European Psychiatric Association (EPA) guidelines. Although both propose psychotherapy (in particular, CBT) with or without family intervention and pharmacological interventions (NCCMH 2013), more rigorous evaluations of treatment efficacy are still needed.

Pharmacological Interventions

A source of substantial debate and controversy is that the most recently published guidelines, the Canadian Treatment Guidelines, have recommended short-term, low-dose, second-generation antipsychotics if CHR-P individuals are not responsive to psychological interventions, and there are severe and progressive attenuated psychotic symptoms that could signal an impending transition to psychosis (Addington et al. 2017). These recommendations are controversial due to the numerous side effects and stigma associated with antipsychotic use. For example, studies have suggested that young people are more prone to having neuroleptic side effects (Fraguas et al. 2008) and that possible brain shrinkage is associated with long-term medication use (Ziermans et al. 2010). Highlighting the unresolved nature of this controversy, two recent reviews of randomized controlled trials (RCTs) that assessed the efficacy of antipsychotics in CHR-P treatment failed to present conclusive evidence for this approach (Stafford et al. 2013; Woodberry et al. 2016). These studies did not provide sufficient evidence owing to frequent confounding of the effects of psychosocial treatment with pharmacological treatment, poor medication adherence, and high dropout rates (Becker et al. 2015; Stafford et al. 2013). The latter two factors signaled very poor tolerability of these medications in the CHR-P population. In sum, given the inconclusive evidence and the demonstrated efficacy of more tolerable psychosocial treatments (below), and because the recommendation for the selective use of antipsychotics has yet to be adopted outside of Canada, further evidence is necessary to support an evidence-based approach concerning antipsychotic use.

Psychosocial Interventions

Numerous psychosocial interventions exist for CHR-P: CBT, family-focused therapy, case management, assertive community treatment, multifamily group psychoeducation, cognitive remediation/enhancement, social skills training, supported employment/education, supportive therapy, needs-based intervention, and crisis intervention (Woodberry et al. 2016). Similar effects have been evidenced in the treatment of CHR-P across existing psychosocial treatments. Cognitive and cognitive behavioral approaches are the most studied psychosocial interventions. Stafford et al. (2013) reviewed nine CBT intervention studies and determined that CBT has a moderate effect on reducing the likelihood of transition at 12 and 18 months. Although European Psychiatric Association guidelines do not include a recommendation for family intervention, the most recently developed treatment guidelines, citing one RCT of a family-focused treatment, recommend CBT with or without family intervention as first treatment after evaluation (Addington et al. 2017). Additionally, one study demonstrated that family-aided assertive community treatment (FACT) is significantly more effective than community care in reducing positive symptoms and improving work and school participation among CHR-P youth at two-year follow-up (McFarlane et al. 2014). Accordingly, the family component should be considered for inclusion in future treatment recommendations.

Nutrition Supplementation

Because deficits in vitamins and polyunsaturated fatty acids are associated with poorer outcomes (e.g., greater symptom severity, reduced neural integrity, and neurocognitive impairments in individuals with FEP), the value of nutrition supplementation (i.e., adjunctive vitamin or antioxidant supplementation) has been examined (Firth et al. 2018). One prominent study showed that intake of omega-3 polyunsaturated fatty acids (FA) was significantly associated with reduced positive, negative, and general symptoms as well as improved functioning (Amminger et al. 2010). Moreover, 93.8% of participants completed this study, compared with the 20% to 66% completion rates for antipsychotics (Amminger et al. 2010). A recent replication study (Cadenhead et al. 2017), however, found that while the experimental group did not significantly differ from the placebo group, there was a significant association between a baseline diet low in omega-3 FA-rich foods and increased symptoms, decreased functioning, and higher likelihood of conversion to psychosis. Because this study was underpowered to detect effects (Cadenhead et al. 2017; Markulev et al. 2017), a subsequent multisite RCT was conducted to assess the efficacy of omega-3 FAs and CBT case management (McGorry et al. 2017). Results again failed to replicate previous findings found in the original Amminger et al. (2010) study, as no significant difference was found in transition rates between the experimental group receiving omega-3 FA plus cognitive behavioral case management (CBCM) and the control group which received a placebo plus CBCM. Because both groups received CBCM as well as focal medication as needed (i.e., selective serotonin reuptake inhibitors for major depression, benzodiazepine therapy for anxiety), and good-quality psychosocial supports have been shown to decrease transition rates thus leading to symptomatic and functional improvement in both groups, conclusions about the specific role of omega-3 FAs were difficult to reach (McGorry et al. 2017). More research is thus required to clarify its role in potentially decreasing rates of transition.

Exercise Interventions

More recently, attention has focused on the use of exercise interventions as adjunctive treatments for individuals with psychosis. In persons with schizophrenia, exercise interventions have been effective in improving physical fitness, reducing cardiometabolic risk, and decreasing psychiatric symptoms (Firth et al. 2015). For CHR-P, research has found that individuals identified as CHR-P are more likely to be physically inactive and to have higher rates of sedentary behavior than persons who did not develop psychosis (Koivukangas et al. 2010). Additionally, self-report assessment of physical activity levels in a CHR-P sample concluded that those with CHR-P exercise less frequently, less intensely, and report lower perceived fitness levels than healthy controls. Further, CHR-P participants reported more barriers to exercise and less positive reasons for exercising (Deighton and Addington 2015). While research has reported on the extent of physical activity among CHR-P individuals, limited work has been conducted to test the efficacy or effectiveness of exercise interventions. Given the evidence above regarding the efficacy of exercise interventions with FEP, these interventions might also benefit individuals with CHR-P. To our knowledge, the only published exercise intervention within the CHR-P population assessed the efficacy of a 12-week program of supervised exercise. The intervention improved positive and negative symptoms, social and role functioning, cognitive functioning, as well as functional connectivity between the hippocampus and occipital cortex (Dean et al. 2017). This research presents promise for the use of physical activity interventions in persons with CHR-P.

Future Work

CHR-P constitutes a meaningful risk syndrome for distressed, help-seeking individuals. Identifying it in individuals not only helps us predict the transition to psychosis among converters, it enables us to address impaired functioning among a substantial proportion of nonconverters. A great deal of research into both aspects has been conducted within high-income, Western European societies. As research has proliferated, a more nuanced understanding of CHR-P identification has emerged (e.g., differing transition rates between symptom subgroups), and we expect that further refinement will be needed to enhance understanding in the prediction of psychosis. Better defining the clinical subtypes may help reduce heterogeneity; identifying core characteristics that predict psychosis may result in more targeted, and ultimately effective, treatment approaches and recommendations.

A substantial gap remains however, in that most or nearly all psychosis risk studies have been conducted in Western European, high-income countries, with the exception of Hong Kong and China (see below). Currently, we do not know how well CHR-P states, including the utility of the risk calculator (Cannon et al. 2016), predict transition to psychosis in non-Western, low- and middle-income countries. Addressing this gap could greatly expand applicability of this meaningful risk syndrome and help symptomatic individuals in other income global contexts.

Stigma and Ethical Dimensions of CHR-P Identification

The second set of issues that we address concerns the stigmatizing effects of being identified with a severe mental health disorder. Comprehensive reviews of stigma and early psychosis among youth are available elsewhere (see Gronholm et al. 2017). Here we highlight stigma and ethical considerations of youth identified as CHR-P at an early and critical stage in their development trajectory.

Stigma of CHR-P

Despite the many potential benefits of early CHR-P identification, those who are identified may experience stigma. Risk of stigma is especially important, given that a majority (i.e., approximately 65%) of those identified as CHR-P will not develop a full psychotic disorder, yet may be subject to negative effects from the stigma associated with this psychiatric classification (Fusar-Poli et al. 2012; Yang et al. 2015). Being identified as at-risk for a severe mental illness during critical developmental stages of adolescence and youth—when an individual's concept of "self" consolidates (Eccles et al. 1993) and when social acceptance is key to identity formation (Moses 2009)—can severely threaten a young person's sense of identity and normalcy (Wisdom and Green 2004; Yang et al. 2007). A small qualitative study showed that CHR-P youth expressed concerns about how peers would perceive them if information about their at-risk status was revealed (Welsh and Brown 2013). Recent research has delineated whether differences in stigma are associated with the CHR-P label or with symptoms (Yang et al. 2015). While stigma related to both symptoms and label mattered for CHR-P youth, stigma related to symptoms was more prominent overall and was associated with increased depression (Yang et al. 2015). In contrast, stigma related to the label was associated with anxiety (Yang et al. 2015). Further, research from a multisite study indicated that a little less than one-third of CHR-P youth endorsed their sense of self as being "most impacted" because they were at-risk for a psychotic disorder (i.e., psychosis or schizophrenia) compared to a nonpsychotic disorder such as anxiety or depression (Yang et al. 2019). In examining factors associated with sense of self, Yang et al. found that individuals who reported "being told" that they were at risk by others or who "believed themselves" to be at risk for developing psychosis experienced increased odds of psychosis risk impacting their sense of self (Yang et al. 2019). This indicates that the stigma associated with CHR-P identification is significant for some individuals and linked to negative psychosocial outcomes. It also suggests that interventions to mitigate stigma could further improve CHR-P outcomes. However, it is also important to consider whether stigma related to CHR-P identification may be affected by other information relayed during the process of being told one is at-risk. For example, an "at-risk" state is distinct from a FEP, and there is a relatively low risk of transition to psychosis, particularly if one is engaging in treatment. Beneficial effects of providing accurate information about the "at-risk" state have been shown to mitigate stigma toward CHR-P among community members (Yang et al. 2013) and could possibly provide similar benefits among CHR-P individuals themselves.

Ethical Challenges

The process of and procedures involved in obtaining informed consent for CHR-P youth (<18 years of age) need to be carefully considered before they participate in research or clinical interventions. Children and adolescents have altered risk perceptions, such as heightened focus on short-term risks and benefits (Scott et al. 1995). Therefore, support should be given to ensure that such participants can competently evaluate the risks and benefits of engaging in research. Additionally, because family members often play an important role in recruitment and may be subject to a particular emotional state (e.g., in distress or overly enthusiastic) when providing informed consent for their children, procedures need to incorporate steps to minimize the potential effects of these biases.

Implementing CHR-P Identification and Treatment Globally

To address the challenges and controversies associated with implementing CHR-P identification on a global scale, we begin with a discussion of how it was originally implemented in Australia. Thereafter we move to the context of Hong Kong, where CHR-P services are currently being developed, and conclude with a discussion of costs and benefits.

Implementation in Australia

The first clinic established to treat UHR-P individuals was the Personal Assessment and Crisis Evaluation (PACE) clinic in Melbourne, Australia (Yung et al. 1995). The establishment of PACE led to the development of other UHR-P programs in Australia, many of which are paired with FEP treatment programs (Cannon et al. 2008; Carr et al. 2000; McGorry et al. 2008a; Phillips et al. 2000; Yung et al. 2008), a model that has proliferated worldwide. In Australia, CHR-P identification and treatment is embedded within Orygen Youth Health, a public mental health program that serves young people from 15–24 years of age (Yung et al. 2004, 2008). Additionally, in 2006, the

Australian government invested in the creation of *headspace*, a nationwide policy initiative designed to decrease fragmentation of services and increase access to services for young people (ages 12–25 yr) who were experiencing a range of mental and substance abuse problems (McGorry et al. 2007b). Headspace provides no- or low-cost services, at in-person locations as well as online, and is focused on youth-oriented treatment and in minimizing the stigma associated with treatment.

Implementation in Hong Kong

Hong Kong is currently initiating a new CHR-P program within an established FEP program. Because many challenges of implementing new CHR-P services mirror the implementation of FEP services within new mental health service settings, Hong Kong serves as an appropriate case study for implementation of CHR-P services in new global contexts.

Mental Health Literacy and Identifying an Appropriate Term for CHR-P for Chinese Groups

In Chinese societies, mental health literacy (or knowledge about mental disorders, which aids in its recognition, management, and prevention), especially regarding psychosis, is poor. In a nationally representative study using hypothetical vignettes, only 8.7% of (urban) respondents correctly identified schizophrenia (vs. 38% for depression) (Huang et al. 2019). Low mental health literacy does not arise from a lack of mental health education alone, but stems from the widespread stigma toward mental illness and the presence of culturally specific idioms regarding mental conditions. In Chinese culture, preserving status as a "fully formed human being" is essential to one's ability to work as well as to achieve a marriage to perpetuate one's family lineage—accomplishments that "matter most" for many Chinese people (Yang and Kleinman 2008). Thus, individuals with a severe mental illness are perceived as "not being fully formed human beings." This diminishes one's participation in social exchange networks (known as *guanxi*), where opportunities to work and to locate marriage partners are often situated. Stigma often extends to family members. In a large study of 1,491 relatives of individuals with schizophrenia, >50% reported experiencing adverse effects of stigma (Phillips et al. 2002b).

Because of these factors, particular care has been given to identifying the appropriate term for psychosis diagnoses. The current Chinese term for schizophrenia, *jing-shen-fen-lie*, translates literally to "mind-split disease" (Chiu et al. 2010)—a term that may perpetuate stigma without offering much insight into the disorder's characteristics (Tang et al. 2010). Public awareness campaigns surrounding psychosis in Hong Kong have sought to rename the term for psychosis based on feedback from health professionals to *si-jue-shi-tiao*, which translates to "thought and perceptual dysregulation." Similar efforts to find an appropriate term for the "clinical high risk for psychosis" designation have been made in Hong Kong. A recent study, which used vignettes describing the at-risk CHR-P condition to 149 community members and 51 health-care professionals, found that many (45%) preferred the Chinese diagnostic term of *yun-niang-qi*, meaning "developing period"—a term that does not connote certainty regarding development of a psychotic illness. While a promising first step, it remains to be determined whether this term is recognizable to the general public, is acceptable to CHR-P youth, and to what extent it protects participants from stigma.

FEP Services and Implementing CHR-P Services Globally

The Early Assessment Service for Young People with Early Psychosis (EASY) program, established in 2001, represents efforts by the Hong Kong government to integrate FEP services into broader mental health-care services. EASY targets 15- to 25-year-olds who present with psychotic symptoms and aims to reduce DUP while optimizing treatment in the first two years after FEP (Tang et al. 2010; Wong et al. 2008). EASY[1] includes three components:

1. *Raising public awareness*: As noted above, an educational campaign, conducted through multiple media streams (Wong et al. 2008), made use of the new term for schizophrenia to reduce stigma and encourage public acceptance of psychosis (Wong et al. 2008). A study of 1,217 local newspaper articles found an overall increase in the use of the new term (*si-jue-shi-tiao*) and a decrease in the original "split-mind disease" term (*jing-shen-fen-lie*) from 2002 to 2012 (Chan et al. 2017). However, findings regarding public acceptance for the new psychosis term have been mixed and have yet to focus on the effectiveness of this new terminology in patients' actual experiences (Chan et al. 2017; Yamaguchi et al. 2017). Additional psychoeducation efforts are thus needed before the full benefits of this new terminology are likely to be observed.
2. *Accessibility to FEP services*: To remove barriers to care, a two-stage assessment system was established: a telephone-based initial screening and a diagnostic assessment with an early psychosis clinician within one week (Wong et al. 2008). Referrals from a broad range of sources were accepted, including (but not limited to) hotlines, email, walk-ins, non-governmental organizations, school social workers, outpatient departments, and non-EASY psychiatrists (Wong et al. 2008). While effective for FEP referrals, these channels would require further expansion for CHR-P programs to detect psychosis before it develops to its full state. This would include incorporating even more extensive contacts with

[1] For further information, see https://www3.ha.org.hk/easy/eng/service.html.

nonclinical settings to implement community outreach to detect individuals when they are still in a high-risk state, as described earlier.

3. *Phase-specific intervention*: FEP services in Hong Kong follow a phase-specific outpatient treatment model that includes the use of multidisciplinary teams. Care is provided according to patients' needs and consists of enhancing psychological adjustment to early psychosis, intervention for secondary morbidity, and CBT for drug-resistant psychotic symptoms (Wong et al. 2008). This standardized intervention package provides in-depth engagement, comprehensive psychoeducation, support for medication adherence, coping and stress management, and relapse prevention (Chang et al. 2017). The FEP phase-specific intervention lasts for two years; in year three, patients enter a transitional step-down clinic, with psychiatric treatment but no case management (Chang et al. 2017; Tang et al. 2010). Many elements of the FEP program (e.g., the multidisciplinary team, standardized treatment protocol, and focus on functional recovery) might be applicable to implementing earlier-phase CHR-P treatment.

FEP Program Efficacy

The EASY program, when compared with standard care, showed changes in key clinical and functional outcomes. Regarding functional outcomes, patients enrolled in EASY achieved longer durations of full-time employment (15.2 months) when compared with matched historical controls (10.5 months), and a greater proportion were engaged in full-time positions for ≥6 months (Chen et al. 2011). EASY also improved clinical outcomes and service utilization. EASY participants had fewer positive and negative symptoms than historical controls, and more EASY patients achieved at least a brief period of recovery within three years (Chen et al. 2011). Finally, EASY patients had significantly better outpatient attendance as well as shorter and fewer hospitalizations than historical controls (Chen et al. 2011).

Despite these improvements, EASY did not appear to reduce DUP for participants compared with historical controls; these groups experienced DUP of 239.8 and 232.0 days, respectively (Chen et al. 2011). Accordingly, the program's impact was attributed not to reduced DUP but to the phase-specific intervention (Tang et al. 2010). This may be due to insufficient time for the public awareness program to have influenced public perceptions and care-seeking before the evaluation was conducted (Chen et al. 2011). These findings are relevant to the implementation of CHR-P programs, which are predicated on the capacity to identify the earliest psychotic signs among community members. Taking the example of Hong Kong, an area of emphasis likely lies in public education for psychosis risk and outreach to the nonclinically based community agencies, so that individuals with psychotic signs can be successfully identified prior to FEP in this and similar global contexts.

Implications for Implementing CHR-P Programs

Based on the Hong Kong implementation experience, there are a number of principles that could be further evaluated as other global settings attempt to adopt CHR-P (and FEP) services. Like the EASY program, programs in other settings should assess the impact of adopting an appropriate term for psychosis and CHR-P, for the setting to improve understanding, increase community detection, and reduce stigma. Additionally, as was conducted in EASY, other programs should target youth in the particular age range during which there is the most heightened risk. Following from the EASY program's inability to reduce DUP, despite more accessible referral and assessment channels, other settings should conduct systematic studies of the factors that shorten or lengthen DUP for this group, particularly through community outreach. Because the EASY program involved only hospital-based care, future outreach efforts for CHR-P individuals will likely require extensive contact with nonclinical, community-based agencies (e.g., schools, youth agencies) to locate CHR-P youth before they enter formal mental health services.

Cost-Effectiveness for Early Intervention for Psychosis Globally

An additional controversy arises when the economic benefits of establishing early intervention services for psychosis are considered or when the feasibility of implementing such services is considered in the context of political and structural barriers embedded within health-care systems in various high-income countries.

Globally, studies find that FEP intervention services are not only more effective than standard care, but that they show cost-effectiveness. In addition to the EASY program in Hong Kong, which demonstrated cost-effectiveness in improving outcomes (26.1% savings on average per patient; Wong et al. 2011), studies elsewhere (e.g., Italy, U.K., Denmark, and Australia) have demonstrated similar effects (Bertelsen et al. 2008; Cocchi et al. 2011; Hastrup et al. 2013; Knapp et al. 2014; Mihalopoulos et al. 2009; Serretti et al. 2009). A study of the Recovery After an Initial Schizophrenia Episode-Early Treatment Program and Navigate Intervention Package (NAV) showed mostly consistent results (Rosenheck et al. 2016). This study compared the cost-effectiveness of NAV (a multidisciplinary, team-based treatment approach for FEP) to community treatment. Compared with community treatment, NAV was somewhat more expensive (due to increased outpatient and medication costs), but it produced better clinical and quality of life outcomes, making it a better value particularly among patients with shorter DUP, who showed lowest costs, greatest improvements in quality of life, and greatest cost-effectiveness.

Regarding CHR-P, existing studies find that while early identification services for CHR-P individuals are initially more costly than standard care, over time the costs averted by early detection ultimately result in cost savings (Knapp et al. 2014). An investigation of the Outreach and Support in South London (OASIS) program in the United Kingdom, a service for people with an at-risk mental state with a high-risk of developing psychosis, found that at 24 months, expected service costs were £4313 and £3285 for OASIS and standard care, respectively (Valmaggia et al. 2009). However, when costs related to lost employment were included, total estimated costs per person were £961 less for OASIS than standard care (Valmaggia et al. 2009). Using a model that extends potential cost savings to criminal justice services, suicide, homicide, and lost employment, a study estimated potential savings of £47.6 million associated with U.K. early detection services within 2–5 years and £41.0 million in years 6–10; per person savings were £3,022 and £2,604 in years 2–5 and 6–10, respectively (McCrone et al. 2010).

In addition to cost, substantial political and structural barriers may exist that can impede implementation of early intervention services. Barriers related to a lack of political will include a lack of interest in preventive measures and a lack of recognition of the needs of patients with early psychosis (Csillag et al. 2017). Ineffective coordination among important stakeholder groups is also an obstacle, as treatment is fragmented, with little communication between mental health specialists, primary care providers, welfare services, and educational institutions (Csillag et al. 2017). Structural and administrative barriers include insufficient funding and constraints in public resources (Csillag et al. 2017). The physical spaces themselves may not be integrated into the medical system in a way that minimizes stigma (Arango et al. 2017). In many contexts, the structure of the mental health system itself (e.g., in countries where institutionalization forms a primary treatment) is not conducive to successful implementation of early intervention services and may be poorly adapted to young peoples' needs (Csillag et al. 2017). For example, programs do not commonly use mobile phones and social networks to communicate with the young adult population (Arango et al. 2017). CHR-P programs face many of the same implementation challenges as these early intervention programs.

Conclusion

While the CHR-P status signifies a crucial advance in the identification and treatment of youth experiencing subthreshold signs of psychosis, unresolved controversies remain regarding the early detection state as it is implemented globally. Here we have reviewed the scope of these challenges and controversies, which range from core issues regarding validity of the CHR-P identification state itself, to topics of stigma and ethics as well as the economic, structural, and cultural issues concerning implementation of this early detection state within novel mental health settings. In tandem with the movement toward earlier treatment for psychosis worldwide, the continuing shift toward CHR-P identification will only make resolving these complex challenges more important. In the future, earliest intervention efforts may benefit from a concerted effort to resolve those controversies most salient to that particular setting (e.g., in countries where the CHR-P identification is established, to resolve controversies around its core validity). While CHR-P identification approaches are now primarily situated within Western European, high-income contexts, as the CHR-P identification expands to novel global and cultural settings, new implementation challenges will be identified which will require resolution. Future research to address these controversies will facilitate adoption of the CHR-P identification into mainstream mental health-care systems globally, thus maximizing public health impact.

Acknowledgments

Preparation of this chapter was supported in part by an award from the National Institutes of Mental Health (NIMH R01-MH096027; PI:Yang). We dedicate this chapter to the memory of Shane Columbo, whose presence graced our lives and who left us too soon.

12

Early Intervention for Schizophrenia

Building Systems of Care for Knowledge Translation

Vinod H. Srihari and John D. Cahill

Abstract

Can regional *systems* of care be designed to disseminate best practices *and* drive necessary research? This is a question of generic interest across health-care conditions, and literature from allied fields will be brought to bear here on how this can be done for youth mental health, with the example of early intervention services for psychotic disorders.

This chapter argues that (i) *knowledge translation* should be the organizing goal of such a system; (ii) *population health* can serve as a conceptual basis for reform, which will be facilitated by a shared vocabulary of "*systems, networks*, and *pathways*"; (iii) measuring *value* can guide inevitable trade-offs in regional allocation of resources; (iv) services should be designed to embrace *complexity* and avoid simplistic approaches to *wicked* problems; and (v) *learning health systems* are an optimal framework within which to design systems for knowledge translation.

The heterogeneous group of primary, non-affective, and chronic psychotic disorders that fall under the umbrella term schizophrenia will be used as a stand-in for the chronic mental illnesses of adulthood that typically onset in youth. While this focus has limitations, it should enable vigorous critique of the proposed design of systems of care: both for relevance to psychotic disorders as well as across the wide range of disorders affecting youth.

Introduction

What follows is an argument for a particular kind of heuristic or "ideal type" to guide the design of systems that can best respond to the challenge raised by this Forum. Can we design regionally relevant *systems* of care for youth with mental health needs that are fit to disseminate best practices and drive necessary research? As these systems have yet to be fully constructed or tested for mental illnesses, this remains in large part a pre-empirical proposal. Embedded in what follows is a critical interrogation of current "ideal types" that guide service design, both to consider their usefulness as well as the ways in which they limit progress.

Youth Mental Health: The Nature of the Challenge

There is an urgent need to develop systems of care that are focused specifically on the psychological health of emerging adults (12–25 years of age). Epidemiological studies provide actionable evidence on the needs of this age group, even as we continue to learn more about the neurobiological underpinnings of this important period in neural and social development (Jones 2013). Four populations are worth recognizing for purposes of service design:

1. *Those suffering from the common vicissitudes of adolescence*: These are exemplified by impulse control disorders and the adverse impacts of substance misuse. This broad, amorphous category of problems includes conditions that cause significant distress, disability, and even premature mortality (e.g., campus binge drinking, unplanned pregnancies, sexually transmitted diseases) while not usually resulting in mental illnesses that will persist into adulthood. Since these disturbances often surface during the transition to adulthood, their impact can reverberate well beyond this period if not addressed in an age-appropriate and timely manner. Examples of such derailments include entanglements with the legal system (which can permanently foreclose future employment opportunities) or, more commonly, setbacks in educational achievement, which can have a long-term impact in labor markets that disfavor those without a college degree or specialized vocational training. This is by far the largest subpopulation in terms of numbers, but not in terms of illness burden.
2. *Emerging serious and chronic mental illnesses*: This often neglected subgroup justifies the claim that "mental disorders are the chronic diseases of the young" (Insel and Fenton 2005). The epidemiological findings here are striking, as summarized by Kessler et al. (2007:359): "Roughly half of all lifetime mental disorders...start by the mid-teens and three-fourths by the mid-20s....Severe disorders are typically preceded by less severe disorders that seldom are brought to clinical attention." The reality that youth and young adulthood are the highest risk period for the onset of mental illness and that treatment access is usually delayed for years after onset supports the formulation of the

12–25 yr age range as a critical focus for testing early interventions to protect long-term adult functioning. Mature models have been developed for early intervention in psychotic disorders (focused mostly on the period of 16–35 yr) and these have survived experimental tests around the world (Correll et al. 2018). These models are also ripe for adaptation to target other emerging serious and persistent mental illnesses including bipolar disorder, obsessive-compulsive disorder, and major depression.

3. *Children and youth with deprived or adverse developmental environments*: Deviations from healthy development can emerge during childhood in the absence of mental illness and are linked to a variety of deprivations (e.g., poverty, neglect, abuse) that can have serious and persistent effects. Those who enter adolescence with inadequate care for and planning around the psychological impact of these deprivations can fall further behind during this challenging phase of life, when poor decisions can have an outsized impact on long-term vocational and social trajectories.
4. *Disorders arising from the first phase of neurodevelopment* (i.e., in infancy): These disorders emerge from abnormal neonatal or early brain development and manifest in childhood, including autism spectrum disorders, attention deficit hyperactivity disorder, various learning disorders, and more severe cognitive impairments. The needs of this group, while ideally identified and treated prior to adulthood, require continued, careful, and specific attention during the transition to adulthood.

An important detail that emerged from these studies is that some of the disorders which first manifest in the period of emerging adulthood are *homotypic* (i.e., look the same at onset in childhood or adolescence as in later adulthood, e.g., antisocial disorders) while others are *heterotypic* (e.g., schizophrenia, which in its earliest phenotypic expression is often indistinguishable from mood and anxiety disorders, or of the normative social distress and dysfunction typical of late adolescence) (Jones 2013; McGorry et al. 2018c). This supports the need for specialized services, targeting the so-called transitional age (late adolescence through early adulthood), that develop the capacity (human and infrastructure) to expertly evaluate, engage, and treat these populations.

Emerging neurobiological understanding of the "second" phase (i.e., between 12–25 years of age) of neurodevelopment provides a rich, textured, and dynamic narrative (Kessler et al. 2007). Much has already been learned that has implications for service design and policy but much more needs to be learned about how these processes can go awry in illness. Such investigations can be supported by service systems that can engage, care for, and thereby recruit subjects with new onset illnesses. The emergence of the mature adult brain is a culmination of a process that begins before puberty and typically proceeds until the third decade of life. The particular sequence of this development suggests why this is commonly a period of psychological turbulence, risk taking, and vulnerability for the emergence of mental illness, substance use disorders, and personality dysfunction. The present system of dividing care between adult and pediatric models of care presents a further challenge to individuals at one of their most vulnerable periods. These system transitions can impede clinical efforts to identify, follow-up, or treat individuals as well as research efforts to fill knowledge gaps about this important developmental period.

Addressing Service Gaps for Schizophrenia: Reform or Reengineer?

From a public health perspective, all four populations described above deserve sustained policy attention, with appropriately tailored solutions. For example, models to extend and carefully transition services and natural supports for those entering adolescence with an already diagnosed childhood-onset illness (population 4) or identified social deprivation (population 3) will not fully meet the needs of the largest population of emerging adults with more diffuse and temporary needs (population 1). Finally, for those with a serious and chronic mental illness that becomes apparent only during their transition from pediatric to adult life (population 2), no specific services may exist. While the choice to reform (an existing set of services) or reengineer (where none exist) services is often dependent on budgetary or regional exigencies, our focus here is on articulating a strategic response. We focus on population 2 and, within this, those with primary psychotic or schizophrenia spectrum disorders (henceforth, schizophrenia).

There are several reasons to use schizophrenia as the target population around which to construct a heuristic system for youth mental health care. First, early intervention service models are most mature in this area (McGorry et al. 2018c). This makes it feasible to consider dissemination and system design. Second, these disorders impact multiple sectors (e.g., health-care, legal, educational), raising the complexity but also the opportunity to consider how to enact shared societal responses. Third, these disorders exact a huge toll in terms of premature mortality, chronic disability, and caregiver burden, all measurable in terms of societal economic cost (Cloutier et al. 2016). Empirically based interventions that target several modifiable contributors are primed for dissemination. Finally, as an archetypal disorder of new onset in the young (population 2), schizophrenia illustrates the need to think beyond refinement and toward reengineering of care that is better attuned to the needs of emerging adults. This is an exercise that will likely provide lessons relevant for many mental illnesses.

While much about the etiology and pathophysiology of schizophrenia remains unclear and as yet of limited applicability to care, much is known about modifiable prognostic variables and effective treatments and services. We must therefore imagine a way of "doing what we know" with best practices to help as many individuals as we can now, while also "learning what to do" (Glasziou et al. 2011), by building research capacity into the design of these services. The notion of *knowledge translation* is often invoked to hasten the application of research-derived knowledge into practice, but the connections between the bench, bedside, community, and policy are best viewed as bidirectional (Dougherty and Conway 2008). Indeed, the often implicit notion of completing research before implementation (Chambers and Norton 2016), or divorcing implementation from the need to ask and answer relevant research questions, is worth challenging. Especially for this heterogeneous group of disorders, with varying responses to available treatments, it is essential for services to not only be open to changing practices as evidence emerges, but to contribute proactively to knowledge generation across the continuum: from discovery-oriented biological research, to clinical trials, to implementation and services research and policy. Such services would be best positioned to refine interventions developed in research settings as well as to highlight knowledge gaps to inform research agendas.

Knowledge Translation: Beginning with the End in Mind

With this goal of building systems of care that are primed for bidirectional knowledge translation (Figure 12.1), two broad categories of resistance must be recognized. First, practical tensions exist between the workflows of clinical care and research. In the face of limited time and resources, implicit allocations may favor one mission to the detriment of the other and reinforce a prevalent but nevertheless conceptually indefensible split between clinical care and research (Kass et al. 2013). An effective response to this inevitable tension

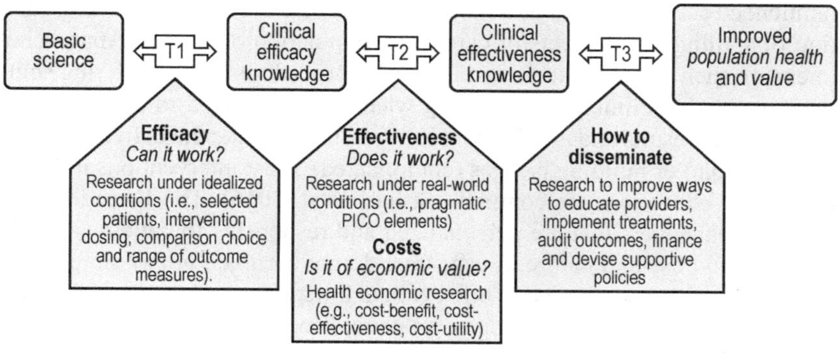

Figure 12.1 Knowledge translation as a goal for systems of care. PICO elements: problem/patient/population, intervention/indicator, comparison, and outcome of interest. Adapted from Dougherty and Conway (2008).

requires a design that can incentivize the agendas of research and care, within a culture that values both missions and enables this with robust informatics. This is detailed below in the description of learning health systems.

Second, it is important to expose an implicit allegiance to what we term a "pipeline model" of knowledge translation. This borrows from a compelling and useful metaphor for transmitting evidence-based information (Glasziou and Haynes 2005), but we use it here to label a misleading heuristic that all too often guides and derails service reform. This heuristic is best presented in mythologic form: pure and potent interventions are developed in research settings, distilled to their "active ingredients," and then channeled to "real-world" settings. On arrival, however, these interventions are subject to local practice distortions ("leakage in potency") that require various forms of policing to ensure application of the active ingredients with appropriate procedural "fidelity" to the original model of intervention. As with most myths, there are a few embedded truths (efficacious treatments or models of care are often misapplied or ignored in practice settings while, conversely, practices refuted by robust research persist), but this glosses over a key distinction between simple (e.g., three drops of polio vaccine) and complex (e.g., psychotherapy, service models) interventions, and leads to ineffective dissemination.

While the impact of a "simple" (but certainly not easy) intervention (e.g., the use of a vaccine or medication) can, in principle, be improved by monitoring for fidelity to research-derived dosing protocols, it is well understood, even here, that variability in pharmacokinetics (how each individual metabolizes a drug) and pharmacodynamics (how each individual is variably impacted by the same dose of the drug) should temper enthusiasm for such protocols. The pipeline model, however, uncritically extends this approach to psychosocial or service-level interventions. For example, efforts to disseminate empirically validated first-episode services (FES) (Srihari et al. 2012) will be misdirected by emphasizing process measures (e.g., delivery of a recommended set of component treatments, at some arbitrary "dose," configuration of staffing, or elements of care) over population outcomes. Approaches to ensure such "fidelity" to research-derived procedures, while offering some reassurance that clinicians are "doing what they are tasked to do," privilege activity over results and are ripe for reality testing. Unlike the delivery of vaccines (simple) or building bridges (complicated), most interventions in health care, as in education, are complex (Srihari et al. 2016). The latter involves iterative maneuvers that are personalized and responsive to patients and can thus vary in dose and nature in ways that do not correlate in any simple way with need or illness severity. While detailed blueprints executed carefully are vital to the construction of bridges, an equivalent fantasy for complex interventions requires disillusionment, not collusion. The practice of monitoring the "fidelity" of service interventions to ensure adherence to mostly process-based measures of research-derived models of care diverts limited resources and exacts excessive opportunity costs. A more realistic focus on the careful measurement of valued outcomes can offer more reliable milestones toward the goal of reduced morbidity and mortality for the target population. We will return to this more concretely after a necessary detour into the population health perspective.

Population Health

The term *population health* has acquired varied uses (Kindig and Stoddart 2003). We prefer "the measurable improvement in the health of a defined population" using "the health outcomes of a group of individuals, including the distribution of such outcomes within the group" with the added qualifier that "geopolitical areas" (Jacobson and Teutsch 2012) be used to define target populations. This latter guidance was originally proposed to acknowledge that funding decisions are often based on political maps, but for our vision of population health for early psychosis, it allows a focus on a relevant network of regional stakeholders (see below). Population health (Figure 12.2) focuses critical attention on both the determinants and the desired outcomes of proposed interventions.

First, we are reminded that medical care is only one of several contributors (*determinants*) to improved health. While psychiatric services might be ahead of general medicine in including behavioral factors and basic needs into standard care models for severe mental illnesses, there remains a clear need to pay more attention to social determinants of health and, relatedly, to include a wider set of stakeholders (beyond traditional health-care agencies) in mounting responses. Second, the rubric to measure success (*population health outcomes*), within the domains of mortality and morbidity, requires assessment and action on disparities across subgroups (e.g., race, class, gender). Social justice aspirations for equitable distribution of the benefits of care provide the

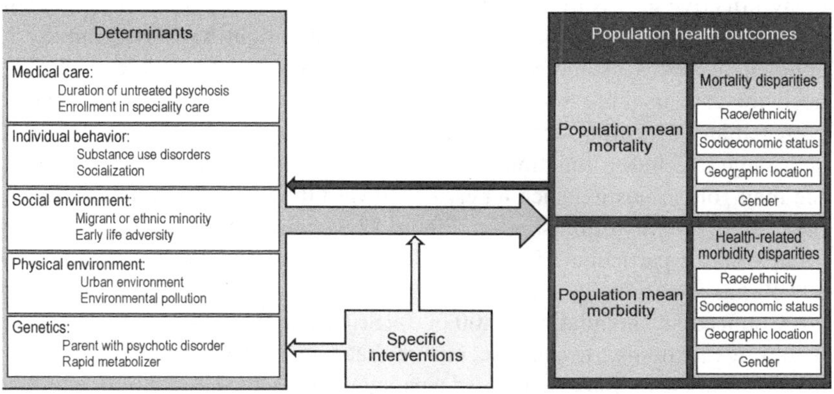

Figure 12.2 Population health for early intervention services for schizophrenia. Adapted from Kindig et al. (2008).

imperative to assess and intervene on the causes of these disparities. These are not an afterthought; they are integral to this model of population health.

How can such a population health framework organize care for recent onset schizophrenia? For those of us working in health-care agencies, this requires both a broader consideration of our role, with respect to the populations we treat, and a reconsideration of some of the terms we use.

Systems, Networks, Pathways: A Vocabulary for Enacting Population Health

> A *system* of care for complex health conditions is a set of activities with a common set of objectives. A *network* is a set of organizations and individuals that deliver the system of care. *Pathways* are the routes that patients follow through the network. —Srihari et al. (2016)

A *system* of care is thus differentiated from its colloquial use, as in some notional aggregation of health-care agencies. After all, health-care agencies represent only a few of the several stakeholders in any region and have a limited, albeit important, impact on overall health outcomes (Schroeder 2007). Added to these agencies are the teachers, friends, family members, clergy, police, and many others who (in ways often unknown to each other) by their responses to psychotic illnesses create the de facto *network* that determines the nature of the *pathways* experienced by young people and their families as they access and engage with the formal health-care sector and community supports.

Designing a population health-based early intervention system for new onset psychosis requires the identification of a target geopolitical region for a defined population (e.g., first-episode psychosis). The various actors in the region can be recognized not simply as facilitators or barriers but rather as active *filters* (O'Sullivan et al. 2007; Srihari et al. 2014) who act to facilitate or delay effective access to care, depending on the characteristics of the patient or situation. For example, agitated male patients might be ferried rapidly to emergency rooms by the same police officers who might underestimate the need for care in those socially isolated by deficit symptoms. With targeted outreach and education, these police officers (stakeholders) can be mobilized and integrated into a functional *network*. Established or nascent FESs might see their role in hosting such a network toward the goal of population health-based care. By way of illustration, Figure 12.3 shows a network of stakeholder groups that a particular FES (Specialized Treatment in Early Psychosis, or STEP) has intentionally sought to integrate across a 10-town region in southern Connecticut (population ~ 400,000) (Srihari et al. 2014). Such a network would, if functioning to purpose, ensure that *every* individual with new onset psychosis in the region experienced a pathway to the local best practice service (STEP), and in a matter that reflects the work of an organized and humane *system* of care, as illustrated in the following case:

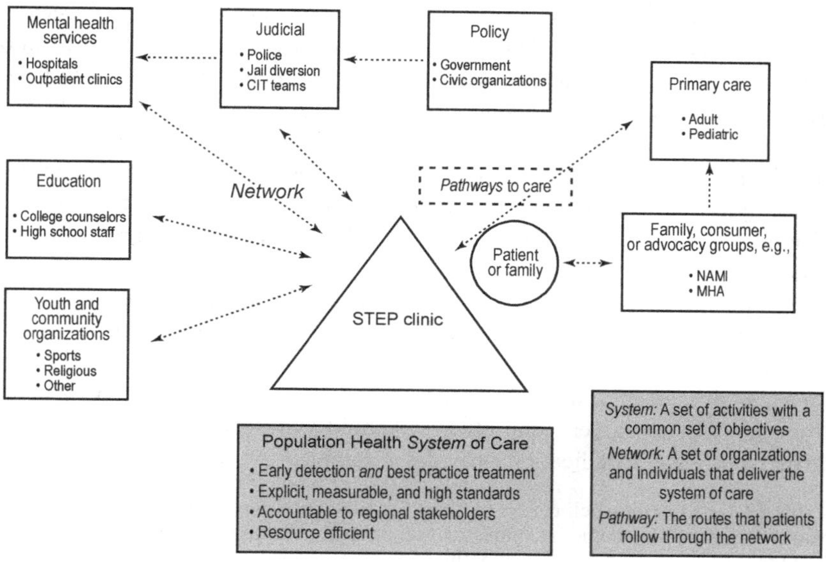

Figure 12.3 Early intervention services as integrators of regional access to care for psychosis: crisis intervention teams (CIT), National Alliance on Mental Illness (NAMI), Mental Health America (MHA).

> Anton is a 17-year-old African-American resident from a nearby town, who was noted to be increasingly suspicious and disheveled over a period of several months. School security staff was called one afternoon to intervene when he was seen brandishing a stick in a busy corridor, and shouting "I hear you" to no one in sight. The staff summoned one of his teachers, who was able to convince him to travel with her in a squad car to the local emergency room. There, rapid assessment determined the presence of a psychotic illness, and during the ensuing hospital admission, Anton was introduced to an outreach worker from a local FES. Upon discharge and with his permission, Anton's teacher and family were included in the initial assessment and provided valuable collateral information on the pace and development of Anton's symptoms. In addition, the school security guard requested and was provided information on the signs and symptoms of psychotic illnesses, and expressed relief that he had not been instructed to take Anton to jail. He asked the FES manager to give a presentation on the topic to his colleagues at a local recreational club. One month later, Anton was able to return to school and, with the assistance of a vocational counselor, advocated for specific accommodations which enabled him to complete graduation requirements despite the need for frequent medical appointments and one additional hospitalization over the next six months.

All too often, pathways to best practice care for youth with new onset mental illnesses do not reflect the coordinated activities of a *system* such as the one above. Instead, they are marked by long delays, multiple help-seeking attempts or, worse, inappropriate diversions into the criminal justice system (Wasser et al. 2017). Individuals outside mental health-care systems are often thrust into the role of "first responder" to socially disruptive behaviors that ensue from psychiatric illnesses. If not adequately educated and integrated, these observers can feel powerless to reduce the shame and social isolation for patients and their families, and frustration for other onlookers. This represents an opportunity—a network in waiting—wherein activities in response to psychotic distress or disorganization can be coordinated into what can more rightfully be called a system of care.

Such systems can be further organized around a clear goal, or *overall aim*, and include concrete *objectives*, *measures*, and *standards*. Such a "system specification," exemplified by STEP's population health-based system for early psychosis (Table 12.1), should be continuously refined with input from patients, caregivers, and other stakeholders who constitute the regional network. The specification provides a template for dashboards to assess

Table 12.1 System specification in STEP: a population health-based early intervention strategy used in southern Connecticut set up to transform outcomes of all within the first three years of psychosis onset within a catchment zone of 10 surrounding towns.

Objective	Measure	Standard	
		Achievable	Aspirational
Access			
1. Rapidity	DUP 1 < 3 mo	30%	75%
	DUP 2 < 12 mo	50%	75%
2. Equity	Proportion of females	20%	30%
	Ratio of ethnic groups		matches census %
	Ratio of towns of residence		matches % of 10 towns
	Proportion aged < 18	15%	80%
3. Coverage	Number annually offered STEP care/ expected annual incidence in zone	15%	80%
4. Pathways to care	Proportion of patients admitted to STEP after psychiatric hospitalization	60%	30%
Engagement			
1. Overall	FES contact at 12 mo post admission	70%	90%
2. Exposure to family education/ support	Family participation in at least 1 qualifying event in first month	75%	90%
3. Exposure to specialized, empirically based psychotherapy	Engagement in qualifying event in first month	75%	90%

continuously the performance of the system, and annual reports to hold the system accountable to the community. Some implications that can be drawn from this approach to implementing early intervention services for psychotic disorders in a public health framework are summarized below:

- Individualized care is attentive to social determinants of access, quality, and outcomes.
- Care processes are responsive to population outcomes measured across domains of access, disease-related morbidity, and broader determinants of social and vocational functioning.
- Fidelity of the service to recommended care processes is treated as one of several potential mediators of population outcomes and is thereby subject to empirical scrutiny, but is not an end in itself.
- Ownership: regional stakeholders set expectations for the system (i.e., objectives and standards).
- Local control allows for creative resourcing of, and even disinvestment from, standard components of care: if a particular outcome (e.g., employment) exceeds benchmarks, then resources can be allocated away

Table 12.1 (continued). Abbreviations: BMI, body mass index; FES, first-episode service; NEET, not in education, employment, or training; PANSS, positive and negative syndrome scale; GF, global functioning; DUP 1, duration of untreated psychosis (time between psychosis onset and first antipsychotic medication trial; DUP 2, duration of untreated psychosis (time between psychosis onset and enrollment in STEP). Adapted from Srihari et al. (2016).

Objective	Measure	Standard	
		Achievable	Aspirational
Outcomes			
1. Hospitalization	Psychiatric admission in months 1–6	<25%	<10%
	and 7–12	<25%	<10%
2. Suicide prevention	Patients attempt, first yr of admission	<10%	<1%
3. Remission	PANSS positive sub-core <3 at 6 mo	70%	85%
	PANSS positive sub-core <3 at 1 yr	80%	90%
4. Recovery	GF: Role scale level ≥8	70%	85%
	GF: Social scale level ≥8	70%	85%
5. Vocational engagement	NEET nor full-time caregiver	<10%	<5%
6. Cardiovascular risk			
Smoking	New smokers at 6 mo	<20%	<10%
	Smoking rate at 6 mo	<60%	<30%
Overweight or obese	BMI < 25 at 12 mo	30%	75%
	Normal BMIs retained at 12 mo	60%	75%
7. Disposition	Successfully transitioned to mainstream health-care services ≤2 yr	70%	80%

from specific care processes (e.g., supported employment models) to other areas of need (e.g., support for transportation).
- Accountability: annual report focused on outcomes of value to local stakeholders.

Value

> [I]n health care we've allowed "quality" to be defined as compliance with evidence-based practice guidelines rather than as improvement in outcomes.... Billing data...don't capture suffering due to the delays, chaos, confusion, and complications that often characterize health care. —Porter (2010:504, 505)

The health economist, Michael Porter, has championed a particular approach to monetizing the impact of health-care interventions represented by the equation: value = health outcomes achieved per dollar spent, over a meaningful period of care (Porter 2010). This perspective highlights the remarkable lack of reliable health outcome data for much of what is ordinarily reported by health-care agencies. For example, less than 2% of measures listed in the U.S. National Quality Measures Clearinghouse are related to outcomes that can be directly tied to patient health (Porter et al. 2016). The relatively large proportion of process measures will not surprise anyone working in health-care agencies, where the notion of valuing what is most easily measured, rather than measuring what should be valued, sadly dominates administrative practice. This often devolves to a focus on worker productivity and related documentation of service utilization. Quite apart from the limited inferences that can be made from such measures to the health of the populations served, they can exert a corrosive effect on cultures of practice. Measurement becomes associated with irrelevant, tedious "paperwork" that has often migrated into (and even been amplified by) regressive electronic systems, thus becoming a contributor to clinician burnout (Shanafelt et al. 2016). This also degrades the quality of any data collected.

A useful sociological commentary recommended a principle of "negotiated accountability" to counter a growing "cult of efficiency" that is overly focused on narrow measures of productivity and health-care utilization (Stein 2002). In a similar spirit, recent principles published by the International Consortium for Health Outcomes Measurement are worth considering for their relevance to the design of population health-based systems of care (Porter et al. 2016):

- Commit to measuring a minimal set of patient-related outcomes.
- Measure outcomes across a "full care delivery chain" or meaningful cycle of care.
- Use explicit, replicable ways to measure outcomes.
- Consider explicit ways to risk-adjust these outcome measures.

- Standardize sets of outcomes for equivalent services, nationally and globally.
- Maximize value = health outcomes achieved per dollar spent.

Value can be a potentially powerful way to prioritize health-care spending (Gray 2012; Lee 2010). While within the general framework of cost effectiveness, the measures used depart from traditional approaches to economic analyses that privilege omnibus measures, such as quality-adjusted life years (QALYs). While QALYs can be pegged in a standardized way to societal preferences and can inform allocations across health-care conditions, they suffer long-recognized limitations in appropriateness and sensitivity to change for mental illnesses (Brazier 2010; McCrone 2011). More to the point, for our argument here, QALYs are not intuitively accessible and are difficult to use in allocative decisions by stakeholders at a regional level. Funding decisions are often made by particular agencies in particular regions with idiosyncratic prioritizations of outcomes. To illustrate, we asked the question: What is the value derived from the incremental investment necessary to mount a FES in a U.S. public sector setting, in terms of patient-centered outcomes (psychiatric hospitalization), over a meaningful duration (1 year) of care? This was one of many outcomes measured in a randomized trial and assessed with traditional cost-benefit analysis (Murphy et al. 2018). While it would cost about 978 USD for one psychiatric inpatient day, an investment of <$100 in the tested FES per patient would help avoid one psychiatric inpatient day over a year of care. Similarly, $152 was the cost of one jail day, whereas $6.6 was the per-patient investment in FES care to prevent one jail day over a year. These were the outcome domains of particular decisional salience to funders of this FES. Sensitivity analyses accommodated expected variability in such costs articulated by this stakeholder. The value approach can thus make clearer, in a more modular way, what the FES could deliver to the local system in terms of improvement in specific outcomes of interest, for the dollars spent. Our estimates were idiosyncratic to the additional cost of mounting the FES within our community mental health center, thus limiting the generalizability of the results, but they made transparent the "return on investment" on an outcome that local decision makers happen to value (see Table 12.1, Hospitalization). While a full presentation of the use of such value-based analyses is beyond the scope of this chapter, it helps make the point that population health-based systems of care for youth mental health can be coherently tied to economic analyses and payment models (Porter and Kaplan 2015) for the transparent consideration of a variety of regional stakeholders. Of course, while the above example focuses on one stakeholder (public sector funder), the population health approach proposed here envisions vigorous input from all relevant stakeholders (Figure 12.3) in specifying the overall system (Table 12.1).

Embracing Complexity

How can services be designed to deliver population health-based care that delivers measurable value to stakeholders? Traditional approaches for dissemination of evidence-based practices for severe mental illnesses have emphasized fidelity to procedures developed at research sites (Addington et al. 2007; Bond et al. 2000). Historically, these have had a variable and, at best, modest impact in moving research into practice, most notably evident in persistently reported gaps in schizophrenia care (Dixon et al. 2010). Fidelity-based approaches, however, do not address well-known barriers to knowledge translation (Jensen 2008; Lane and Flagg 2010): the diverse and evolving needs of implementation sites for leadership, clinical ownership of the problems addressed, and the overall culture of practice (Torrey et al. 2001). Indeed, these barriers to "doing what we know works" (Glasziou et al. 2011) have long been recognized as pervasive across health-care settings and conditions (Institute of Medicine's Quality of Health Care in America 2001).

Another way to describe this problem is that extant models of dissemination are fundamentally ill-suited to *complex* interventions and to the complex adaptive systems into which they must be integrated (Hawe et al. 2004; Mackenzie et al. 2010). The implicit presumption of a research to practice "pipeline" (Glasziou and Haynes 2005), which aspires to deliver identifiable "active ingredients" with high fidelity, may apply for conceptually simple (albeit, not easy) interventions (e.g., polio vaccines) but can reduce the potency of complex interventions. The latter include several interacting components, require variable integration of these in response to the needs of patients, and thus require a great deal of flexibility and variability in their conceptualization, even if this is sadly ignored in simple-minded, fidelity-driven efforts at dissemination.

Additionally, variations across implementation sites in patient samples, clinical and rehabilitative resources, and desired outcomes make straightforward applications of research-based service models inappropriate (Plsek and Greenhalgh 2001). The logistical challenges of delivering team-based, multicomponent care in environments with myriad regulatory demands, inefficient medical record systems, and limited reimbursement for psychosocial services means that standards based on some notion of "minimal dosing" of treatment components cannot be persistently met. More usually, cultural norms determine trade-offs that should be made in the service of patient/population outcomes rather than bureaucratic allegiance to procedures. In addition to the treatment packages or services, the context in which they are to be implemented is often also complex (Plsek and Greenhalgh 2001:625):

> A complex adaptive system is a collection of individual agents with freedom to act in ways that are not always totally predictable, and whose actions are interconnected so that the action of one part changes the context for other agents.

Table 12.2 Comparing simple, complicated, and complex problems. Adapted from Glouberman and Zimmerman (2002).

Simple: Following a Recipe	Complicated: Sending a Rocket to the Moon	Complex: Raising a Child
The recipe is essential	Formulae are critical and necessary	Formulae have a limited application
Recipes are tested to assure easy replication	Sending one rocket increases assurance that the next will be OK	Raising one child provides experience but no assurance of success with the next
No particular expertise is required. But cooking expertise increases success rate	High levels of expertise in a variety of fields are necessary for success	Expertise can contribute but is neither necessary nor sufficient to assure success
Recipes produce standardized products	Rockets are similar in critical ways	Every child is unique and must be understood as an individual
The best recipes give good results every time	There is a high degree of certainty of outcome	Uncertainty of outcome remains
Optimistic approach to problem possible	Optimistic approach to problem possible	Optimistic approach to problem possible

Accepting such complexity includes embracing inherent nonlinear change, tension, creativity, and emergent phenomena (Shiell et al. 2008). Glouberman and Zimmerman (2002) outline some differences between approaching complex problems (versus simple or complicated problems) by evoking the metaphor of raising a child (Table 12.2).

For a related perspective, let us consider elements of problems which Rittel and Webber (1973) term as "wicked":

- Problem framing, not problem solving is often the main task.
- No stopping rule: limits are resources aimed at "good enough" responses.
- (Re)solutions are not true/false but good/bad.
- There are no "permissible" limits on what is worth trying.
- Every wicked problem is unique: real but limited transfer of processes across cases.
- A problem may not be solved (in a generalizable manner) but rather "resolved" within a community of stakeholders and may need to be revisited as conditions or priorities change.

These elements are easy to invoke when considering this typical case presenting to a FES:

> Jack is a 21-year-old high school student who was recently asked to leave his college dormitory after repeatedly threatening his roommate who he accused of

"spying on his thoughts" by "using radio waves." He refused to inform his parents and thus had to live in a homeless shelter, which he described as very stressful. He arrived at the FES refusing to accept treatment but demanded assistance in finding better housing and a "doctor's letter" which he said was necessary for him to return to college. He displayed an obvious thought disorder, and at times it was very difficult for the assessor to follow his line of thinking. He demonstrated no insight into any of his psychotic symptoms and denied need for any kind of clinical treatment.

Which problem should be addressed first? Would insistence on antipsychotic medication treatment reduce his symptomatic burden enough to allow him to participate in informed decision making? Would this instead alienate him and lead him to drop out from the service? Would a return to college simply expose him to more public ridicule and negative academic consequences, or would it improve the FES's alliance with him and thereby facilitate his acceptance of treatment?

These questions are but a small subset of those presented in ordinary practice and cannot be resolved with reference to a standard set of procedures. Rather, an iterative set of options may be pursued, failure may lead to retraction or refinement even as the target problem is changed or specified more clearly as the patient's preferences (the utility he attaches to different component of the service), the disease process (severity of symptoms), or environmental constraints (college's requirements for his return) evolve over time, and in response to interventions. Complex (rather than merely complicated) problems are thus commonplace in the implementation of multicomponent services like FES. This reality has implications for how best practices might be disseminated effectively, while also enabling continued research focused on addressing persistent challenges, whether amenable to simple, complicated, or complex interventions.

Complex problems in complex systems require continual observation of the systems on multiple levels, problem-framing rather than problem-solving, fostering conditions for change by exerting "influence" rather than futile "command and control" (Rouse 2008). At the level of mental health services, this would mean influencing cultures of practice toward achieving patient-centered outcomes rather than overly specifying processes of care (Pollard et al. 2016).

Learning Health Systems for Knowledge Translation

A learning health system occurs when "science, informatics, incentives, and culture are aligned for continuous improvement and innovation...and new knowledge is captured as an integral by-product of the care experience. —Institute of Medicine (2013)

How can such population health-oriented services be enabled to participate in a multisite system for knowledge translation? The notion of a learning health system offered by the Institute of Medicine (2013) provides a useful framework. These systems must be designed to attend simultaneously to

- *science,* through the collection of valid and reliable measures, innovative statistical and translational research methodologies, and the identification, generation, and free exchange of knowledge and expertise between researchers and clinicians,
- *informatics,* robust, user-friendly and collaboratively designed software that allows for a range of data collection methods, integrating with existing databases/health records and interfacing with all stakeholders,
- *incentives,* by facilitating accountability to key stakeholders, fostering creativity, growth and optimism, and empowering members with support, tools and resources, and
- *culture,* via the formation of nonjudgmental, diverse communities of agencies which embrace both local ownership of care and a shared core mission of measuring and learning from patient outcomes.

For early intervention models for schizophrenia, we have specified many details of a system that would meet these design principles. Existing FESs could serve as catalytic nodes within regional networks that share a commitment to a core set of outcomes within a shared system specification, as exemplified in Table 12.1 and detailed in Srihari et al. (2016), and which share lessons across sites to support cultures that are consistent with these principles. Member services of such a network would commit to measuring and reporting a minimum core set of benchmarked, patient-centered outcomes (rather than simply process or fidelity measures) to guide continuous quality improvement. Customized informatics and communication infrastructures can provide user-friendly functionality, such as modular practice management functionality, centralized structured assessments (as needed by under-resourced clinics), as well as integrated and passive data collection from extant electronic medical record systems. Multi-stakeholder groups within local communities would be periodically engaged to validate the objectives or range of outcome domains and review overall system performance. This relevant and rigorous data from the sites within this system would also be available to researchers to better understand and deliver new approaches to persistent challenges. This alignment of practice-relevant research and informatics within a culture that supports measurement and provides the necessary supports and incentives would model a learning health system for early psychosis.

There is a dual reality for schizophrenia care today. On one hand is the considerable public health impact that can be derived by implementing existing interventions. On the other, there is too much that remains mysterious about the causes and physiologic bases of these illnesses. Services that are designed for knowledge translation, as we have argued here, will be in a good position to contribute to these two tasks. The success of pediatric oncology in wedding the two missions of best practice delivery and quality improvement ("doing what we know") with research ("learning what to do") offers a useful precedent (Unguru 2011). The development of learning health-care systems for new onset psychotic disorders is a good place to start and may provide a compelling prototype for other mental illnesses.

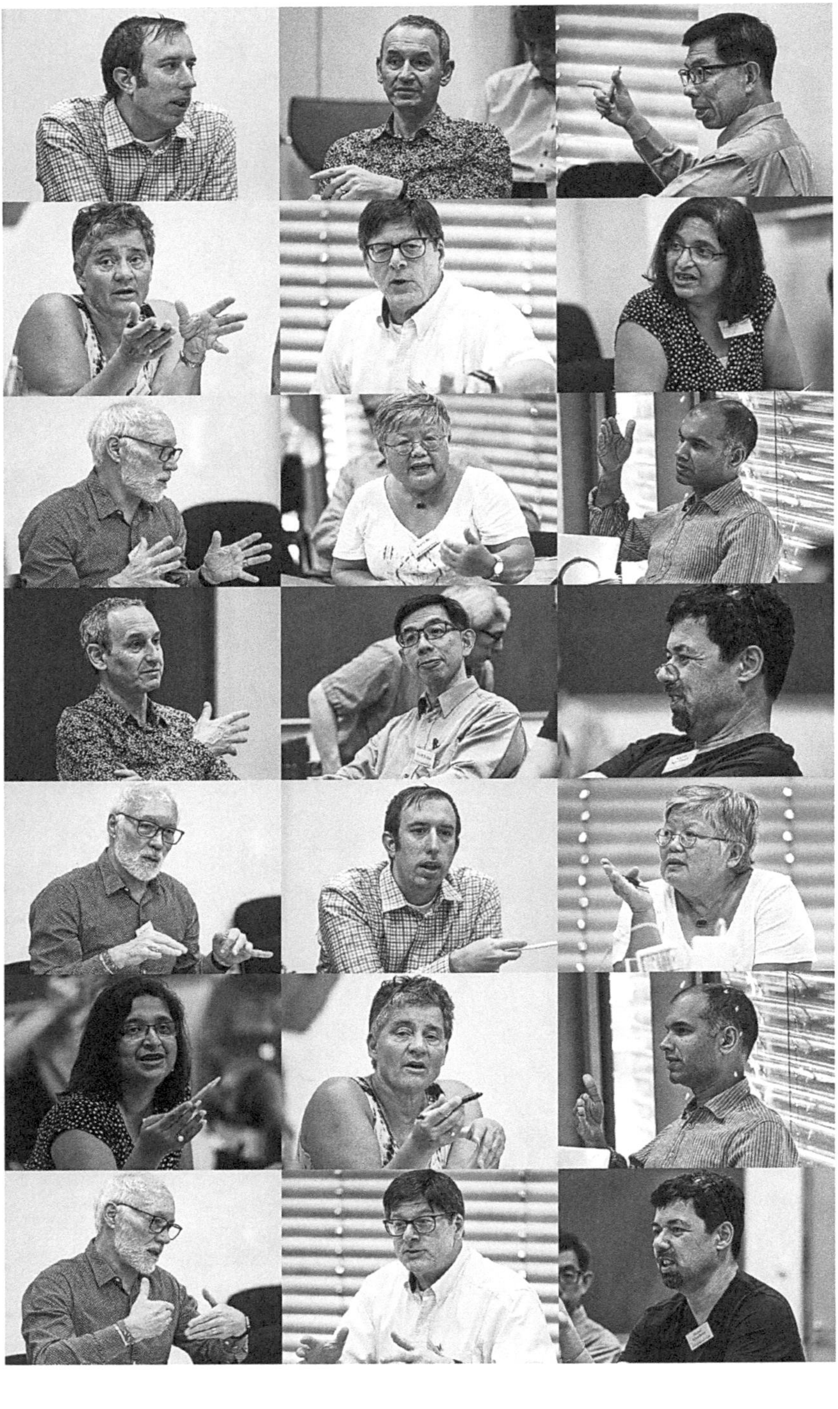

13

Developing and Implementing Tools for Prevention and Early Intervention

John Torous, Andrew M. Chanen, Eric Y. H. Chen, Kim Q. Do, Robert K. Heinssen, Patrick D. McGorry, Merete Nordentoft, Michael Schoenbaum, Vinod H. Srihari, and Swapna K. Verma

Abstract

Mental ill-health poses the greatest threat worldwide to the survival, fulfillment, and productivity of young people. Implementation of prevention and early intervention services during adolescence and youth offers the best opportunity for health and productivity gains, as 75% of all mental and substance use disorders emerge before the age of 25 years. Our vision is that all young people will be better protected from the major risk factors that threaten their mental health and well-being so that they will be able to access freely, without stigma, mental health care that is as expert and evidence-based as possible—care that is continuously shaped by new research knowledge as well as perspectives and needs of young people, their families, and their communities.

Case History of Optimal Care

Daniel, 19, a first-year university student, has been struggling with his studies since commencing an economics degree at a major university. He had moved away from home and was in unfamiliar surroundings, though some of his high school friends were attending the same university. They noticed he had become increasingly withdrawn and irritable and was using cannabis in greater amounts. One of his friends, Michelle, reached out to him and carefully explored what he

Group photos (top left to bottom right) John Torous, Andrew Chanen, Eric Chen, Merete Nordentoft, Bob Heinssen, Swapna Verma, Pat McGorry, Kim Do, Vinod Srihari, Andrew Chanen, Eric Chen, Michael Schoenbaum, Pat McGorry, John Torous, Kim Do, Swapna Verma, Merete Nordentoft, Vinod Srihari, Pat McGorry, Bob Heinssen, Michael Schoenbaum

was experiencing. Daniel was guarded at first but Michelle persisted, and he was able to confide that he was feeling very anxious and low in mood and energy. He also said he did not feel safe going out and was unable to sleep well. After a few conversations, he agreed to accompany Michelle and talk to the local integrated youth health service, which operated a suite of services on campus. The open plan design and informal, welcoming attitude of the reception/concierge staff put him at ease, and he was able to share his story with Amy, a clinician at the service. Further sessions led to a shared understanding that Daniel had developed relatively severe depression complicated by warning signs of psychosis. A holistic recovery plan was devised, involving cessation of cannabis use, sensitive support from Amy and one other male friend, liaison with his course coordinator regarding course pressures, and involvement of Daniel's parents, who visited and received support and information with Daniel's permission. While antidepressants were not prescribed initially, pending a trial of psychotherapy (cognitive behavioral therapy, CBT), they were added after several weeks as Daniel had not responded quickly enough to the other interventions. Despite subthreshold psychotic symptoms, antipsychotic medication was not necessary and the former faded away as Daniel slowly improved. Within a few months he had recovered fully and was able to complete his first year of university successfully, albeit with somewhat lower grades than he would otherwise have expected. His friendships strengthened and his relationship with his parents improved. His teachers also gained a better understanding of how to support students impacted by mental ill-health.

Case History of Modal or Suboptimal Care or Failure of Care

Jodie, 17, experienced a steady increase of problems at school. She was in conflict with teachers and her peer relationships were unstable and short-lived. Having been bullied earlier in high school, she was often low in mood with episodes of explosive anger. She also suffered from anxiety and, more recently, panic attacks. Her parents were extremely worried, especially by recent episodes of self-harm during which she inflicted cuts on her forearms. Jodie went to see the local doctor who, after 7 mins of strained discussion, prescribed antidepressants and arranged to see her again in 3 weeks. He did not contact her parents due to privacy issues. Several days later, Jodie made a series of deep cuts to her left thigh and was taken by ambulance to the local emergency department. There she was met with a deeply unsympathetic response and informed that she was wasting the time of the staff, who needed to attend to "real" medical problems. One staff member even said not to come back unless she was "serious" about killing herself. She was discharged without a follow-up appointment. Her parents sought to make an appointment with the local specialist mental health service but were told that she "did not meet the criteria" for serious mental illness and would not be offered a service. She was referred back to her local doctor. Private psychiatric help was only available at high cost in a different part of the city. Jodie became more angry, hopeless, and disengaged. Six months later she threw herself in front of a train at her local station.

Realizing The Vision for Optimal Care

To ensure that the type of care represented in the first case history is available to all, a paradigm shift is needed—one marked by innovation and change on three levels (Figure 13.1) that interact and synergize each other:

1. *Diagnosis with utility*: Utility for early intervention and youth mental health means harnessing the principles of staging and precision medicine in mental health care across all stages of illness to guide treatment and discovery.
2. *Mechanisms of risk and protection*: Discovery and deeper understanding are needed of the malleable neurobiological mechanisms involved in the emergence, persistence, recurrence, and progression of mental ill-health in youth. Similarly, we need to characterize the developmental trajectories during transition to adulthood as well as the risk and protective factors that influence the emergence of ill-health, caseness, and need for care. Ideally this will enable interventions (biological or psychosocial) to be synchronized with both developmental and clinical stages.

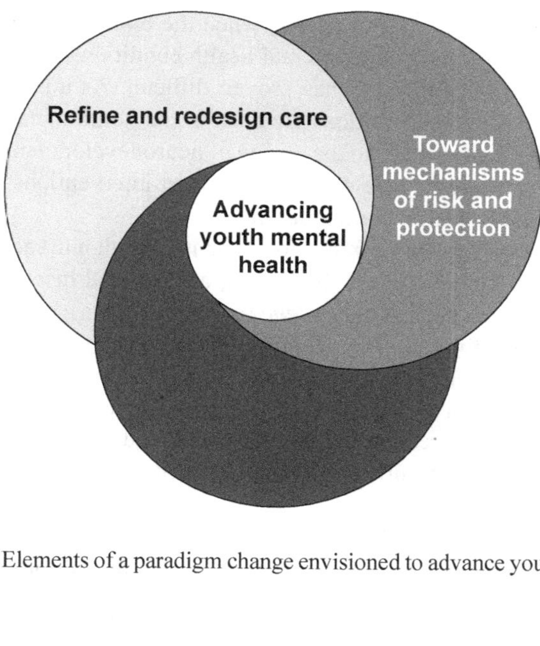

Figure 13.1 Elements of a paradigm change envisioned to advance youth mental health.

3. *Refine and redesign*: Existing evidence needs to be translated and effective models scaled up into routine care that aims for universal access and optimal quality. Design and construction of models of care need to ensure early diagnosis and sustained intervention for as long as required.

Over the past two decades, genuine progress in early intervention has been made. This began with early psychosis and has now expanded to a wider range of mental disorders. New models of care that place a premium on early diagnosis, hope, and recovery have been developed and are being expanded (Hetrick et al. 2017; Kane et al. 2016; Malla et al. 2017; McGorry 2015; McGorry et al. 2014a). Substantial progress has been made and principles clarified. However, adaptation is required for various levels of resourcing and different cultures, and there is a need to integrate primary care with specialized care to manage complexity, acuity, and persistence.

The Target Population in Youth Mental Health: Refine versus Redefine

The move toward a transdiagnostic and dimensional conceptualization of severe mental illnesses offers the opportunity to advance a framework that facilities a more unified model of prevention and early intervention. Evidence that many, although not all, mental disorders emerge post puberty (Merikangas et al. 2009) indicates that there is a critical time in development to which efforts should be targeted. However, the actual delineation of this critical period—that is, defining the specific time frame when the brain is maturing and most susceptible to risk of developing mental health conditions, and likewise most receptive to preventive efforts—has proven difficult. As a result, poor, variable, and often arbitrary definitions are used in the youth mental health field, resulting in unique challenges to the design of neurodevelopmentally appropriate prevention and (neuro)scientifically informed interventions, as well as in the delivery of high-quality continuous care.

Any discussion that aims to frame youth mental health must acknowledge the challenges posed by the cultural, biological, and societal heterogeneity that is embedded in concepts such as *adolescence* and *youth*. Even a seemingly straightforward definition of youth—the period of time between sexual maturation and the assumption of adult roles and responsibilities conferred by culture—underscores the challenges of drawing boundaries. The absence of an operational definition for youth sets up real barriers to prevention and intervention efforts, as it creates an overreliance on current definitions, which are largely based on chronological age.

The most commonly utilized standard for defining youth mental health, chronological age, imposes artificial boundaries on clinical care during critical periods of brain development. Across the world, different definitions of youth are used: 12–18 years of age is frequently utilized for administrative and service delivery purposes. There is some merit to this definition, as it is widely recognized that many mental illnesses first manifest during the sensitive period of brain development surrounding puberty (see Allen, this volume). Thus, puberty provides a common starting point for many mental illnesses and often falls within the 12- to 18-year range. However, overwhelming evidence and consensus among all authors of this chapter hold that this definition is wrong. In particular, we are most concerned with the upper age cutoff point. Given the convenience of chronological age, we believe that there is a need to create more epidemiological and neurodevelopmentally appropriate definitions of scope.

While there is no simple solution to help define the scope of youth mental health, recognizing the challenge is a practical first step. From a neurological perspective, the age of 18 years is not an appropriate cutoff point, given the overwhelming evidence of continued brain maturation and onset of new illnesses (Kessler et al. 2007) like schizophrenia, bipolar disorders, and alcohol use disorders, as of this point in life. Yet while 18 years is too early, it is not clear what should constitute a more appropriate upper limit, as there remains a lack of strong evidence of an individual biomarker that would signify the end of adolescence on personal, social, and brain development. Neuroimaging-based definitions of brain development offer some clues but currently do not provide a practical or scalable solution. This, in part, explains the continuing reliance on chronological age as a default: there is simply no other alternative. Recognizing that chronological age will continue to be utilized, if only for administrative reasons, we suggest that it is more appropriate to set the upper limit at age 25 years. This better reflects the underlying neurodevelopmental risk period for youth mental health and, as will be outlined below, confers additional benefits through the creation of new opportunities in support of primary as well as secondary prevention efforts.

The direct harm that results from current definitions of scope are exemplified in challenges encountered by some early intervention service programs. For example, despite robust evidence that cost savings occur when prevention and early intervention programs are in place, the very structure of mental health services causes ineligibility for care once an individual surpasses the system's age limit. As of age 18, for instance, an individual is no longer part of child/adolescent services and is covered only by adult services. While there must be a transition, the age of 18 is less than optimal. Forced termination of coverage by adolescent services often precludes optimal implementation of much-needed care, such that individuals no longer receive the longitudinal care they need toward recovery and society is unable to benefit from the projected cost savings commitment with delivery of that care. Compounding the issue, limiting the scope of youth mental health to

18 years creates a loophole for insurance companies, which may opt not to provide "adult" mental health patients over the age of 18 with access to early intervention services.

Thus, a more ideal definition of the scope of youth mental health will not reflect chronological age, but rather be framed in the context of clinical services designed to meet the needs of the population at risk and which require interventions. This includes creating services that integrate mental, physical, and sexual health with alcohol and other drugs expertise, vocational interventions, and online/digital health platforms (McGorry et al. 2014a; Rickwood et al. 2019). This functional definition moves discussion away from chronological age and more toward service delivery. It also raises important questions for consideration: What service delivery model should now be used to define youth mental health? Is it necessary to create a new model or clinical specialty?

One example of a clinical service-based definition that offers opportunity for improvement is to link youth mental health to child and adolescent psychiatry. For many patients, the transition from child/adolescent/youth to adult services creates an abrupt transition of care, commensurate with loss of strong therapeutic relationships and access to specialized care. For example, in the same clinic, the needs of a 19-year-old with recent onset of psychosis in an adult clinic are radically different than those of a 45-year-old with chronic schizophrenia, in terms of required psychosocial support, medical needs, employment assistance, and more. This raises the potential need for a new branch of mental health services—one that extends across the current boundary imposed by age (18 years) and connects the child/adolescent/youth psychiatry and adult psychiatry systems, with a flexible boundary between each system to enable seamless care across the lifespan. The concept of less rigid borders is already accepted in mental health service delivery, as the transition between geriatric and adult psychiatry is often fluid, based on the needs of the patient at hand. Yet even if a new youth mental health specialty were to be created, it is unclear how "appropriate transitions" would be defined. For this, we need a research agenda focused on two broad domains (see, e.g., Shah et al. as well as Bitanihirwe and Woo, this volume): biomarkers and clinical decision making. Until research is able to provide guidance on the optimal time for transitions to adult services, a focus prioritizing continuity of care is most appropriate. This functional definition allows consideration for local resources and cultural practices while aiming to support optimal care for youth mental health.

Even without a more concrete definition, it is still critical to plan for and conceptualize the scope of youth mental health in terms of evolving care systems. Such plans create the foundation upon which further support can be solidified, research efforts can be directed, and around which communities can unite and direct their efforts. Conceptualizing youth mental health as prevention for the general population as well as an early intervention mechanism for those with acute needs offers a practical starting point to frame future steps. This definition also broadens the scope of youth mental health: it acknowledges that to reach the general population as well as serve those in need, youth mental health services must operate beyond the clinic and become embedded in the community, marked by strong collaborations with the educational, judicial, and social services where at-risk youth may first present.

How Can Knowledge Exchange Improve Both Science and Clinical Care?

The bench to bedside mantra is a staple of biomedical research. In youth mental health, can this bidirectional exchange be accelerated to effect much-needed solutions in both prevention and early intervention? Can we employ the rigor and methods of scientific research in clinical care and use the priorities of patients to drive the research agenda?

To account for the unique aspects of youth mental health, we propose that the bidirectional knowledge exchange be reframed as a three-way interaction between researchers, clinicians, and patients/families. Targets for this tridirectional knowledge exchange would include the discovery of risk factors, mechanisms, and clinical responses to existing interventions in youth mental health. These multiple stakeholders and targets must also be considered within the context of prevention, early intervention, and ongoing care. Further, new strategies must be framed from the perspective of brain development so that interventions can take place at the right time during the right stage of neurological maturation. Given the complexity of multiple stakeholders, targets, domains, and time frames, it is easy to understand why unified research has progressed slowly, despite a number of pioneering advances in individual areas of research. Equally, however, there is great potential embedded within this complexity. To harness it, we propose a learning health-care system for youth mental health (see Figure 13.2).

The Institute of Medicine (IOM) has presented a vision for twenty-first century health care based on the principles of efficacy, safety, and equity. Accordingly, characteristics of an ideal health system include science-based intervention, easy and timely access to services, and person-centered care. Measurement-based treatment plays a key role in assuring the quality, effectiveness, and responsiveness of therapies provided to individual patients. Medical informatics and data science specialties provide powerful tools for aggregating and mining clinical data, which in turn can be used to discern lessons about current practice, areas of uncertainty, and opportunities for new research. The learning health-care system envisioned by IOM is an ideal platform for practice-based studies in youth mental health, aimed at improving patient care and driving the process of scientific discovery.

Developing a common framework for data collection, analysis, and reporting is a necessary step. Key global initiatives to facilitate this process have already been formed. The International Youth Mental Health Research Network (IYMHRN), currently represented by over 30 academic and other organizations involved in youth mental health research, has produced a set of research priorities for youth mental health, in consultation with funding bodies (C. Mei et al., in prep.). These priorities include developing a global standardized toolkit of assessment and outcome measures for youth mental health that can be used to evaluate and compare services and identify effective service features. Further proposed activities of the IYMHRN include linking clinical research with data analysts to support the utilization and interpretation of large data sets. Overall, the priorities developed by IYMHRN aim to provide a youth-specific framework to enable a systematic and global strategy for new and innovative research as well as the translation and implementation of existing evidence, in collaboration with key stakeholders, including young people and their families, mental health clinicians and service providers, and policy makers. This is facilitated by IYMHRN's strong links with other youth-focused initiatives such as Frayme, a Canadian-based international knowledge translation platform. A key focus of Frayme is to synthesize evidence, translate knowledge, and support the global implementation of integrated youth services (Halsall et al. 2019). These recent initiatives are supported by a range of established platforms, including the International Association for Youth Mental Health, IEPA Early Intervention in Mental Health, and the journal, *Early Intervention in Psychiatry*, which supports evidence-based practice in youth mental health as well as research innovation and translation.

With a specific focus on the early psychosis spectrum, the National Institute of Mental Health (NIMH) has expressed strong interest in a subset of measures that could bridge clinical and academic programs, thereby supporting implementation, quality improvement, health services, and translational research. The immediate goal of this multisite research approach, the Early Psychosis Intervention Network (EPINET), is to improve early identification, diagnosis, clinical assessment, intervention effectiveness, service delivery, and health outcomes in clinics that offer evidence-based specialty care to persons in the early stages of psychotic illness. EPINET will link community clinics and academic research programs through core measures of clinical phenotypes, service delivery, and functional outcomes as well as a uniform informatics approach for aggregating and analyzing pooled data. Data analytics will allow individual clinics to monitor treatment fidelity, quality, and outcome metrics in real time, and to compare local performance to results obtained across all network sites. With standard clinical measures as its *lingua franca,* EPINET will facilitate communication and collaboration among participating clinicians, academic researchers, and early psychosis service users, thus setting the stage for a large practice-based research program aimed at establishing new standards for care

Table 13.1 Interactions in the Early Psychosis Intervention Network (EPINET), a learning health-care model for youth mental health. Discovery in basic sciences can inform translational research and, in turn, clinical service delivery, which then can inform the agenda for basic discovery science

	Clinical Service Delivery System	Translational Research Clinics	Discovery Science Research Centers
Conceptual Framework	Measurement-based treatment	Experimental therapeutics	Neuroscience molecular biology genomics
Methodology	Clinical staging, treatment to target, step-wise care	Experimental manipulation of putative mechanism	Network, circuitry, morphological, and functional profiling in experimental models with genetic or environmental risks
Principal Responsibilities	Implement, refine, and optimize evidence-based interventions	Establish target engagement and treatment efficacy	Identify disorder mechanisms and therapeutic targets

and accelerating studies of psychosis risk factors, biomarkers of illness, and preemptive intervention. Table 13.1 illustrates "upstream" interactions among discovery science centers and research-oriented clinical programs. Standard measures of these dimensions will create a "data bridge" across research and clinical settings:

1. Common data elements will be used to identify potential research participants among those enrolled in early psychosis programs.
2. Using these common measures as end points in diverse studies, translation and implementation of findings will be accelerated into clinical practice settings.

EPINET will create a national laboratory to address important practice issues as well as emerging scientific questions. EPINET stakeholders anticipate a national forum to promote active sharing of experience, data, and new ideas about the nature and optimal treatment of early psychosis. Expertise within the network will accelerate progress in several areas, including practice innovations for reducing the duration of untreated psychosis, mitigating medical comorbidities in first-episode psychosis, and optimizing the effectiveness of existing treatments. Scientifically, EPINET will support a range of precision medicine approaches to early psychosis, including observational and experimental studies of underlying mechanisms and novel interventions. Working in collaboration with national partners and international colleagues, such as the Australian Early Psychosis Research Network, NIMH imagines a new era of early psychosis treatment that fully realizes the IOM vision of effective, continuously improving, and science-driven health care for the future.

Building a Tridirectional Partnership

The success of any learning health-care system will be reliant on an effective exchange of knowledge, within and between stakeholder groups, as well as on fruitful collaborations and cooperation. We hold that the unique aspects of youth mental health require a partnership between three general groups of stakeholders: researchers, clinicians, as well as patients and their families. Notwithstanding the presence of various hurdles within each stakeholder group, which must be addressed and overcome, multiple factors will hinder effective collaboration between the groups. Here we highlight challenges as well as opportunities for synergy within and between each stakeholder group.

Within the research community, there is an overall need for more transdisciplinary collaborations. Emergent knowledge from multiple disciplines (e.g., molecular, genetic, social, and behavioral science) is required to understand the complexities involved in youth mental health. Within each research domain, well-honed specialization is needed, yet this in itself can create barriers to experts from other domains, thus pointing to the need for effective cross-disciplinary communication.

Effective communication and collaboration must also be secured between the research and clinical communities (bench to bedside and back again). Figure 13.2 illustrates a fully integrated translational approach that links clinical and discovery science in accordance to the learning health-care model proposed above. Interactions between clinical and preclinical research—at various levels of investigation (genetic, molecular, cellular, circuitry, psychic, cognitive, and behavioral phenotyping), performed with state-of-the-art methodologies—are applicable to both patients and animal models. At various stages of disease, patient assessments together with epidemiological, ecological momentary investigations lead to the development of preclinical models that are closely linked to the pathophysiology of the disease. To test the interaction between genetic and environmental risk factors during the critical period of peripuberty/adolescence, insults derived from epidemiological studies could be applied in appropriate animal models at various periods of brain development. Wherever possible, assessment end points of preclinical models should be aligned with the ones used in clinical studies. Besides demonstrating new pathological mechanisms involved in the progression and modification of disease, this integrated translational approach should lead to the identification of sensitive and accurate biomarker profiles that are essential for early diagnostics, for monitoring therapeutic efficacy, as well as for potential drug targets, to be tested and validated in clinical settings.

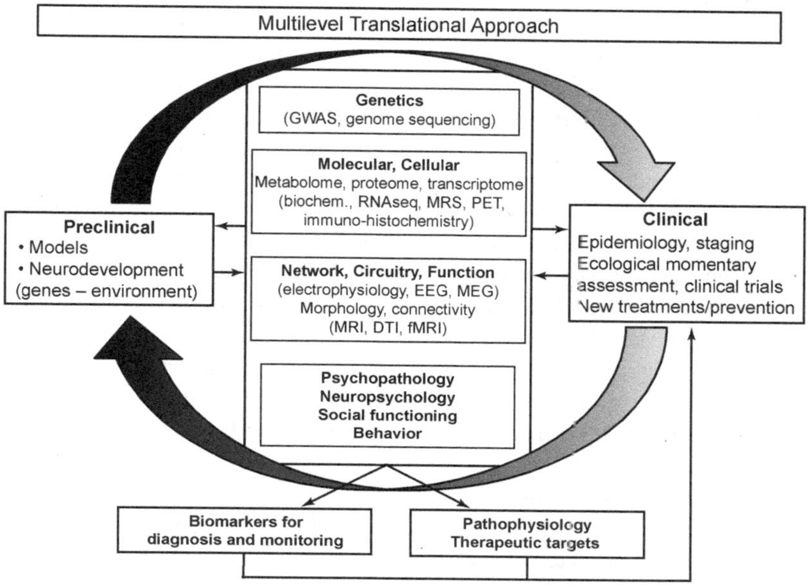

Figure 13.2 Framework by which mechanisms suggested by clinical observations can be tested and preclinical models in patients validated. Risk assessments gained from genome-wide association studies (GWAS) and whole genome sequencing are used to generate novel experimental models. Biochemical and RNA deep sequencing methodologies establish profiles (metabolomic, proteomic, and transcriptomic) on specific biological materials (blood, fibroblasts, olfactory tissue, stem cells, nervous tissues). Noninvasive brain magnetic resonance spectroscopy (MRS) and positron emission tomography (PET) are methods of choice for translation to assess molecular and cellular alterations in specific structures in both patients and models. Histochemistry (immunolabeling, *in situ* hybridization) applied to patients' postmortem brain and nervous tissue allows specific altered cell types to be identified. At the circuitry and network connectivity levels, electroencephalography (EEG), magnetic encephalography (MEG), and functional and diffusion magnetic resonance imaging (fMRI, DTI)—combined with classical electrophysiology—enable specific dysfunctions to be characterized at high time and spatial resolutions. Finally, psychopathology profiling and cognitive/affective and social impairments can be studied in both patients and experimental models.

Applying such a translational approach within early intervention programs, researchers have demonstrated that effective links could be established between clinical and discovery science (Baumann et al. 2013; Föcking et al. 2016). For instance, the role of a glutathione brain deficit in schizophrenia pathophysiology, first observed in patients (Do et al. 2000; Gysin et al. 2007; Tosic et al. 2006; Xin et al. 2016), was investigated in rodent models to allow characterization of its role in inducing numerous relevant schizophrenia phenotypes, such as inflammation, NMDA receptor hypofunction, and dopamine dysregulation (Dwir et al. 2016; Hardingham and Do 2016; Steullet et al. 2016). Interestingly, the experimental model of gene–environment interactions showed that additional insults at peripuberty, but not in adulthood, led to permanent excitatory-inhibitory cortical imbalance, which is known to underlie cognitive deficits (Cabungcal et al. 2013a). This finding highlights childhood and peripuberty as critical periods of high vulnerability for environmental adverse insults, and has led to the study of the differential impact of traumatic early- versus late-life events in patients (Alameda et al. 2016) and the contribution of redox imbalance (Alameda et al. 2018).

The same complexity that can isolate researchers from each other, however, can also occur with clinicians as well as patients and families. For clinicians, co-designing research platforms within clinical services, joint journal clubs, and joint meetings offer possible solutions. For patients and families, synergistic collaborations offer opportunities to better characterize the phenomenology of youth mental health and build support for the research agenda among a more cognizant general public.

Apart from translational neuroscientific approaches, an important knowledge domain in youth mental health is descriptive psychopathology. Current initiatives for early detection are limited by a lack of psychopathological knowledge for the early evolution of symptoms. Existing psychopathological knowledge is mostly based on patients with established illnesses. Efforts to extend this knowledge base have thus far come from two approaches: (a) simple epidemiological tools (such as self-administered questionnaires), developed for large population surveys with acknowledged limitations for capturing subtle early psychopathology, and (b) methods extending from established illnesses (such as the CAARMS). Neither method addresses the possibility of new complexities and forms of experiences, which may not simply be diluted forms of psychopathological experiences from established illnesses. Recent research has emphasized external empirical brain measurements and tended to under-recognize the value of information provided by subjective experiences. Yet in general, symptoms still contribute most of the predictive powers in outcome determination. To what extent a refined psychopathological information may help to provide diagnostic and prognostic information to guide treatment is an empirical question that will only be answered once we have the right approaches and tools—such as those offered by the learning health-care model for youth mental health.

Ignoring patients and families from the knowledge exchange network would be a critical oversight. Traditionally there have been many heterogeneous voices from the patient/family communities, and at times critical voices from those who may have had poor experiences with the current system. However, supporting those who have had good experiences and coalescing their voice through youth research councils or leadership roles in mental health service organizations can help ensure that their voice is better recognized—and that we learn from it. As youth are increasingly being approached by researchers, especially in an era of digital and technology-based monitoring, it is important that they be allowed the opportunity to set their agenda and demand that research suit their personal and ethical considerations. The initial challenges of the first wave of digital interventions may be related to poorly developed collaborations (Torous et al. 2019). Finally, the evidence for youth mental health prevention increasingly suggests the necessary role of families and environments in promoting mental wellness. Patient/family synergies with clinicians to develop more comprehensive treatment plans that deliver clinical services where needed but also engage the family unit and local community offer high potential for improved youth mental health outcomes.

Neuroscience research can also directly inform novel interventions for youth mental health and learn from what they seek. Patient interest in biofeedback offers one example of a bridge between neuroscience and care that has great potential. For instance, understanding how functional connectivity between the prefrontal cortex and amygdala supports (as well as disrupts, in several conditions) cognitive control offers the potential of neurocircuit-specific interventions (e.g., biofeedback and CBT) optimized to these targets. However, to date such specific efforts directed toward youth mental health are scarce and should be prioritized in the research agenda.

To advance this tridirectional knowledge exchange requires removing barriers and gathering of new support. One primary barrier that currently impacts all stakeholders is the chronological age determination used in child and adolescent services. As discussed, chronological age determination often removes patients and families at a time when their involvement is most crucial. In terms of support, specific funds for intergroup collaborations (e.g., clinicians who wish to pursue research) are often limited in resources-limited mental health settings.

How Can Effective Prevention and Early Intervention Efforts Be Refined or Redesigned?

Delivering effective preventions and interventions for youth mental health requires a synthesis between scientific and care delivery systems. Primary prevention remains the goal and a research priority, although currently there is more actionable evidence for secondary and tertiary prevention efforts. Lack of primary prevention, however, curtails our ability to act. Priority needs to be given to activate the support necessary to advance research and engage the family unit, public policy, and clinical systems, not merely to support but also to implement preventive efforts.

One immediate challenge is the blurring of current definitions of prevention and intervention in youth mental health. Because risk factors, triggers, onset, and course of many youth mental health conditions are the focus of active research, prevention programs themselves are still evolving. Current prevention efforts target mainly nonspecific risk factors, and quantifying their success remains a challenge as this must occur over the course of years to even decades. In addition, many current prevention strategies do not take into account considerations of the temporal development and progression of risk across different neurodevelopmental stages unique to youth mental health conditions. However, as discussed below, clinical staging has emerged as a promising framework to guide service delivery and research given its focus on the continuum of mental disorders from asymptomatic to chronic illness and its conceptualization of the transdiagnostic trajectories of mental disorders. This focus facilitates the selection of interventions that are proportionate to need and risk of illness progression and provides a framework for evaluating the pathophysiology and biomarkers for each illness stage that can then inform innovative neurobiological and psychosocial interventions (McGorry and Hickie 2019). The universal, selective, and indicated preventive mental health framework reviewed by Arango et al. (2018) offers a series of strategies aimed toward prevention (Figure 13.3).

We wish to point out, however, that disagreement (both local and global) exists as to what constitutes a triad of universal, selective, and indicated strategies as well as when and where it should actually be implemented. A further challenge to implementing prevention programs relates to the epidemiological uncertainty of how many youths are actually at risk of developing mental health conditions, let alone understanding their degree of risk. Without better quantification of risk, it is difficult to plan or promote funds for the appropriate scale and scope of required services.

Likewise, interventions today are limited by an evolving understanding of youth mental disorders and often do not take into account considerations of the temporal development and progression of these conditions related to underlying brain changes. Some youth mental health interventions, like the Recovery After an Initial Schizophrenia Episode (RAISE) program at NIMH, do offer

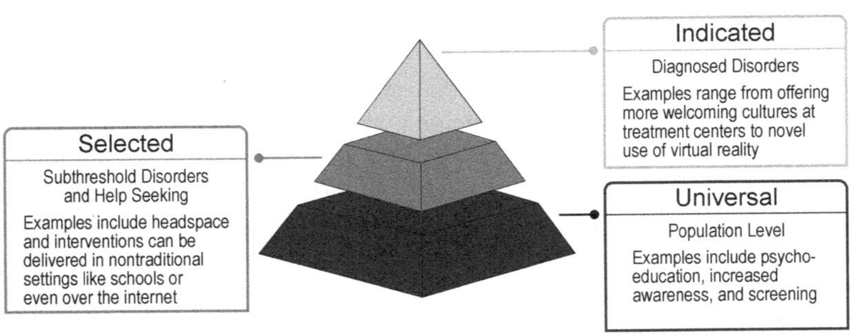

Figure 13.3 Selected, universal, and indicated strategies for a preventive youth mental health framework.

a more neurodevelopmentally informed approach toward intervention, in this case for schizophrenia. One potential reason may be that the relatively low prevalence of schizophrenia compared to other youth mental health disorders, such as depression, makes early intervention efforts for schizophrenia feasible to fund and support. Programs that target young people with early phases of psychosis include OPUS in Denmark, EPPIC in Australia, PIANO in Italy, and PEPP in Canada.

More broadly, a number of youth mental health services that target a range of mental disorders have emerged over the last decade, initiating in Australia through the development of headspace and flowing to other parts of the globe (McGorry and Mei 2018). These integrated models of care have shown positive outcomes across access to care, symptomatic and functional recovery, and client satisfaction (Fusar-Poli 2019; Hetrick et al. 2017). Available services span the United Kingdom (Youthspace), Ireland (Jigsaw), Canada (Foundry, ACCESS Open Minds), the United States (allcove), the Middle East (headspace in Israel), and Europe (headspace in Denmark and Iceland; @ease in The Netherlands). Youth mental health services, such as headspace in Australia, deliver treatment within a preventive framework that provides evidence-informed stepped care guided by risk-benefit considerations and shared decision making (McGorry et al. 2014a). A key component of the headspace model is ensuring that the delivery of evidence-based treatment is matched to the patient's current need as well as the risk of illness persistence and progression. This preventive focus is essential given that the majority of headspace clients present during the early stages of illness and often experience risk of self-harm and suicidal ideation, significant distress, functional impairment, and substance abuse (Rickwood et al. 2014, 2015; Scott et al. 2012b). Simple and brief psychosocial interventions are typically offered as first-line treatments, with pharmaceutical approaches provided to those who do not benefit from initial psychosocial interventions or who present with increased severity or risk (McGorry et al. 2014a). This is in line with the clinical staging model (McGorry et al. 2006).

Across the diagnostic spectrum, clinical staging offers a way forward to bridge current gaps in linking diagnostic models to more personalized and effective intervention, prognosis, neurobiological markers, and psychosocial outcomes (McGorry and Hickie 2019). The clinical staging model currently provides a useful heuristic transdiagnostic framework to guide early intervention and prevention. To achieve its full potential, the model aims to evolve into an evidence-based clinicopathological framework, whereby each stage is linked to neurobiological, psychological, and clinical phenotyping (McGorry et al. 2014b). To date, a number of neurobiological markers have been linked to stage of illness, with findings indicating that established mental disorders are associated with more severe neurobiological and neurocognitive markers compared to attenuated syndromes (Bartholomeusz et al. 2017; Hermens et al. 2013; Lagopoulos et al. 2012; Naismith et al. 2012). This aligns with the potential progression of mental illness proposed by the clinical staging model and supports the applicability of staging to prognosis, early intervention, and prevention, particularly in the context of youth mental health.

Meeting the need for a more transdiagnostic framework—one that offers appropriate intervention and prevention strategies—is further impaired by a lack of disease-specific staging with which these strategies could be coupled. Concern for nonspecificity and a lack of validity with current diagnostic schemes, represented often by the DSM or ICD, have recently given rise to efforts that seek to reconceptualize or reclassify mental illnesses. Resulting efforts (e.g., clinical staging, RDoC, or HITOP) reflect research-directed projects to increase the validity of diagnostics. Whether these and other efforts will transfer well into pathways of care, and how they may be able to guide appropriate service delivery, remains a research priority; currently, clinical staging offers greater clinical utility, particularly in guiding treatment selection and models of care (McGorry and Hickie 2019). Closing the treatment gap through better implementation and utilization of today's service and interventions constitutes another.

This discussion on radical changes to nosology presents a broader question of whether the underlying youth mental health system itself must radically change. Can progress toward effective prevention and early intervention be obtained through incremental improvement, refinement, and a more radical redesign of how we scientifically study and clinically approach youth mental health? One argument for refinement is that current patients need ongoing services and support. Since many evidence-based practices, especially around access to services and screening, are not always implemented in youth mental health, actualizing current knowledge and interventions appropriately may be a way to effect rapid improvement. A redesign argument considers the current unmet need, paired with today's poor clinical outcomes in youth mental health, and suggests that new approaches are necessary. Further, it suggests that the structure, funding, and support of today's youth mental health services, as well as current model of illnesses, may impede adoption of evidence-based practices today as well as the development of new ones tomorrow. One advantage of redesigned systems is that they provide an opportunity for low- and middle-income countries to develop initial youth mental health systems that are adaptive and often better received by patients.

It is clear that the process of redesign must be accomplished together with young people (Rickwood et al. 2019). Feedback from youth shows that they want mental health clinics to be different: open during hours that suit their lifestyle and a better setting, one that is more welcoming and less clinical. The headspace program in Australia, which has been scaled up to 110 national centers and replicated internationally, suggests that simply lowering the barriers to entry, to simply the need to talk, creates a better, stigma-free entry point for youth to access mental health services. This has been confirmed by an independent evaluation of headspace, which revealed improved access to care for young people with high levels of satisfaction (Hilferty et al. 2015). It also suggests the potential of positioning mental health services in less traditional environments, such as shopping malls, schools, or community centers. Likewise, there is support for increasing the appeal of youth mental health services when they are co-located within primary care/general practices or pediatric clinics. Neuroscience-focused language can be employed to frame the biological basis of youth mental health to patients/families; this can help reduce stigma and enable patients/families to better understand the nature of these conditions. In addition, minimizing the use of mental health diagnoses and instead explaining conditions in terms of features may help youth better accept and engage with services. The role of online/mobile technology and smartphones will be critical in the redesign of programs, as seen already through headspace's online service (eheadspace), which offers access to information, support, and mental health care for young people, including those who might otherwise not access professional help (Rickwood et al. 2016). The current success of suicide text messages services (e.g., CrisisTextLine in the United States) likely foreshadows a new way to deliver mental health services.

Normal neurodevelopmental progression associated with stages of youth (e.g., exploration, risk taking, peer approval, and autonomy) provides a context to increase the acceptability, uptake, and support for youth mental health services by patients. For example, matching the desire for peer support with peer-led treatments (e.g., peer support services offered at headspace, ACCESS Open Minds, Foundry, and the Wellness Recovery Action Planning in schizophrenia) offers potential. Although more evidence exists for adults than youth (Cook et al. 2012), peer support is a key component of youth mental health services that is acceptable to young people and potentially cost-effective (Hamilton et al. 2017). Some interventions which have been validated in adults (e.g., use of peer interpersonal contact to decrease stigma) may not be as effective when applied to youth. To inform applicability of existing services and guide the development of novel prevention and intervention strategies focused on youth mental health, a research agenda that accounts for normal developmental as well as dynamic pathological processes is necessary.

What Principles Might Guide the Development and Accelerate Clinical Deployment of Digital Technologies in Youth Mental Health?

The recent rise in interest in digital mental health technologies (e.g., smartphone apps and virtual reality) represents an evolving frontier for youth mental health. With direct applicability to prevention and interventions efforts, digital mental health offers a relevant example that can be explored to highlight current successes as well as failures in a vision for the field, refining versus redesigning care, implementing learning health-care systems to support tridirectional knowledge exchange, and creating the support to overcome barriers.

A useful starting point is to consider both the benefits and risks of new digital technologies, along with their unique relevance to youth mental health. Potential benefits include scalability, novel monitoring, real-time interventions, and new investment:

1. Because prevalence of ownership and access to smartphones and computers is high in youth, a foundation for scalability of any digital mental health program is already given.
2. A myriad of sensors on today's smartphones (e.g., GPS, accelerometer, gyroscope, microphone, screen touch, proximity, Bluetooth, wifi, and more) offers a window into real time and often functional outcomes (Torous et al. 2016). A patient's phone, for instance, can record how many hours a person slept, exercised, or spent calling peers. Real-time collection of smartphone signals requires no active engagement from an individual and is often labeled passive data. Active data refers to more traditional ecological momentary assessment, or surveys, which can also be offered via a smartphone. Together, active and passive smartphone data, as well as a host of wearable sensors (e.g., smartwatches), provide an opportunity to collect low-cost longitudinal data at a previously unprecedented level of detail.
3. Digital technologies like smartphones and sensors not only collect data, they can process it, implement decision support algorithms, and provide real-time interventions via app-based exercises, peer support, and connection to care. Virtual reality headsets already possess a strong evidence base for delivering effective exposure therapy and are well accepted among youth.
4. Because of broad support for digital mental health, new funding resources, from both philanthropy and pharmaceuticals, can be used to advance the field.

However, the unique advantages of digital mental health must also be considered in light of several, also unique, risks:

1. Clinical evidence for the efficacy of digital mental health tools (e.g., smartphone apps) is currently minimal, although there is a growing wealth of feasibility studies. A recent systematic review of mental health apps targeting preadolescent and adolescent mental health identified 24 studies, of which only 7% featured patients with a mental health diagnosis (Grist et al. 2017).
2. Real-time monitoring raises privacy and ethical concerns.

3. There is growing concern that few mental health patients actually adhere to smartphone apps and may instead use them only for a limited time before deleting.
4. There is risk that digital mental health tools may fragment youth mental health if data is not appropriately shared with clinical systems, thus isolating mental health from general health.

The unique elements of digital mental health offer numerous visions for the future of youth mental health. From a practical standpoint, digital tools fulfill two roles: (a) to augment and integrate with care systems and (b) to push toward more self-care. Currently, there is a plethora of mental health apps that promote a self-responsibility and self-care vision for the field (Parker et al. 2018). They also provide a novel approach for peer support and create easily accessible networks for youth trained to support each other. Digital health tools can be designed to offer youth a customized treatment delivery platform that can be adapted to their unique needs. On a design level, the user interface, user experience, social experience, and external reinforcements can be co-designed by youth to drive engagement with care. While currently under-researched, there is a need to understand how certain deficits in diseases such as schizophrenia (e.g., working memory or attention) may need to be offset in the design of these digital tools.

The issue of refining versus redesigning care also emerges in digital mental health. In lower- and middle-income countries, where minimal investment is often allocated to basic health-care services, can digital technologies jump-start efforts and deliver new models of digital psychiatry that are effective and accessible? In all areas of the world, can digital mental health tools be used to quantify a patient's environment and then use that data to recommend appropriate interventions (e.g., sleep, exercise, diet)?

The redesign of the approval process by the U.S. Food and Drug Administration (FDA) for medical software (covering apps and virtual reality) represents a radical departure from the past. On the youth mental health side, digital tools have not yet forced the issue of refining versus redefining care, although the issue will be accelerated with the pending (as of 2019) FDA approval of the first video game for attention deficit hyperactivity disorder. Although telemedicine has not caused a redesign of youth mental health, increased access and expansion of the digital age through mobile technology now needs to be addressed. We need to reconsider how to assess the efficacy of these new digital tools. Randomized controlled trials do offer benefits, and will be necessary, but they may not necessarily capture the potential of these technologies to offer individual and personalized interventions. More importantly, digital technologies will require continual improvement and iterations that evolve both with technology and user demand. Evaluation models, such as A/B design, and partnerships with experts in the game industry may offer a novel way to isolate the currently elusive active ingredient in digital mental health tools.

The necessity of a learning health-care system to support tridirectional knowledge exchange is also relevant in digital mental health. Many existing evidenced-based CBT apps, supported by on-demand clinicians or coaches, have failed because they did not consider patient/family perspectives. Increasingly, research has shown that apps designed without the input of users suffer from poor engagement (Torous et al. 2019). Patient/family viewpoints need to be considered through the co-design of apps and informed consent. However, little evidence exists on the co-design of apps for youth with mental health needs, and even less about what is needed to build trust and deliver informed consent. Privacy issues remain a top concern when surveying users about smartphone apps. If a smartphone, for example, can capture a digital signature of an underlying endophenotype, it may be possible to design studies to assess both longitudinal outcomes as well as causal inference. Theories such as how the adolescent brain is cued to respond to social reward could then be tested at scale across multiple countries in a uniform manner. Whether digital phenotyping will prove capable of predicting clinical outcomes or identifying risky behavioral patterns, amidst digital noise and the natural variation in human behavior, remains an open research question.

Finally, as with other aspects of youth mental health, creating the support to overcome barriers remains an important focal point for discussion. Little is known about how digital psychiatry should interface with the technology industry in terms of partnerships, privacy, cost models, data ownership, data access, and ethics. While there is no simple solution, there is an urgent need for increased transparency. For example, the privacy policies of many mental health smartphone apps require a college level education for comprehension, which not all youth with mental health issues possess (Powell et al. 2018). Increasingly, patients are turning to clinicians to ask whether technology itself poses a risk to youth mental health through internet addiction. The current lack of knowledge on the topic and need for an informed response is a pressing issue, as are questions regarding legal access to youth mental health data: When should parents, police, and clinicians be able to obtain legally the digital data collected on an individual? Data from digital devices will clearly offer an important new tool in the future of youth mental health, but addressing these ethical and legal questions around its use must be a first priority.

How Can We Build Support and Overcome Barriers to Ensure Successful Implementation of Youth Mental Health Services?

All mental health systems across the globe are under-resourced. Lack of adequate resources is especially true for youth mental health services, which further is impacted by the arbitrary definitions that often remove support for necessary services when a person reaches the age of 18. In campaigns to increase support, prior efforts have framed deficits in youth mental health as a human rights violation or called for cost redistribution of resources within health-care systems. Neither approach has yielded substantial results. Thus, to increase support and overcome barriers in youth mental health, we advocate pursuing a new vision, approach, and societal investment strategy.

Focusing on support, we present the "model, mobilize, and momentum" mantra as a scaffold for the field to optimize opportunities. One way to build support is to model youth mental health services in a particular area around successful examples from other regions or countries. Careful comparison to successful models can create a convincing argument for support at home. In addition, it is important to mobilize evidence and build youth mental services on solid scientific backing. Seizing momentum, it may be beneficial to expand a certain domain or service when the opportunity arises, rather than wait for broad scope funding to improve all aspects of care. Together the "model, mobilize, and momentum" mantra allows youth mental health services to be poised to act and advocate for support at the right moment.

Opportunities for support are more likely to emerge when stakeholders are well aligned. This includes improving relationships within as well as outside of the mental health field. Within the mental health field, there is a need for continual education and training around youth mental health interventions (e.g., headspace model, individual placement and support, RAISE, EPPIC, OPUS, and PIANO). Medical students and mental health clinicians need to read about youth mental health interventions and service models (e.g., headspace, RAISE) in textbooks, lectures, and clinical guidelines because without exposure, they will never turn to or demand more research on these evidence-based programs. Outside of the mental health field, better alignment is needed (e.g., with NGOs) to ensure that the perspectives of all patients (not just those who are engaged) are heard. In Denmark, for example, the organization PsykiatriAlliancen (psychiatry alliance), comprised of 33 organizations, has developed a core program to promote mental health services and to campaign for and present a unified voice, similar to current efforts in cancer advocacy. Acknowledging that some individuals may have a negative experience with the current youth mental health system, it is important to also ensure that the vast majority who do have good experiences are also heard.

In addition, it is important to mobilize individuals as well as entire communities. Outreach must go beyond families and political leaders: engaging police departments, schools, and social services can build powerful partnerships that are often overlooked. Framing youth mental health as a net gain at the community level, by explaining long-term health and cost savings and focusing on high prevalence disorders (e.g., depression), can garner broad support. However, unifying community support around more prevalent conditions carries the risk of reducing support for serious mental illnesses, thus creating inadvertent competition for support between different illnesses. One potential solution is to utilize a hybrid approach—one that offers both primary and specialist mental health care in a single package.

Even when community support is optimal, the youth mental health field itself can cause barriers if services or programs are not designed properly or adequately funded to meet the scale of need (McGorry et al. 2019). The key to any successful program is to ensure access and efficacy of an intervention, so that functional outcomes can be delivered to all stakeholders. When there is a bottleneck in access or efficacy, the probability of failure increases greatly. Another common stumbling block occurs when the field is held to an unduly high standard for evidence; in reality, a plethora of evidence-based interventions already exist just waiting for implementation, such as around access to services and screening. Furthermore, ensuring that an intervention delivers functional outcomes (e.g., increased employment or social skills), as opposed to a mere change in symptom measures, is important for creating the necessary impact to build continued support. Primary prevention efforts in the community, modeled after successful efforts in the cancer and cardiology communities, offer a practical starting point. It is important to set realistic expectations, realizing that a successful youth mental health intervention will require many years of follow-up. While early returns on investments, such as in RAISE, OPUS, and youth mental health care more broadly are possible, this should not be seen as the norm.

Finally, the design of services in conjunction with users provides another means to reduce barriers and garner support. Here, digital mental health offers a tremendous opportunity for collaboration. Utilizing the digital expertise of youth mental health patients offers potential for co-design of new online and connected tools.

Conclusion

The youth mental health field has many advantages working in its favor, as nearly all societies offer broad support for youth. Harnessing that support into (a) diagnosis with utility, (b) mechanisms of risk and protection, and (c) the refinement and redesign of care models will advance the field and improve lifelong outcomes. New tools from genetics to digital phenotyping and advanced models of partnerships from learning health-care systems to community collaborations will help. What is lacking, however, is an effective research agenda to address many of the unanswered questions that remain:

- How should the youth mental health field best communicate with the public?
- How can effective interventions be implemented and scaled up?
- What standards for evidence are needed?
- How can the co-design of effective interventions be optimized?

- What is the best way to identify the functional outcomes that matter most to stakeholders?
- Which research and clinical priorities need to be addressed to maximize clinical impact?

Our vision is for all young people to be better protected from the major risk factors that threaten their mental health and well-being, so that they can freely access, without stigma, mental health care that is as expert and evidence-based as possible. Achieving this vision will require a massive focus on research focused on

- identifying targets for early prevention and longitudinal data on trajectories of illness,
- establishing nationwide programs that ensure early access to care,
- implementing today's important evidence-based interventions,
- furthering efforts to bridge basic science and clinical practices, and
- activating communities.

Future Directions for Youth Mental Health

14

Lessons Learned and Future Directions for Early Intervention and Youth Mental Health Paradigms

Research for Reform

Patrick D. McGorry

Abstract

Until recent decades, early intervention seemed like a Utopian ideal, hopelessly out of reach. One of the prerequisites for intervening early is the availability of effective treatment. However, even when effective treatments for the major mental disorders emerged in the 1950s, the weight of pessimism, neglect, and discrimination in the care of the mentally ill buried all realistic notions of intervening early to modify the course of serious mental illness. In the 1980s, research began to focus on first-episode psychosis to seek greater clarity of the underlying etiopathology. The long delays in accessing initial treatment became immediately apparent, as did the fact that the treatment needs of early-stage patients and their families were dramatically different from those with long-term chronic illness. The harm suffered by patients through these delays and the crudeness of standard care was exposed and demanded a new approach. The therapeutic value of hope was rediscovered, and the erroneous nature of the nineteenth-century belief of inevitable deterioration or degeneration, also captured in the 1980s phrase "doomed from the womb," became clear. Short- to medium-range outcomes were improved and shown to be heterogeneous and malleable. The world of schizophrenia research was transformed, and several stages of illness, each with their own treatment needs, were defined, from the earliest clinical features to enduring chronic illness. This paradigm shift paved the way for the creation of a transdiagnostic model of clinical staging that was capable of catalyzing early intervention across other diagnostic landscapes and congruent reform of systems of mental health care. An international scientific movement emerged under the banner of the International Early Psychosis Association (IEPA) in 1997, and a new journal, *Early Intervention in Psychiatry*, was established in 2007 to sustain and extend the growth of knowledge in early intervention. With 75% of mental and substance use disorders emerging before the age of 25 years, this reform has focused especially on young people in transition to adult life, where the consequences of delayed and poor quality of care are greatest. Despite overwhelming logic, a compelling body of evidence, including cost-effectiveness data, reform, and investment, has been hampered by inertia, structural stigma, and a rearguard action, aimed at seeding doubt, by a small number of academic critics. The other major missing element is public engagement and mobilization in support of change. Reform is best informed by science, but it is in the end a sociopolitical process, and there are signs that this is becoming better understood. Early intervention provides a blueprint and launch pad to radically change the wider landscape of mental health care, to prioritize youth mental health, and to dissolve many of the barriers that have constrained progress for so long. This chapter captures the lessons learned and indicates avenues for further progress.

Introduction

For many decades, early intervention has been a central pillar of treatment in all the major physical noncommunicable disease areas. Early intervention can be defined as diagnosis at the earliest possible point, even presymptomatically, followed by proportional or stage-specific intervention, adapted and sustained for as long as necessary and effective. This strategy has been a major factor in the increased survival and better outcomes seen notably in cancer and cardiovascular disease. Mental illness is increasingly recognized as the noncommunicable disease with the greatest impact on human potential and economic productivity since, due to its timing early in the life span and consequent long period of impact, it results directly, and indirectly via physical illness, in a substantial reduction of life expectancy and is responsible for *the* most significant contribution to disability-linked disease burden (Bloom et al. 2011). Yet the curve of mortality and morbidity has not changed, even in developed countries. Given the lessons from cancer and cardiovascular disease, why has early intervention in mental health *not* been an absolutely top priority? We have effective treatments, but they are typically deployed late and without the strategic goal of reducing progression of illness. Provided that at each stage of illness, treatment is proportional (i.e., adapted to maximize benefits and minimize risks), early intervention in mental health care more than qualifies for a green light. This means offering psychosocial and safer biotherapies at earlier undifferentiated stages of illness, where diagnostic and therapeutic specificity has yet to be identified and indeed where it may or may not actually exist. On the other hand, while balancing risks and benefits, as in cancer, treatment should aim to be preemptive rather than reactive to worsening status. Our aim must be to achieve remission and recovery and then to sustain this. While it has been a long hard road to build momentum to make early intervention a standard feature of mental health care, there is a sense that we are at a tipping point. Only high-quality translational research and advocacy will ensure that this is not a mirage or false dawn.

What Is Early Intervention?

In psychiatry, the term early intervention has been interpreted in various ways. Some use it to characterize interventions early in life, many of which are preventive rather than therapeutic. Others use it in relation to relapse prevention, where early means early in an episode of illness, not necessarily the initial one. Still others use it to focus on the early diagnosis and treatment of emerging mental disorders. Early intervention sits within a preventive psychiatry framework. Clearly, prevention is better than cure; however until prevention has been 100% successful, early intervention is the next best thing. When would early intervention not be a good thing? If there are no effective treatments or if the cure was worse than the disease (i.e., the treatments caused more harm than good, as in "the treatment was successful but the patient died"), then early intervention could be useless or worse. In diseases like Alzheimer, where unfortunately there is no effective treatment, early diagnosis is still justified so that the patient and family can be better prepared and supported in relation to the progress of the illness. In psychiatry, even after the discovery of much more effective treatments, a range of factors conspired to create the impression that they might do more harm than good, thus undermining any momentum for early intervention until the past two decades.

Origins of Early Intervention

Despite the overhang of nineteenth-century thinking, embedded in concepts like "degeneration," "dementia praecox," and even "schizophrenia" itself, there were some early pioneers who dared to dream of early intervention. For example, the American social psychiatrist, Harry Stack Sullivan, stated: "I feel certain that many incipient cases might be arrested before the efficient contact with reality is suspended, and a long stay in institutions made necessary" (Sullivan 1927:106–107). Such pioneers were stymied by the lack of effective treatments, but even so, there was a level of naturalistic remission and recovery that began to challenge the Kraepelinian paradigm, even in the latter's own lifetime. Recovery, almost despite contemporary treatment, was clearly possible in schizophrenia, though partially concealed by the *clinician's illusion* (Bleuler et al. 1976; Cohen and Cohen 1984). The clinician's illusion refers to the fact that clinicians' perception of any illness and its prognosis is powerfully shaped by the setting in which they work. In particular, since clinicians are typically more heavily exposed to the more severely and persistently ill subgroup of patients, they form a much more pessimistic mind-set than accords with the true spectrum of outcomes. The advent of effective antipsychotic drugs, developed in the 1950s and the rise of first-generation community psychiatry should have been much more potent in dispelling pessimism and paving the way for early intervention; however, the immature and divided state of psychiatry, the deep stigma and discrimination, the disastrous mismanagement of deinstitutionalization, and the crude way that new medications were used in routine practice combined to sink this possibility. It was not to be until the 1980s when the focus of schizophrenia research would turn to the early stages of psychotic illness and the notion of early diagnosis would become a realistic proposition. Initially, this was driven purely by a research agenda, which proposed that studying first-episode patients who were free of the many confounding variables present in chronic and multi-episode samples would shed more light on etiopathological questions. However, the establishment of streamed, or discrete, early psychosis programs (McGorry 1985; McGorry et al. 1996), intended to facilitate such research, starkly revealed the clinical imperatives both from a harm reduction perspective and as an opportunity to reduce premature death and disability, and enable more complete functional recovery. The value of hope was rediscovered, and although traditionalists dubbed the new approach a "rescue fantasy" (suggesting an unrealistic optimism deriving from the needs of the clinician), an increasing number of rescues were successfully and routinely performed as care evolved, supported by hope and a growing research base.

Progress: Research for Reform

During the 1990s, early intervention for psychosis became a new paradigm. I have previously described in detail how this scientific paradigm developed and spread (McGorry 2015). A phalanx of like-minded and collegial leaders in Australia, Europe, North America, and Asia developed streamed early detection and intensive early intervention programs for psychotic patients, which also functioned as innovation platforms for new research in both neurobiology and novel therapies. Many focused on schizophrenia, but the most successful programs included all forms of early psychosis, presaging the wider transdiagnostic shift that is now underway in early intervention. Factors that enabled this successful paradigm shift were that it

- became a "movement," albeit scientifically grounded;
- was patient and family centered;
- was led by clinician-scientists and not pure researchers or pure clinicians, but was highly inclusive;
- created platforms like the IEPA and later a journal, *Early Intervention in Psychiatry*, to organize the field and build interest, commitment, talent, and careers; and

- engaged in the process of advocacy and reform, and could be characterized as "research for reform," not merely for publication success (which nevertheless certainly occurred as a by-product as the field expanded exponentially).

In addition to the limited lateral expansion beyond schizophrenia into psychotic mood disorders, the focus was extended: earlier than the first episode into the subthreshold or prodromal stage, and later through the "critical period" (Birchwood and Fiorillo 2000) of the first 2–5 years after the first episode, where the major impact of the illness was understood to occur and set the course over the long term. This formed the foundation of our later transdiagnostic clinical staging model (McGorry et al. 2006), which has the potential to reorient all mental health care and research and facilitate prevention, early intervention, and indeed long-term and palliative care.

Lessons Learned

Lesson 1: The need for mental health care precedes the emergence of the major DSM syndromes of interest, and proportional, preemptive treatment is safe and effective

"The onset of a mental illness is generally a gradual one..." (Kraepelin 1909). "Schizophrenia rolls in like a slow fog, becoming imperceptibly thicker as time goes on." (Saks 2007)

Sullivan (1927) and later Meares (1959) wrote eloquently about the prodromal phase of schizophrenia, and Häfner et al. (1992) mapped the evolution of the onset phase of schizophrenia and depression, showing that subthreshold symptoms preceded the current diagnostic threshold in most patients for months or even many years. As early psychosis programs developed, the breakthrough, therapeutically speaking, was to recognize that this subthreshold state caused distress and functional impairment, and therefore a "need for care," and that a subset at least of people in this stage of illness sought help or were prepared to do so. This led to a *prospective* definition of what was termed an "at-risk mental state" (McGorry and Singh 1995; Yung and McGorry 1996), which indicated both the current need for intervention as well as the risk of a more severe stage of illness. Special clinics in stigma-free locations were established to provide care and to study this stage of illness (Phillips et al. 2002a; Yung et al. 1995). An essential feature of this at-risk or ultra-high risk (UHR) concept was that it did not connote *inevitable* risk for a more severe stage psychosis or for schizophrenia. There was a lateral and future valence for other syndromes as well as stasis and remission.

This looser linkage with schizophrenia allowed critics to question the value of the concept from two perspectives. Some misrepresented the whole notion by stating that patients were not ill at all, implying their symptoms were absent or trivial, and that they were not functionally impaired, thus raising the issue of the boundary of mental health care with "normality." These critics used data from population health surveys to suggest that since the lower reaches of the psychosis phenotype appeared to be benign, there was a risk of inappropriate treatment of "normal" people (Frances 2012; van Os and Guloksuz 2017). It has now become clear, however, that low-grade psychotic symptoms, if persistent and associated with anxiety and depression, represent a poor prognostic sign (Kelleher et al. 2012a; van Os et al. 2009). Other critics focused on the partial specificity or valence that the syndrome possessed for future sustained psychotic disorder and argued the "false positive" rate was too high, especially as the rate of transition to psychosis steadily fell. This was one of the key reasons why the endeavor to embed a specific psychosis risk syndrome ultimately failed. However, the false positive rate for psychosis transition not only varies with the degree of serial enrichment of the sample, but when the false positive rate for *any* current or future disorder was revealed (Lin et al. 2015); this turned out to be very low, since those who failed to develop a psychotic illness frequently developed another disorder or comorbid blends. This partial specificity and low false positive rate for any disorder, with overlap of psychosis with other syndromal outcomes, has opened the door to a broad concept of initial common pathways and stages and the clinical staging model (for a recent review of this issue, see McGorry et al. 2018a).

There are two pathways for future research. The first, which appeals especially to those still with confidence in the validity and utility of the schizophrenia concept, is to seek greater precision in prediction of the single syndromal outcome of psychosis or schizophrenia using serial enrichment, biomarkers, and more potent statistical tools (Clark et al. 2016). The second, which is compatible with the first, is to move to a transdiagnostic approach with a broad set of entry criteria (Hartmann et al. 2019) and look at progression rates to several late phenotypes. This has major advantages in terms of yield or power to predict as well as treatment capacity and reflects the major progress that has been achieved in this field: we now have Cochrane level 1 evidence revealing that it is possible to achieve better symptomatic and functional outcomes in the subthreshold or prepsychotic UHR stage and to reduce the one- to two-year risk of progression to full threshold psychosis (Schmidt et al. 2015; van der Gaag et al. 2013, 2019).

The at-risk mental state or UHR concept stimulated great controversy as it revived old controversies around labeling and the risks of overtreatment (Frances 2012). This, in turn, raises key questions of obvious interest in early intervention: When can we say a mental disorder is present? How do mental disorders emerge and evolve? Defining some kind of boundary is necessary, because it is linked to a categorical decision of whether treatment or at least some kind of help is indicated and should be offered. I argue that this should be a fuzzy boundary in which the patient also has a major say, not only health professionals, funders, and polemicists (Frances 2013; Greenberg 2013). There should be a soft entry policy but safeguards linked to proportional treatment, balancing benefits versus risks, guided by the maxim *primum non nocere*. Clinical staging enables this to occur.

Defining a boundary or border zone must be complemented by an understanding of the dynamics of how people move from being "well" to "ill" (Scott 1973). Eaton (2001) has described how this occurs in very clear terms: People develop symptoms through the intensification of existing traits or features within the normal range of experience (e.g., anxiety or sadness), the acquisition of novel subjective experiences (e.g., hallucinations or obsessional thoughts), or a combination of the two. Syndromes or constellations of symptoms develop through the concurrent or sequential accumulation of such experiences and behaviors as well as when they manifest some coherence and stability.

Severity and persistence are the key characteristics for determining whether there is a disorder (McGorry and van Os 2013), although some argue that distress and/or functional impairment must also be present. In real life, these phenomena emerge in sporadic or gradual ways, often ebbing and flowing, sometimes following familiar trajectories and sequences, other times in a more fluid and reversible manner. How they stabilize or fade, and how they attract other features, comorbid patterns, and behaviors has not yet been systematically studied.

In the early stages of mental ill-health, diffuse and unstable subthreshold states of anxiety and depression are common, but often comingle with other features (including psychotic-like disturbances of salience and perception) and emotional dysregulation to produce a kaleidoscopic series of microphenotypes (McGorry and van Os 2013). We have not yet defined which set of variables to include in systematic studies of this stage of illness development, but they could include traditional symptom concepts, momentary emotional and perceptual states, self or corporeal disturbances, and sleep and motor activity changes. Prospective studies can reveal exactly how these microphenotypes resolve or intensify, cohere, and evolve into macrophenotypes such as mania, psychosis, major depression, borderline personality disorder, or blends of these.

In addition to the emergence and evolution of symptoms and syndromes, patienthood, help-seeking, and need for care are influenced and defined by sociological factors, notably prejudice, stigma, and illness behavior (Pilowsky 1969, 1978). Financial constraints can have a strong influence on where the bar is set by governments, social welfare agencies, and health insurers for access to financial coverage for care. Ideological forces also seek to deny the reality of need for care by asserting against all available evidence that mental ill-health is actually part of the human condition (the "worried well") and naturally heals through "resilience." The same could be said about limb fractures, which are common, subject to a natural healing process, and yet require professional intervention for optimal healing. These factors are arguably more potent in the mental health field in distorting the definition of need for care and the boundary between health and illness. More subtle variants of this invalidation involve the unhelpful distinction between high- and low-prevalence disorders. Neglect is common to both. The former are trivialized, the latter sold short.

Lesson 2: There are long delays or failure of access to care, despite reaching diagnostic threshold for serious mental illness, and these can be reduced by community education and early detection

In an influential paper, Wyatt (1991) showed that not only were long delays in access to treatment the norm in schizophrenia but there was a correlation between the length of the duration of untreated psychosis and outcome. The new information that in high-income countries people with fully fledged psychosis had not been able to access treatment for an average of one to two years (Loebel et al. 1992) created a profound effect. It seemed obvious to all that in view of the suffering and obvious risks of untreated illness that access time to treatment should be reduced. Yet some appeared to question this and debated the direction of causality in relation to the link of duration of untreated psychosis (DUP) with outcome. While treatment delay could allow the illness to exert damaging psychosocial effects and possibly neurobiological damage as well, the worse outcome associated with treatment delay could also be explained by those patients with an intrinsically more severe illness presenting later, due to features such as an insidious onset which was more difficult to detect. The latter view arose within the fatalistic mind-set of inevitable deterioration, and essentially suggested that earlier treatment was only justified if longer-term outcomes could be shown to be improved. Systematic reviews and meta-analyses of nonexperimental studies were conducted to try to resolve the issue (Marshall et al. 2005; Perkins et al. 2005); however, only an experimental design in which the DUP variable was manipulated was capable of doing this. From 1992 onward, we have shown at the Early Psychosis Prevention and Intervention Centre in Melbourne that if an early detection team was established and referral sources in the community were educated, then the DUP could be reduced to a matter of weeks (McGorry et al. 1996). Importantly, the Stavanger group—led by Jan-Olav Johannessen, Thomas McGlashan, and T. K. Larsen, who used a quasi-experimental design and employed intensive and sustained community education and detection teams—found that a major reduction of DUP produced better outcomes that were maintained over a long-term period of ten years (Hegelstad et al. 2012). The amount of outcome variance that DUP accounts for is only around 10–15%, but around twice as many patients were found to have achieved recovery at ten years in the experimental group whose DUP was reduced to a matter of weeks. When this experimental intervention was withdrawn at the end of the study, the DUP once again lengthened (Joa et al. 2007). Both community education and mobile case detection were shown to be necessary to achieve a reduction in DUP. If DUP reduction had been combined with sustained intensive stage-specific care, then further improvements could have been expected. What is notable is that despite this issue having been resolved, few services, even early psychosis programs, invest in community education and mobile case detection. This is an excellent example of a failure to implement hard won scientific evidence. Long delays are also seen in other serious mental disorders, notably bipolar disorder, anorexia nervosa, and borderline personality disorder (Chanen 2015; Dagani et al. 2017; de Girolamo et al. 2012; Neubauer et al. 2014).

Lesson 3: Stage-specific interventions are needed in the critical early years post diagnosis

There are numerous examples of this principle (McGorry et al. 2008a). An array of randomized control trials have demonstrated that antipsychotic medication is not appropriate as a first-line treatment during the subthreshold or UHR stage of illness. First-episode psychosis studies have shown that substantially lower doses of antipsychotic medications are effective in achieving remission in drug-naïve patients than are required in multi-episode patients (McGorry et al. 2011; Merlo et al. 2002). The evidence base for maintaining remission and recovery during the critical period post first-episode psychosis is incomplete and a current focus of research attention (Alvarez-Jimenez et al. 2013). When to reduce dosage, in whom, and what other psychosocial interventions support such dose reduction and discontinuation strategies are unclear. The role of long-acting injectables and the timing of clozapine therapy are both active areas of focus within a staged model of treatment (O'Donoghue et al. 2019). Psychosocial interventions have similar stage-related features. The needs of patients and families vary according to illness stage. Family interventions are very different early in the course of illness, and vocational interventions have a more central place and are more effective in the "critical period" in early psychosis (Killackey et al. 2008). Similar issues exist in mood disorders, where less stage-specific research has been conducted (Berk et al. 2017).

Lesson 4: A streamed and flexible early intervention culture of care for first-episode psychosis, with tenure of at least two years for all and up to at least five years for most, is essential to optimize and sustain remission and functional recovery

In contrast to treatment as usual for first-episode psychosis, the value of specialized early psychosis services in producing better outcomes across a wide range of indicators is now fully supported by Cochrane level 1 evidence (Correll et al. 2018). The potency of this effect has probably been underestimated (McGorry et al. 2018c). The studies captured by Correll et al. (2018) in their meta-analysis, while valuable and demonstrative of the genuine value of this approach, may not have revealed the full potential of early intervention. Timeliness, dose, stage specificity, and tenure could all be enhanced. The RAISE study (Kane et al. 2016) illustrated that early intervention is time sensitive and more effective than treatment as usual only if the DUP was less than a median of 74 weeks, which represents a very long DUP. It is likely that much better early remissions and functional recoveries are achievable if DUP can be reduced to a matter of weeks. The median DUP for the Correll et al. (2018) meta-analysis was lower than in RAISE, but further reductions must be possible because few of these models did what is necessary to reduce DUP to a matter of weeks; namely, intensive community education and mobile detection teams. Timing can also be optimized if a clinical high-risk or, better still, a youth-friendly enhanced primary care service is included in the new system of care and a higher percentage of patients can be engaged at this stage of illness. This helps to delay onset, reduce DUP, and ensure patients are well engaged with clinicians at the point of transition, should it occur, or even in some cases to prevent full expression of the vulnerability to psychotic disorder and other comorbidity.

Many of the early intervention programs included in the Correll et al. (2018) meta-analysis were not well separated in terms of clinical pathways or culture from treatment as usual and chronic mental health settings. The dose and tenure of care was variable, and some programs failed to adapt interventions to stage of illness, merely increasing intervention "dose." Another way that outcomes could be improved in early psychosis is by extending the tenure of care from two to at least five years. Two recent studies have shown that if better quality care is delivered for up to five years, the outcome benefits can be safeguarded (Albert et al. 2017; Malla et al. 2017). Finally, we should be able to optimize outcomes and survival by ensuring that physical and sexual health and substance use are integral components of early intervention services.

In summary, it is conceivable that larger effect sizes favoring early intervention could be observed if all components of early intervention services were optimized. In Australia, six such fully-fledged early psychosis systems linked to the headspace primary care system are now in operation and are under evaluation. This body of research should be transformative for health systems everywhere, because it shows that even with existing knowledge and treatments we can "bend the curve" of outcome in a positive direction, reduce suicide rates, and potentially reduce the risk of premature mortality through medical causes. This approach has not yet been extended to other variants of potentially severe and persistent mental illness, but should be the focus of future research.

Lesson 5: Vocational interventions are essential for functional and social recovery

Forty-eight percent of people who ultimately develop a serious mental illness, especially psychosis, will have failed to complete secondary education (Jablensky et al. 1999). A much higher proportion of young people who are seeking help for emerging mental disorders from the general population will already be "not in education, employment or training" (O'Dea et al. 2014). Without specialized individual placement and support interventions, offered within the clinical governance of the mental health service, there will be little or no improvement in vocational outcomes. Clinical trials have shown that safeguarding or restoring vocational trajectories is a highly successful strategy within early intervention services focused on young people (Killackey et al. 2008). Once again, funding models to integrate such approaches horizontally within multidisciplinary teams remain weak and piecemeal; however there are major opportunities for better outcomes and greater cost-effectiveness.

Lesson 6: Early intervention is the best buy in mental health reform

Campion and Knapp (2018) recently reported on the return on investment for various evidence-based elements of mental health care. For both depression and psychosis, early intervention was prominent among the best buys, with early psychosis intervention returning £17.97 for every £1 invested. Many other studies have produced similar results, with savings flowing from direct health care as well as, even more strongly, from indirect savings, notably reduced welfare, prison, suicide, homicide, and housing costs, and increased taxation receipts (Hamilton et al. 2017).

Lesson 7: Early intervention is effective in other mental disorders, not solely psychosis

Evidence from depression, borderline personality disorder, and other diagnoses suggests that there is merit in extending this paradigm across the board in mental health care (Chanen and McCutcheon 2013; Clarke et al. 1995; Hetrick et al. 2017; Stockings et al. 2016). What is striking, however, is the apparent inertia and ambivalence in doing so despite the success of the paradigm in psychosis. In depression, there is a strong appetite for prevention and for increasing the coverage for people with established illness. Early intervention or indicated/targeted intervention for subthreshold depression has been successfully developed (Beardslee et al. 1993; Clarke et al. 2001; Garber et al. 2009) but not widely implemented. The reasons for this may have to do with the extent of unmet need in depression, which obscures the value and undermines the capacity for early intervention. The higher incidence and prevalence of depression means that systems of primary care with high throughput capacity will be a central feature of early intervention for mood disorders. Strangely, although bipolar disorder is a low incidence condition, there is ambivalence in that field regarding the feasibility of early intervention, even though there are long delays before it is diagnosed (for recent discussion, see Duffy 2018; Malhi et al. 2017; McGorry et al. 2018b). A possible solution, one that is transdiagnostic, is outlined in the next two sections.

Lesson 8: Clinical staging provides a heuristic tool for safe, preemptive intervention and etiological research

One of the urgent challenges for psychiatry is to create a simpler, more useful approach to diagnosis. Our traditional diagnostic systems are categorical and siloed, consisting of polythetic operational definitions of clinical phenotypes. The boundaries between syndromes and phenotypes are not clear and comorbidity is the rule rather than the exception. We know that dimensionality underlies most of these phenotypes and that distress, impairment, and need for care are not limited to the full threshold versions of these phenotypes. All of this points to the necessity of establishing a transdiagnostic approach. The dynamics of early psychopathology are complex; emerging microphenotypes ebb and flow, and evolve in numerous patterns that do not follow rigid train tracks to discrete macrophenotypes, such as schizophrenia or bipolar disorder. The reification of these macrophenotypes has led to a spurious certainty about the indications, specificity, and timing of drug therapies, with risks of premature and overtreatment, undertreatment, and mismatched treatment. Emerging psychopathology is a fluid mixture of anxiety, affective dysregulation, aberrant salience, motivational changes, and other features that dynamically influence one another over time, creating a range of clinical patterns. Network analysis, supported by frequent sampling of experience and behavior over time, is well placed as an approach to study emerging psychopathology (Borsboom 2017; Borsboom and Cramer 2013).

In large transdiagnostic samples there is a general psychopathology factor (the "p" factor) that has good predictive validity (Caspi et al. 2014); most domains of psychopathology appear to conform to dimensional rather than categorical models and seem to favor a unitary or at least a noncategorical approach. This thinking is compatible with the creation of the Research Domain Criteria (RDoC) project, which has embraced a transdiagnostic approach in research, attempting to base psychiatric nosology on neuroscience and behavioral science rather than on DSM-defined diagnostic categories (Sanislow 2016).

In my view, these approaches downplay the role of clinical phenotype-based classification and overstate the role of neuroscience and behavioral constructs. Part of the frustration with phenotype-based classification, and the perceived roadblock that it is believed to have introduced to progress in research, may be attributable not to phenotype-based classification per se but rather to the oversimplified and broad nature of contemporary psychopathological descriptions that are present from DSM-III onward, and in many of the instruments used to measure psychopathology in research studies. To adopt geological terminology, focusing on plate tectonics (underlying neurobiology) should not replace or compensate for poor characterization of topography (phenomenology). In addition, the RDoC approach as yet confers no diagnostic benefit to clinical care, and its feasibility in many clinical settings is questionable, because care systems in the U.S.A. and elsewhere are typically structured according to traditional diagnostic categories and block transdiagnostic research. A lack of clinical utility also applies to the Hierarchical Taxonomy of Psychopathology (HiTOP) project, which seeks to provide a hierarchical dimensional approach to psychiatric classification (Kotov et al. 2018). Based in quantitative nosology, HiTOP is promising and has greater intrinsic phenotypic validity; however, like the RDoC model, it is currently cross-sectional and static, lacking a dynamic or longitudinal dimension. While there is a lively debate between proponents of HiTOP and network analysis (Borsboom et al. 2017; Forbes et al. 2017), the latter may have a greater capacity to contribute to the development of new diagnostic approaches. Other dynamic prediction approaches may also come to be of value (Nelson et al. 2017).

Despite the complexity, fluidity, and dimensionality of clinical phenotypes, treatment decisions are binary, and clinicians need categories, however arbitrary (as in hypertension and cancer), to guide their decisions. This is why clinical staging has emerged as a potentially useful model: one that is especially suited to early interventions that seek to preempt progression of illness and enhance understanding of psychopathology over the long-term course of illness across the diagnostic spectrum. To shed further light on the relevancy of this model, a series of papers over the past decade have described its features and reported on findings to date (Cross et al. 2018a; Hickie et al. 2013b; McGorry et al. 2006, 2014b, 2018a; Purcell et al. 2015).

The primary goal of clinical staging is to provide a more accurate guide to treatment selection as well as to prognosis. It also serves to organize research into psychosocial risk factors, neurocognitive variables, and biomarkers (both of current stage and risk for stage development). The model attempts to determine the position of an individual along a continuum of illness (see Figure 14.1), defined according to stages:

Stage 0 = no current symptoms
Stage 1a = help-seeking with distress
Stage 1b = attenuated (i.e., subthreshold) syndrome
Stages 2–4 = full threshold disorder with varying degrees of recurrence and severity

The best known application of clinical staging has been in oncology. One could argue that the progression or resolution of cancer is also a dimensional issue, but we have imposed categories or stages in a successful effort to intervene proportionally and preventively, to reduce the risk of extension of the disease and ultimately death. The risk-benefit ratio is a guide to how aggressively to intervene, with the balance in favor of proactive treatment at each stage, rather than waiting for treatment failure and then stepping up the intensity, as with "stepped care" in mental health, which responds often very belatedly to treatment resistance. Examples of this are dynamic vocational salvage and recovery efforts early in the course of illness, and early use of clozapine in psychosis

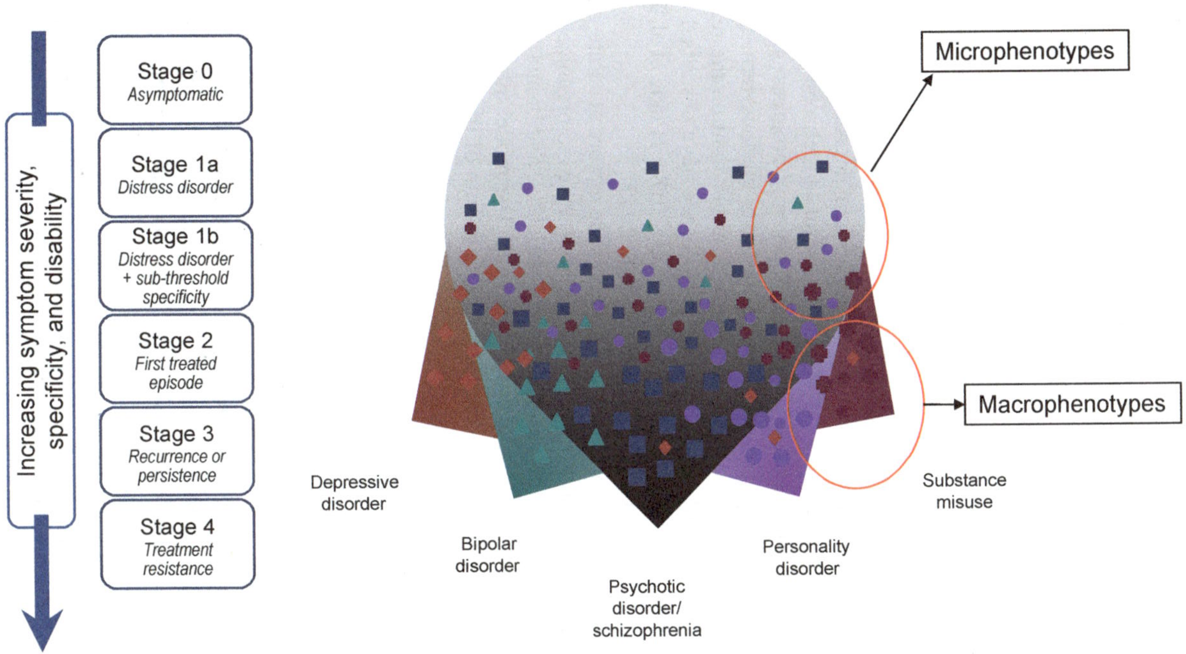

Figure 14.1 Clinical staging model for psychiatry (McGorry et al. 2018a). Reproduced with permission.

(Edwards et al. 2011; Homan and Kane 2018; Killackey et al. 2008, 2019; Okhuijsen-Pfeifer et al. 2018; Thien et al. 2018).

Lesson 9: New stigma-free, developmentally appropriate models of care focused on young people across the peak age of risk for the mental disorders of adult life must be designed and scaled up if early intervention is to be feasible and optimized

The peak incidence and prevalence of mental ill-health among young people in transition to adulthood calls for a new approach to service provision: one that can handle high volumes, allows a role for new technologies, and offers the depth and expertise necessary to manage the diversity, complexity, and persistence of this need. The capacity to cope with the extent of the need for care is crucial if early intervention is to be feasible. Different service levels that cover the entire spectrum of illness complexity and severity are required: from e-health, primary care services, or enhanced primary care services, for those with earlier mild to moderate forms or stages of mental ill-health, to specialized "back-up" services for those with complex presentations or more severe illness. The key principles of such systems can be summarized as follows:

- Youth participation is necessary at all levels to enable the creation of youth-friendly, stigma-free cultures of care that will provide what young people and their families really need, while acknowledging the evolving developmental culture of emerging adults.
- A preventive and optimistic framework must emphasize early intervention and offer holistic, evidence-informed, staged care governed by risk-benefit considerations and shared decision making. Social and vocational outcomes are among the key targets.
- A "one-stop shop" or "integrated practice unit" (Porter and Lee 2013) is integral: multidisciplinary teams of providers need to be organized around the customer (the young person and their family) and their needs, and a dedicated team of clinical and nonclinical personnel will provide the full care cycle for the young person's condition. This fundamentally changes the way clinicians are organized to deliver care. The ideal version involves both horizontal and vertical integration.
- Discontinuity of care at age 18 must be eliminated, because peak periods of care are needed during this crucial developmental transition.
- Positive and seamless linkages with services for younger children and older adults must be secured.
- Flexible tenure and reentry to care, as needed, are required during the critical period of transition to adulthood.

These principles and the models that flow from them to provide care for young people are highly congruent with the perspective of Porter and Lee (2013), who stressed the need for value for patients (the best outcomes at the lowest cost) as the overarching goal in health care. To date, this has been a hallmark of both early intervention and youth mental health reform.

The first and now most extensive example of the development of integrated care for young people began in Australia. In 2006, the Australian Federal Government established *headspace*, a national youth mental health service stream designed to provide highly accessible, youth-friendly centers that promote and support early intervention for mental and substance use disorders in young people through four core service streams: mental health, drug and alcohol services, primary care (general health), and vocational/educational assistance (McGorry et al. 2007b, 2014a). Operating on an enhanced primary care model, headspace provides a multidisciplinary care structure with close links to local specialist services, schools, and other community-based organizations, and offers evidence-based care within a clinical staging framework. In addition to the four core service streams, each headspace center delivers local community awareness campaigns to enhance young peoples' help-seeking behavior, the ability of families and local service providers to identify emerging mental health concerns in young people early, and to strengthen the referral pathways into the service. In addition to these face-to-face services, headspace also runs a 24/7 nationwide online support service (eheadspace) where young people can "chat" with a mental health professional either online or by telephone and access assessment and therapeutic care. In recognition of the issue of youth suicide in Australia, headspace also provides a support service for schools affected by student suicide (headspace school support), which offers a wide range of services.

From the original ten centers in 2006, headspace has been successfully scaled up to reach over 110 Australian communities and many more via eheadspace. The bulk of the young people using headspace services, even when highly distressed, are experiencing mild to moderate levels of mental ill-health and are in the early stages of illness (Rickwood et al. 2014); however, at most headspace sites there is also a substantial subset of young people with more complex, severe, and enduring problems who currently are unable to gain access to the traditional child and adolescent/adult mental health system. An independent evaluation has shown that in addition to greatly improved access, there are modest short-term improvements in outcome in contrast to standard primary care, including reduced self-harm and improved role functioning (Hilferty et al. 2015).

However, headspace is still a work in progress and important gaps remain. The most serious gap lies in its capacity for vertically integrated specialized care. While headspace provides a valuable entry to the health and welfare system and can address the needs of perhaps two-thirds of its clientele through its enhanced primary care capacity, the remainder need a more expert, specialized, and at times more intensive approach, which may include mobile, home-based and outreach care or acute and subacute residential care. To begin to address this gap, the Australian Government has funded the creation of six "enhanced headspace" services, which will be resourced to deliver fully fledged evidence-based early psychosis services and a modest but more flexible stream of funds for nonpsychotic yet complex presentations. These centers will ideally be integrated with and act as the portal for such care. Similar models to headspace have been implemented in other countries, such as Canada, Ireland, Denmark, Israel, the Netherlands, and Singapore. Similar services are being developed in some parts of the U.S.A. and the U.K. A common sequence is for initial catalytic philanthropic funding to develop services and demonstrate effectiveness, which is then followed by government funding to scale up and sustain the venture.

The long-term aim of these reforms is to develop a nationwide youth mental health stream that fully integrates care for young people, so as to provide seamless coverage of mental health care from puberty to mature adulthood (at around 25 years of age), with soft transitions between child and adult mental health care. Distinctions between the tiers of primary and specialist care will be blurred to utilize a staging approach aimed at preempting the progression of illness. This means youth-friendly, stigma-free primary care portals for young people with undifferentiated needs, backed up with intensive community education, mobile detection and assertive treatment teams, and specialized streams of expert care. The latter streams would cover not only early psychosis but also the other major macrophenotypes that emerge, notably complex mood, borderline personality, substance use, and eating disorders. Such vertical integration of care could deliver early intervention and secure tenure of care during the critical period of transition to adulthood, when major mental disorders emerge and embed. Clearly, the success of these reforms will ultimately only be able to be assessed after careful evaluation, and more health services research is necessary to develop, refine, adapt, and evaluate new service models, both within their individual contexts and across sectors.

Lesson 10: Challenges to transformational reform: Evidence is necessary but not sufficient

Mental health remains the poor cousin in health care and medical research. Despite its much greater projected impact on human suffering and productivity over the next 20 years, it continues to be seriously underfunded in comparison with cancer, cardiovascular disease, diabetes, and other noncommunicable diseases. This shortfall is even more dramatic in the developing world. However, in both high-income and low- to middle-income countries, current and future generations of young people are being consigned to the social and economic scrapheap because of the neglect of their major health and social needs. Meanwhile, health expenditures continue to balloon worldwide, with little rationality, thoughts of value for money, or even humanity to guide this. Most people agree that this needs a major rethink (Gawande 2017), and while it will be challenging to contain expenditure in emotionally sensitive areas, we must channel future growth in health expenditure to areas that will benefit people and society most. As Porter and Lee (2013) point out, this will require a reorganization of the health-care system that makes value (meaning the best outcomes for clients at the lowest cost) the overarching goal. Since approaches that deliver better mental health are best positioned to deliver enhanced value at a lower cost than other health expenditures, they should be strongly prioritized. This means affirmative action and preferential investment in the "best buy" of mental health care. However, this does not mean more of the same. In the post-deinstitutionalization era, mental health care itself needs to be reorganized: it must extract itself from many of the unhelpful constraints and perverse incentives that have flowed through its marriage with mainstream medical care, as identified by Porter and Lee (2013). Specifically, we must identify priorities that will result in health gain and value both to the patient and the funder. Obvious low-hanging fruit includes achievable prevention that targets younger children and parenting as well as early intervention strategies for emerging mental ill-health in young people. How can this be achieved? Key steps involve innovation as well as the translation of existing knowledge, effective advocacy, and sociopolitical activism.

Innovators and early adopters need to be nurtured as we seek progress in mental health care. Late adopters should be respected, listened to, persuaded, and convinced on the basis of logic and scientific evidence wherever possible. Skepticism and debate are crucial processes to guide and safeguard effective reform. However, extreme or excessive skepticism should prompt an analysis of motives, since vested interests and ideological groups have been known to misuse science to undermine valid change and reform (Oreskes and Conway 2010). These sociological forces must be understood, recognized and responded to quite differently on their merits within the cycle of innovation and reform. Finally, engaging with the general public and helping them to mobilize in their own self-interest are missing ingredients in securing a fair deal for the mentally ill and to promote reform and investment.

Even in the absence of new therapeutic discoveries, we can still substantially reduce the "avertable burden of disease" (Andrews et al. 2004) by increasing the scale, coverage, and value of mental health care and by reengineering the timing and culture of the provision of services. The related concepts of implementation science and "scaling up" of innovations, especially of service models, are particularly relevant. The scaling up literature (Bradach 2003; Cooley and Kohl 2006), a body of knowledge that cuts across many fields, contains the key elements that are required for success.

We now have Cochrane level 1 evidence for the value of early intervention services for psychosis (Correll et al. 2018; van der Gaag et al. 2013), which is capable of even greater potency. These services have been scaled up in many places worldwide, but coverage is piecemeal, program fidelity patchy, and momentum still too slow. Conversely, integrated primary youth mental health care has been scaled up more rapidly, despite the fact that supporting evidence has followed rather than led the reform. This may be because the value to communities is so palpable that the requirement for disease-modifying evidence is less, because access and engagement have so obviously been improved, the product on offer is so appreciated, and modestly better outcomes are also occurring. Implementation failure is a genuine risk in health services reform and arises from a range of sources. Even when reform has been well funded, threats have arisen from devolved commissioning and poor model fidelity, from mission creep (as seen in the U.K. when early psychosis services were extended across the life span without new resources or evidence), and resistance from clinicians to implementing key evidence-based elements of the model (e.g., community education, mobile detection, and home-based treatment). Additional challenges involve engaging the wider community, creating political will, building the right cultural and physical settings, and attracting a dynamic, skilled, and optimistic workforce.

Conclusion

Early intervention and youth mental health are twin paradigms that have the potential to transform the landscape of mental health over the coming decade. An overarching enabler will be the creation of a professional field of knowledge and expertise to be known as "youth mental health" or even "youth health," which is quite distinct from child and adolescent psychiatry or pediatrics. The concept of adolescent health falls short because it retains the outmoded concept of adolescence, has failed to capture the full extent of the developmental processes in play in the current era, and has minimized the salience of mental ill-health as the major health threat to a flourishing generation and productive society. This new endeavor must draw on a wide range of disciplines and skills, which may help to redefine the emergent field in a way that we can currently not imagine.

Abbreviations

ADHD	attention deficit hyperactivity disorder
ALSPAC	Avon Longitudinal study of parents and children
APSS	attenuated positive symptom syndrome
ASD	autism spectrum disorder
BDNF	brain-derived neurotrophic factor
BIPS	brief intermittent psychotic syndrome
BLA	basolateral amygdala
BMI	body mass index
BPRS	brief psychiatric rating scale
B-SNIP	bipolar and schizophrenia network for intermediate phenotypes
CAARMS	comprehensive assessment of at-risk mental state
CB1R	cannabinoid 1 receptors
CBCM	cognitive behavioral case management
CBT	cognitive behavioral therapy
CCK	cholecystokinin
CHR-P	clinical high-risk for psychosis
CIT	crisis intervention teams
CNS	central nervous system
CNV	copy number variation
COGDIS	cognitive disturbance
DHA	docosahexaenoic
DSM	Diagnostic and Statistical Manual
DTI	diffusion tensor imaging
DUP	duration of untreated psychosis
DZ	dizygotic
EASY	Early Assessment Service for Young (people with psychosis)
EEG	electroencephalography
E-I balance	excitatory-inhibitory balance
EMA	ecological momentary assessment
EPA	eicosapentanoic acid
EPINET	Early Psychosis Intervention Network
EPPIC	Early Psychosis Prevention and Intervention Centre
ESM	experience sampling methodology
FA	fatty acids
FDA	Food and Drug Administration
FEP	first episode of psychosis
FES	first-episode service
fMRI	functional magnetic resonance imaging
GAF	global assessment of functioning
GM	gray matter
GRD	genetic risk and decline
GWAS	genome-wide association studies
HiTOP	Hierarchical Taxonomy of Psychopathology project
HLA	human leucocyte antigen

HPA	hypothalamic pituitary adrenal
HPC	hippocampus
HPG	hypothalamic pituitary axes
ICD	International Classification of Diseases
IEPA	International Early Psychosis Association
IOM	Institute of Medicine
IQR	interquartile
IYMHRN	International Youth Mental Health Research Network
LTD	long-term depression
LTP	long-term potentiation
MEG	magnetic encephalography
MRI	magnetic resonance imaging
MRS	magnetic resonance spectroscopy
MZ	monozygotic
NAMI	National Alliance on Mental Illness
NAPLS	North American Prodrome Longitudinal Study
NAV	Navigate Intervention Package
NEET	not in education, employment, or training
NIMH	National Institute of Mental Health
NMDA	N-methyl-D-aspartate
NVHL	neonatal ventral hippocampal lesion
OASIS	Outreach and Support in South London
PET	positron emission tomography
PFC	prefrontal cortex
PIER	Portland Identification and Early Referral program
PNN	perineuronal net
PUFA	polyunsaturated fatty acids
PV	parvalbumin
QALYs	quality-adjusted life years
RAISE	recovery after an initial schizophrenia episode
RCTs	randomized control trials
RDoC	research domain criteria
SIPS	Structured Interview for Prodromal Symptoms
SOFAS	Social and Occupational Functioning Assessment Scale
SOPS	Scale of Prodromal Symptoms
STEP	Specialized Treatment in Early Psychosis
tDCS	transcranial direct current stimulation
THC	tetrahydrocannabinol
TMS	transcranial magnetic stimulation
UHR-P	ultra-high risk for psychosis
VTA	ventral tegmental area
WM	white matter

Bibliography

Abrahám, H., A. Vincze, I. Jewgenow, et al. 2010. Myelination in the Human Hippocampal Formation from Midgestation to Adulthood. *Int. J. Dev. Neurosci.* **28**:401–410. [9]

Adachi, P. J. C., and T. Willoughby. 2013. Do Video Games Promote Positive Youth Development? *J. Adolesc. Res.* **28**:155–165. [6]

Adams, R. B., R. G. Franklin, N. O. Rule, et al. 2010. Culture, Gaze and the Neural Processing of Fear Expressions. *Soc. Cogn. Affect. Neurosci.* **5**:340–348. [6]

Addington, D. E., E. McKenzie, J. Addington, et al. 2007. Performance Measures for Evaluating Services for People with a First Episode of Psychosis. *Early Interv. Psychiatry* **1**:157–167. [12]

Addington, J., D. Addington, S. Abidi, T. Raedler, and G. Remington. 2017. Canadian Treatment Guidelines for Individuals at Clinical High Risk of Psychosis. *Can. J. of Psychiatry* **62**:656–661. [11]

Addington, J., B. A. Cornblatt, K. S. Cadenhead, et al. 2011. At Clinical High Risk for Psychosis: Outcome for Nonconverters. *Am. J. Psychiatry* **168**:800–805. [11]

Addington, J., and R. K. Heinssen. 2012. Prediction and Prevention of Psychosis in Youth at Clinical High Risk. *Annu. Rev. Clin. Psych.* **8**:269–289. [11]

Addington, J., R. K. Heinssen, D. G. Robinson, et al. 2015. Duration of Untreated Psychosis in Community Treatment Settings in the United States. *Psychiatric Serv.* **66**:753–756. [11]

Agius, M., C. Goh, S. Ulhaq, and P. D. McGorry. 2010. The Staging Model in Schizophrenia, and Its Clinical Implications. *Psychiatria Danub.* **22**:211–220. [2]

Aguzzi, A., B. A. Barres, and M. L. Bennett. 2013. Microglia: Scapegoat, Saboteur, or Something Else? *Science* **339**:156–161. [7]

Akbarian, S., C. Liu, J. A. Knowles, et al. 2015. The Psychencode Project. *Nat. Neurosci.* **18**:1707–1712. [8]

Alameda, L., M. Fournier, I. Khadimallah, et al. 2018. Childhood Trauma Engages Oxidative Stress, Hippocampus Alterations, and Poorer Clinical Outcome in Early Psychosis Patients. *Schizophr. Bull.* **44**:S25–S26. [13]

Alameda, L., P. Golay, P. S. Baumann, et al. 2016. Age at the Time of Exposure to Trauma Modulates the Psychopathological Profile in Patients with Early Psychosis. *J. Clin. Psychiatry* **77**:e612–618. [13]

Albert, N., M. Melau, H. Jensen, et al. 2017. Five Years of Specialised Early Intervention Versus Two Years of Specialised Early Intervention Followed by Three Years of Standard Treatment for Patients with a First Episode Psychosis: Randomised, Superiority, Parallel Group Trial in Denmark (OPUS II). *BMJ* **356**:i6681. [14]

Albrecht, D. S., C. Granziera, J. M. Hooker, and M. L. Loggia. 2016. *In Vivo* Imaging of Human Neuroinflammation. *ACS Chem. Neurosci.* **7**:470–483. [7]

Aldridge, J. M., and K. McChesney. 2018. The Relationships between School Climate and Adolescent Mental Health and Wellbeing: A Systematic Literature Review. *Int. J. Educat. Res.* **88**:121–145. [6]

Alexander, G. E., M. R. DeLong, and P. L. Strick. 1986. Parallel Organization of Functionally Segregated Circuits Linking Basal Ganglia and Cortex. *Annu. Rev. Neurosci.* **9**:357–381. [9]

Alfano, C. A., A. A. Pina, I. K. Villalta, et al. 2009. Mediators and Moderators of Outcome in the Behavioral Treatment of Childhood Social Phobia. *J. Am. Acad. Child Adolesc. Psychiatry* **48**:945. [4]

Ali, S. 2007. "Go West Young Man": The Culture of Migration among Muslims in Hyderabad, India. *J. Ethnic Migration Stud.* **33**:37–58. [6]

Allen, N. B., and P. B. T. Badcock. 2003. The Social Risk Hypothesis of Depressed Mood: Evolutionary, Psychosocial, and Neurobiological Perspectives. *Psychol. Bull.* **129**:887–913. [4]

Allis, C. D., T. Jenuwein, and D. Reinberg. 2007. Overview and Concepts. In: Epigenetics, ed. C. D. Allis et al., pp. 23–62. Cold Spring Harbor: Cold Spring Harbor Laboratory Press. [8]

Alnæs, D., T. Kaufmann, N. T. Doan, et al. 2018. Association of Heritable Cognitive Ability and Psychopathology with White Matter Properties in Children and Adolescents. *JAMA Psychiatry* **75**:287. [4]

Alvarez-Jimenez, M., S. Bendall, P. Koval, et al. 2019. Horyzons Trial: Protocol for a Randomised Controlled Trial of a Moderated Online Social Therapy to Maintain Treatment Effects from First-Episode Psychosis Services. *BMJ Open* **9**:e024104. [10]

Alvarez-Jimenez, M., S. Bendall, R. Lederman, et al. 2013. On the Horyzon: Moderated Online Social Therapy for Long-Term Recovery in First Episode Psychosis. *Schizophr. Res.* **143**:143–149. [14]

Alvarez-Jimenez, M., J. F. Gleeson, S. Bendall, et al. 2018. Enhancing Social Functioning in Young People at Ultra High Risk (UHR) for Psychosis: A Pilot Study of a Novel Strengths and Mindfulness-Based Online Social Therapy. *Schizophr. Res.* **202**:369–337. [10]

Alvarez-Jimenez, M., A. G. Parker, S. E. Hetrick, P. D. McGorry, and J. F. Gleeson. 2011. Preventing the Second Episode: A Systematic Review and Meta-Analysis of Psychosocial and Pharmacological Trials in First-Episode Psychosis. Schizophr Bull. *Schizophr. Bull.* **37**:619–630. [10]

Alvarez-Jimenez, M., A. Priede, S. E. Hetrick, et al. 2012. Risk Factors for Relapse Following Treatment for First Episode Psychosis: A Systematic Review and Meta-Analysis of Longitudinal Studies. *Schizophr. Res.* **139**:116–128. [10]

Amminger, G. P., M. Berger, S. M. Rice, et al. 2017. Novel Biotherapies Are Needed in Youth Mental Health. *Australas. Psychiatry* **25**:117–120. [10]

Amminger, G. P., B. Nelson, C. Markulev, et al. 2018. Neurapro Revisited: Increases in Long-Chain Omega-3 Fatty Acids Improve Functional and Symptomatic Outcomes in Ultrahigh Risk Patients. *Schizophr. Bull.* **44**:228. [10]

Amminger, G. P., M. R. Schäfer, K. Papageorgiou, et al. 2010. Long-Chain Omega-3 Fatty Acids for Indicated Prevention of Psychotic Disorders: A Randomized, Placebo-Controlled Trial. *Arch. Gen. Psychiatry* **67**:146–154. [10, 11]

Amminger, G. P., M. R. Schäfer, M. Schlögelhofer, C. M. Klier, and P. D. McGorry. 2015. Longer-Term Outcome in the Prevention of Psychotic Disorders by the Vienna Omega-3 Study. *Nat. Commun.* **6**:7934. [10]

Andersen, S. L., and M. H. Teicher. 2009. Desperately Driven and No Brakes: Developmental Stress Exposure and Subsequent Risk for Substance Abuse. *Neurosci. Biobehav. Rev.* **33**:516–524. [5]

Anderson, S. A., J. D. Classey, F. Conde, J. S. Lund, and D. A. Lewis. 1995. Synchronous Development of Pyramidal Neuron Dendritic Spines and Parvalbumin-Immunoreactive Chandelier Neuron Axon Terminals in Layer III of Monkey Prefrontal Cortex. *Neuroscience* **67**:7–22. [7]

Andrews, G., C. Issakidis, K. Sanderson, J. Corry, and H. Lapsley. 2004. Utilising Survey Data to Inform Public Policy: Comparison of the Cost-Effectiveness of Treatment of Ten Mental Disorders. *Br. J. Psychiatry* **184**:526–533. [14]

Anticevic, A., M. S. Brumbaugh, A. M. Winkler, et al. 2013. Global Prefrontal and Fronto-Amygdala Dysconnectivity in Bipolar I Disorder with Psychosis History. *Biol. Psychiatry* **73**:565–573. [9]

Arango, C., M. Bernardo, P. Bonet, et al. 2017. When the Healthcare Does Not Follow the Evidence: The Case of the Lack of Early Intervention Programs for Psychosis in Spain. *Revista de Psiquiatría y Salud Mental* **10**:78–86. [11]

Arango, C., C. M. Díaz-Caneja, P. D. McGorry, et al. 2018. Preventive Strategies for Mental Health. *Lancet Psychiatry* **5**:591–604. [13]

Arnold, A. P., and S. M. Breedlove. 1985. Organizational and Activational Effects of Sex Steroids on Brain and Behavior: A Reanalysis. *Horm. Behav.* **19**:469–498. [7]

Arruda-Carvalho, M., W.-C. Wu, K. A. Cummings, and R. L. Clem. 2017. Optogenetic Examination of Prefrontal-Amygdala Synaptic Development. *J. Neurosci.* **37**:2976–2985. [9]

Assies, J., F. Pouwer, A. Lok, et al. 2010. Plasma and Erythrocyte Fatty Acid Patterns in Patients with Recurrent Depression: A Matched Case-Control Study. *PLoS ONE* **5**:e10635. [10]

Atilola, O. 2015. Cross-Cultural Child and Adolescent Psychiatry Research in Developing Countries. *Glob. Mental Health* **2**:1–12. [5]

Australian Government Department of Health and Ageing. 2012. E-Mental Health Strategy for Australia. https://www1.health.gov.au/internet/main/publishing.nsf/content/7C7B0BFEB985D0EBCA257BF0001BB0A6/$File/emstrat.pdf. (accessed July 22, 2019). [10]

Avner, P., and E. Heard. 2001. X-Chromosome Inactivation: Counting, Choice and Initiation. *Nat. Rev. Genet.* **2**:59–67. [8]

Bagge, C. L., C. R. Glenn, and H.-J. Lee. 2013. Quantifying the Impact of Recent Negative Life Events on Suicide Attempts. *J. Abnorm. Psycholog.* **122**:359–368. [3]

Bailey, R. C., and B. F. S. Grenyer. 2014. Supporting a Person with Personality Disorder: A Study of Carer Burden and Well-Being. *J. Pers. Disord.* **28**:796–809. [10]

Bailey, S., and M. Dolan, eds. 2004. Adolescent Forensic Psychiatry, vol. London: Arnold. [6]

Baker, K. D., M. L. Den, B. M. Graham, and R. Richardson. 2014. A Window of Vulnerability: Impaired Fear Extinction in Adolescence. *Neurobiol. Learn. Mem.* **113**:90–100. [9]

Bannerman, D. M., M. Grubb, R. M. Deacon, et al. 2003. Ventral Hippocampal Lesions Affect Anxiety but Not Spatial Learning. *Behav. Brain Res.* **139**:197–213. [9]

Bannerman, D. M., J. N. Rawlins, S. B. McHugh, et al. 2004. Regional Dissociations within the Hippocampus: Memory and Anxiety. *Neurosci. Biobehav. Rev.* **28**:273–283. [9]

Bannerman, D. M., R. Sprengel, D. J. Sanderson, et al. 2014. Hippocampal Synaptic Plasticity, Spatial Memory and Anxiety. *Nature reviews. Neuroscience* **15**:181–192. [9]

Bányai, F., Á. Zsila, O. Király, et al. 2017. Problematic Social Media Use: Results from a Large-Scale Nationally Representative Adolescent Sample. *PLoS ONE* **12**:e0169839. [6]

Barnea-Goraly, N., V. Menon, M. Eckert, et al. 2005. White Matter Development During Childhood and Adolescence: A Cross-Sectional Diffusion Tensor Imaging Study. *Cereb. Cortex* **15**:1848–1854. [7]

Bartholomeusz, C. F., V. L. Cropley, C. Wannan, et al. 2017. Structural Neuroimaging across Early-Stage Psychosis: Aberrations in Neurobiological Trajectories and Implications for the Staging Model. *Aust. N. Z. J. Psychiatry* **51**:455–476. [13]

Bartholomeusz, C. F., E. Killacky, A. Thompson, and S. J. Wood. 2011. Interventions Targeting Social and Vocational Dysfunction in Individuals with a Schizophrenia Spectrum Disorder. In: Handbook of Schizophrenia Spectrum Disorders, ed. M. S. Ritsner, vol. 3. Heidelberg: Springer. [1]

Baum, G. L., R. Ciric, D. R. Roalf, et al. 2017. Modular Segregation of Structural Brain Networks Supports the Development of Executive Function in Youth. *Curr. Biol.* **27**:1561. [4]

Baumann, P. S., S. Crespi, R. Marion-Veyron, et al. 2013. Treatment and Early Intervention in Psychosis Program (Tipp-Lausanne): Implementation of an Early Intervention Programme for Psychosis in Switzerland. *Early Interv. Psychiatry* **7**:322–328. [13]

Bays, H. E. 2007. Safety Considerations with Omega-3 Fatty Acid Therapy. *Am. J. Cardiol.* **99**:35C–43C. [10]

Beardslee, W. R., P. Salt, K. Porterfield, et al. 1993. Comparison of Preventive Interventions for Families with Parental Affective Disorder. *J. Am. Acad. Child Adolesc. Psychiatry* **32**:254–263. [14]

Becker, K. D., S. L. Buckingham, L. R. Najarian, and E. R. Kline. 2015. The Common Elements of Treatment Engagement for Clinically High-Risk Youth and Youth with First-Episode Psychosis. *Early Interv. Psychiatry* **10**:455–467. [11]

Bedi, G., F. Carrillo, G. A. Cecchi, et al. 2015. Automated Analysis of Free Speech Predicts Psychosis Onset in High-Risk Youths. *npj Schizophrenia* **1**:15030. [6]

Bedrosian, T. A., and R. J. Nelson. 2013. Influence of the Modern Light Environment on Mood. *Mol. Psychiatr.* **18**:751–757. [6]

———. 2017. Timing of Light Exposure Affects Mood and Brain Circuits. *Transl. Psychiatry* **7**:e1017–e1017. [6]

Bedrosian, T. A., C. A. Vaughn, A. Galan, et al. 2013. Nocturnal Light Exposure Impairs Affective Responses in a Wavelength-Dependent Manner. *J. Neurosci.* **33**:13081–13087. [6]

Benca, R. M., W. H. Obermeyer, R. A. Thisted, and J. C. Gillin. 1992. Sleep and Psychiatric Disorders: A Meta-Analysis. *Arch. Gen. Psychiatry* **49**:651–668. [2]

Benes, F. M. 1989. Myelination of Cortical-Hippocampal Relays During Late Adolescence. *Schizophr. Bull.* **15**:585–593. [7, 9]

Benes, F. M., M. Turtle, Y. Khan, and P. Farol. 1994. Myelination of a Key Relay Zone in the Hippocampal Formation Occurs in the Human Brain During Childhood, Adolescence, and Adulthood. *Arch. Gen. Psychiatry* **51**:477–484. [9]

Benros, M. E., P. R. Nielsen, M. Nordentoft, et al. 2011. Autoimmune Diseases and Severe Infections as Risk Factors for Schizophrenia: A 30-Year Population-Based Register Study. *Am. J. Psychiatry* **168**:1303–1310. [8]

Berardi, N., T. Pizzorusso, and L. Maffei. 2000. Critical Periods During Sensory Development. *Curr Opin. Neurobiol.* **10**:138–145. [7]

Berens, A. E., S. K. G. Jensen, and C. A. Nelson. 2017. Biological Embedding of Childhood Adversity: From Physiological Mechanisms to Clinical Implications. *BMC Med.* **15**:135. [6]

Berger, M. E., S. Smesny, S. W. Kim, et al. 2017. Omega-6 to Omega-3 Polyunsaturated Fatty Acid Ratio and Subsequent Mood Disorders in Young People with At-Risk Mental States: A 7-Year Longitudinal Study. *Transl. Psychiatry* **7**:e1220–1226. [10]

Berk, M., P. Conus, N. Lucas, et al. 2007. Setting the Stage: From Prodrome to Treatment Resistance in Bipolar Disorder. *Bipolar Disord.* **9**:671–678. [2]

Berk, M., F. Kapczinski, A. C. Andreazza, et al. 2011. Pathways Underlying Neuroprogression in Bipolar Disorder: Focus on Inflammation, Oxidative Stress and Neurotrophic Factors. *Neurosci. Biobehav. Rev.* **35**:804–817. [9]

Berk, M., R. Post, A. Ratheesh, et al. 2017. Staging in Bipolar Disorder: From Theoretical Framework to Clinical Utility. *World Psychiatry* **16**:236–244. [14]

Berretta, S., D. W. Munno, and F. M. Benes. 2001. Amygdalar Activation Alters the Hippocampal GABA System: "Partial" Modelling for Postmortem Changes in Schizophrenia. *J. Comput. Neurol.* **431**:129–138. [8]

Bertelsen, M., P. Jeppesen, L. Petersen, et al. 2008. Five-Year Follow-up of a Randomized Multicenter Trial of Intensive Early Intervention vs. Standard Treatment for Patients with a First Episode of Psychotic Illness: The OPUS Trial. *Arch. Gen. Psychiatry* **65**:762–771. [11]

Beurdeley, M., J. Spatazza, H. H. Lee, et al. 2012. Otx2 Binding to Perineuronal Nets Persistently Regulates Plasticity in the Mature Visual Cortex. *J. Neurosci.* **32**:9429–9437. [7]

Bhugra, D., and M. A. Becker. 2005. Migration, Cultural Bereavement and Cultural Identity. *World Psychiatry* **4**:18–24. [6

Biagianti, B., D. Hidalgo-Mazzei, and N. Meyer. 2017. Developing Digital Interventions for People Living with Serious Mental Illness: Perspectives from Three mHealth Studies. *Evid. Based Mental Health* **20**:98–101. [6]

Bickart, K. C., M. C. Hollenbeck, L. F. Barrett, and B. C. Dickerson. 2012. Intrinsic Amygdala-Cortical Functional Connectivity Predicts Social Network Size in Humans. *J. Neurosci.* **32**:14729–14741. [6]

Bickart, K. C., C. I. Wright, R. J. Dautoff, B. C. Dickerson, and L. F. Barrett. 2011. Amygdala Volume and Social Network Size in Humans. *Nat. Neurosci.* **14**:163–164. [6]

Bilbo, S. D., N. J. Newsum, D. B. Sprunger, et al. 2007. Differential Effects of Neonatal Handling on Early Life Infection-Induced Alterations in Cognition in Adulthood. *Brain Behav. Immun.* **21**:332–342. [7]

Bilbo, S. D., and J. M. Schwarz. 2009. Early-Life Programming of Later-Life Brain and Behavior: A Critical Role for the Immune System. *Front. Behav. Neurosci.* **3**:14. [9]

———. 2012. The Immune System and Developmental Programming of Brain and Behavior. *Front. Neuroendocrin.* **33**:267–286. [7]

Birchwood, M., and A. Fiorillo. 2000. The Critical Period for Early Intervention. *Psychiatric Rehabilit. Skills* **4**:182–198. [14]

Bird, V., P. Premkumar, T. Kendall, et al. 2010. Early Intervention Services, Cognitive-Behavioural Therapy and Family Intervention in Early Psychosis: Systematic Review. *Br. J. Psychiatry* **197**:350–356. [10]

Bitanihirwe, B. K., M. P. Lim, and T.-U. W. Woo. 2010a. N-Methyl-D-Aspartate Receptor Expression in Parvalbumin-Containing Inhibitory Neurons in the Prefrontal Cortex in Bipolar Disorder. *Bipolar Disord.* **12**:95–101. [7]

Bitanihirwe, B. K., D. Peleg-Raibstein, F. Mouttet, J. Feldon, and U. Meyer. 2010b. Late Prenatal Immune Activation in Mice Leads to Behavioral and Neurochemical Abnormalities Relevant to the Negative Symptoms of Schizophrenia. *Neuropsychopharmacology* **32**:2462–2478. [7]

Bitanihirwe, B. K., L. Weber, J. Feldon, and U. Meyer. 2010c. Cognitive Impairment Following Prenatal Immune Challenge in Mice Correlates with Prefrontal Cortical Akt1 Deficiency. *Int. J. Neuropsychopharmacol.* **13**:981–996. [7]

Björkqvist, K., K. M. J. Lagerspetz, and A. Kaukiainen. 1992. Do Girls Manipulate and Boys Fight? Developmental Trends in Regard to Direct and Indirect Aggression. *Aggressive Behav.* **18**:117–127. [6]

Blakemore, S. J. 2008. The Social Brain in Adolescence. *Nature reviews. Neuroscience* **9**:267–277. [9]

Blakemore, S. J., S. Burnett, and R. E. Dahl. 2010. The Role of Puberty in the Developing Adolescent Brain. *Hum. Brain Mapp.* **31**:926–933. [4, 7]

Blakemore, S. J., and K. L. Mills. 2014. Is Adolescence a Sensitive Period for Sociocultural Processing? *Annu. Rev. Psychol.* **65**:187–207. [5]

Blank, T., and M. Prinz. 2013. Microglia as Modulators of Cognition and Neuropsychiatric Disorders. *Glia* **61**:62–70. [7]

Blay, S. L., J. Aguiar, and I. C. Passos. 2016. Polycystic Ovary Syndrome and Mental Disorders: A Systematic Review and Exploratory Meta-Analysis. *Neuropsychiatr. Dis. Treat.* **12**:2895–2903. [6]

Bleuler, M., G. Huber, G. Gross, and R. Schüttler. 1976. The Long-Term Course of Schizophrenic Psychoses: The Combined Results of Two Research Studies. *Nervenarzt* **47**:477– 481. [14]

Bloch, M. H., and J. Hannestad. 2012. Omega-3 Fatty Acids for the Treatment of Depression: Systematic Review and Meta-Analysis. Molecular Psychiatry. *Mol. Psychiatr.* **17**:1272–1282. [10]

Blondeau, N., C. Nguemeni, D. N. Debruyne, et al. 2009. Subchronic Alpha-Linolenic Acid Treatment Enhances Brain Plasticity and Exerts an Antidepressant Effect: A Versatile Potential Therapy for Stroke. *Neuropsychopharmacology* **34**:2548–2559. [10]

Bloom, D. E., E. T. Cafiero, E. Jané-Llopis, et al. 2011. The Global Economic Burden of Non-Communicable Diseases. A Report by the World Economic Forum and the Harvard School of Public Health. Geneva: World Economic Forum. [2, 14]

Blum, R. W., F. I. Bastos, C. W. Kabiru, and L. C. Le. 2012. Adolescent Health in the 21st Century. *Lancet* **379**:1567–1568. [5]

Bond, G. R., L. Evans, M. P. Salyers, J. Williams, and H. W. Kim. 2000. Measurement of Fidelity in Psychiatric Rehabilitation. *Ment. Health Serv. Res.* **2**:75–87. [12]

Bondi, C. O., A. Y. Taha, J. L. Tock, et al. 2014. Adolescent Behavior and Dopamine Availability Are Uniquely Sensitive to Dietary Omega-3 Fatty Acid Deficiency. *Biol. Psychiatry* **75**:38–46. [8]

Borison, R. L., and B. I. Diamond. 1978. A New Animal Model for Schizophrenia: Interactions with Adrenergic Mechanisms. *Biol. Psychiatry* **13**:217–225. [8]

Bornstein, M. H. 2013. Parenting and Child Mental Health: A Cross-Cultural Perspective. *World Psychiatry* **12**:258–265. [6]

Borsboom, D. 2017. A Network Theory of Mental Disorders. *World Psychiatry* **16**:5–13. [1, 14]

Borsboom, D., and A. O. J. Cramer. 2013. Network Analysis: An Integrative Approach to the Structure of Psychopathology. *Annu. Rev. Clin. Psych.* **9**:91–121. [14]

Borsboom, D., E. I. Fried, S. Epskamp, et al. 2017. False Alarm? A Comprehensive Reanalysis of "Evidence That Psychopathology Symptom Networks Have Limited Replicability" by Forbes, Wright, Markon, and Krueger (2017). *J. Abnorm. Psycholog.* **126**:989–999. [14]

Bos, P. A., J. Panksepp, R. M. Bluthe, and J. van Honk. 2012. Acute Effects of Steroid Hormones and Neuropeptides on Human Social-Emotional Behavior: A Review of Single Administration Studies. *Front. Neuroendocrin.* **33**:17–35. [4]

Bottjer, S. W., and F. Johnson. 1997. Circuits, Hormones, and Learning: Vocal Behavior in Songbirds. *J. Neurobiol.* **33**:602–618. [4]

Bourc'his, D., and T. H. Bestor. 2004. Meiotic Catastrophe and Retrotransposon Reactivation in Male Germ Cells Lacking Dnmt3L. *Nature* **431**:96–99. [8]

Bourgeois, J. P., P. S. Goldman-Rakic, and P. Rakic. 1994. Synaptogenesis in the Prefrontal Cortex of Rhesus Monkeys. *Cereb. Cortex* **4**:78–96. [9]

Bouwmeester, H., G. Wolterink, and J. M. van Ree. 2002. Neonatal Development of Projections from the Basolateral Amygdala to Prefrontal, Striatal, and Thalamic Structures in the Rat. *J. Comput. Neurol.* **442**:239–249. [9]

Braams, B. R., A. C. van Duijvenvoorde, J. S. Peper, and E. A. Crone. 2015. Longitudinal Changes in Adolescent Risk-Taking: A Comprehensive Study of Neural Responses to Rewards, Pubertal Development, and Risk-Taking Behavior. *J. Neurosci.* **35**:7226–7238. [4, 9]

Bradach, J. L. 2003. Going to Scale: The Challenge of Replicating Social Programs. *Stanford Soc. Innov. Rev.* **1**:19–25. [14]

Braff, D. L., T. A. Greenwood, N. R. Swerdlow, et al. 2008. Advances in Endophenotyping Schizophrenia. *World Psychiatry* **7**:11–18. [8]

Brainstorm Consortium, V. Anttila, B. Bulik-Sullivan, et al. 2018. Analysis of Shared Heritability in Common Disorders of the Brain. *Science* **360**:eaap8757. [6]

Braithwaite, D., D. H. Moore, R. H. Lustig, et al. 2009. Socioeconomic Status in Relation to Early Menarche among Black and White Girls. *Cancer Causes Control* **20**:713–720. [9]

Bramen, J. E., J. A. Hranilovich, R. E. Dahl, et al. 2012. Sex Matters During Adolescence: Testosterone-Related Cortical Thickness Maturation Differs between Boys and Girls. *PLoS ONE* **7**:e33850. [9]

Bratman, G. N., J. P. Hamilton, K. S. Hahn, G. C. Daily, and J. J. Gross. 2015. Nature Experience Reduces Rumination and Subgenual Prefrontal Cortex Activation. *PNAS* **112**:8567–8572. [6]

Brazier, J. 2010. Is the EQ-5D Fit for Purpose in Mental Health? *Br. J. Psychiatry* **197**:348–349. [12]

Brennand, K. J., A. Simone, J. Jou, et al. 2011. Modelling Schizophrenia Using Human Induced Pluripotent Stem Cells. *Nature* **473**:221–225. [8]

Bridge, J. A., S. Iyengar, C. B. Salary, et al. 2007. Clinical Response and Risk for Reported Suicidal Ideation and Suicide Attempts in Pediatric Antidepressant Treatment: A Meta-Analysis of Randomized Controlled Trials. *JAMA* **297**:1683–1696. [10]

Brody, G. H., S. M. Kogan, Y.-F. Chen, and V. McBride Murry. 2008. Long-Term Effects of the Strong African American Families Program on Youths' Conduct Problems. *J. Adolesc. Health* **43**:474–481. [6]

Bronfenbrenner, U. 1994. Ecological Models of Human Development. In: International Encyclopedia of Education, pp. 37–43, vol. 3. Oxford: Elsevier. [5]

———. 1996. The Ecology of Human Development: Experiments by Nature and Design. Cambridge, MA: Harvard Univ. Press. [6]

Brothers, L. 1990. The Social Brain: A Project for Integrating Primate Behavior and Neurophysiology in a New Domain. *Concepts Neurosci.* **1**:27–51. [6]

Brown, A. S. 2006. Prenatal Infection as a Risk Factor for Schizophrenia. *Schizophr. Bull.* **32**:200–202. [8]

———. 2011. The Environment and Susceptibility to Schizophrenia. *Prog. Neurobiol.* **93**:23–58. [8]

Brumbach, B. H., A. J. Figueredo, and B. J. Ellis. 2009. Effects of Harsh and Unpredictable Environments in Adolescence on Development of Life History Strategies: A Longitudinal Test of an Evolutionary Model. *Hum. Nat.* **20**:25–51. [5]

Bruns, R. F., S. N. Mitchell, K. A. Wafford, et al. 2018. Preclinical Profile of a Dopamine D1 Potentiator Suggests Therapeutic Utility in Neurological and Psychiatric Disorders. *Neuropharmacology* **128**:351–365. [7]

Bucci, S., K. Berry, C. Barrowclough, and G. Haddock. 2016. Family Interventions in Psychosis: A Review of the Evidence and Barriers to Implementation. *Aust. Psychol.* **51**:62–68. [10]

Buckholtz, J. W., and A. Meyer-Lindenberg. 2012. Psychopathology and the Human Connectome: Toward a Transdiagnostic Model of Risk for Mental Illness. *Neuron* **74**:990–1004. [2]

Budday, S., P. Steinmann, and E. Kuhl. 2015. Physical Biology of Human Brain Development. *Front. Cell. Neurosci.* **9**:257. [7]

Burns, J. K. 2013. Pathways from Cannabis to Psychosis: A Review of the Evidence. *Front. Psychiatry* **4**:128. [7]

Burt, S. A. 2009. Rethinking Environmental Contributions to Child and Adolescent Psychopathology: A Meta-Analysis of Shared Environmental Influences. *Psychol. Bull.* **135**:608–637. [6]

Busner, J., S. D. Targum, and D. S. Miller. 2009. The Clinical Global Impressions Scale: Errors in Understanding and Use. *Compr. Psychiatry* **50**:257–262. [10]

Butterworth, P., and H. Berry. 2004. Addressing Mental Health Problems as a Strategy to Promote Employment: An Overview of Interventions and Approaches. *Aust. Soc. Policy* **2004**:19–24. [1]

Cabungcal, J. H., D. S. Counotte, E. M. Lewis, et al. 2014. Juvenile Antioxidant Treatment Prevents Adult Deficits in a Developmental Model of Schizophrenia. *Neuron* **83**:1073–1084. [9]

Cabungcal, J. H., P. Steullet, R. Kraftsik, M. Cuenod, and K. Q. Do. 2013a. Early-Life Insults Impair Parvalbumin Interneurons Via Oxidative Stress: Reversal by N-Acetylcysteine. *Biol Psychiat* **73**:574–582. [13]

Cabungcal, J. H., P. Steullet, H. Morishita, et al. 2013b. Perineuronal Nets Protect Fast-Spiking Interneurons against Oxidative Stress. *PNAS* **110**:9130–9135. [7]

Cadenhead, K., J. Addington, T. Cannon, et al. 2017. 23rd Omega-3 Fatty Acid Versus Placebo in a Clinical High-Risk Sample from the North American Prodrome Longitudinal Studies (NAPLS) Consortium. *Schizophr. Bull.* **43**:S16. [10, 11]

Cadenhead, K., and H. Mirzakhanian. 2016. A Case of Attenuated Psychosis Syndrome: A Broad Differential Diagnosis Requires Broad-Spectrum Treatment. Am. J. Psychiatry 173:321–329. [10]

Caira, M. 2008. The Concept of Migration and Clandestinity in the Chinese Culture. *Soc. Sci. Informat.* **47**:623–628. [6]

Call, K. T., and J. T. Mortimer. 2001. Arenas of Comfort in Adolescence: A Study of Adjustment in Context. Mahwah: Lawrence Erlbaum Associates. [5]

Callaghan, T., P. Rochat, A. Lillard, et al. 2005. Synchrony in the Onset of Mental-State Reasoning: Evidence from Five Cultures. *Psychol. Sci.* **16**:378–384. [6]

Campion, J., and M. Knapp. 2018. The Economic Case for Improved Coverage of Public Mental Health Interventions. *Lancet Psychiatry* **5**:103–105. [14]

Cannon, T. D., K. Cadenhead, B. A. Cornblatt, et al. 2008. Prediction of Psychosis in Youth at High Clinical Risk: A Multisite Longitudinal Study in North America. *Arch. Gen. Psychiatry* **65**:28–37. [11]

Cannon, T. D., C. Yu, J. Addington, et al. 2016. An Individualized Risk Calculator for Research in Prodromal Psychosis. *Am. J. Psychiatry* **173**:980-988. [11]

Cantor-Graae, E., and J.-P. Selten. 2005. Schizophrenia and Migration: A Meta-Analysis and Review. *Am. J. Psychiatry* **162**:12–24. [6, 8]

Carballedo, A., J. Scheuerecker, E. Meisenzahl, et al. 2011. Functional Connectivity of Emotional Processing in Depression. *J. Affective Disord.* **134**:272–279. [9]

Cardis, R., J. H. Cabungcal, D. Dwir, K. Q. Do, and P. Steullet. 2018. A Lack of GluN2A-Containing NMDA Receptors Confers a Vulnerability to Redox Dysregulation: Consequences on Parvalbumin Interneurons, and Their Perineuronal Nets. *Neurobiol. Dis.* **109**:64–75. [7]

Cardoos, S. L., A. B. Suleiman, M. Johnson, et al. 2017. Social Status Strategy in Early Adolescent Girls: Testosterone and Value-Based Decision Making. *Psychoneuroendocrinol.* **81**:14–21. [4]

Carpenter, J. S., A. C. Abelmann, S. N. Hatton, et al. 2017a. Pineal Volume and Evening Melatonin in Young People with Affective Disorders. *Brain Imaging Behav.* **11**:1741–1750. [2]

Carpenter, J. S., R. Robillard, D. F. Hermens, et al. 2017b. Sleep-Wake Profiles and Circadian Rhythms of Core Temperature and Melatonin in Young People with Affective Disorders. *J. Psychiatr. Res.* **94**:131–138. [2]

Carpenter, J. S., R. Robillard, and I. B. Hickie. 2015a. Variations in the Sleep-Wake Cycle from Childhood to Adulthood: Chronobiological Perspectives. *ChronoPhysiolo. Therapy* **5**:37–49. [2]

Carpenter, J. S., R. Robillard, R. S. Lee, et al. 2015b. The Relationship between Sleep-Wake Cycle and Cognitive Functioning in Young People with Affective Disorders. *PLoS ONE* **10**:e0124710. [2]

Carr, V., S. Halpin, N. Lau, et al. 2000. A Risk Factor Screening and Assessment Protocol for Schizophrenia and Related Psychosis. *Aust. N. Z. J. Psychiatry* **34**:S170–180. [11]

Carrera Fernández, M. V., M. L. Fernández, Y. R. Castro, J. M. Failde Garrido, and M. C. Otero. 2013. Bullying in Spanish Secondary Schools: Gender-Based Differences. *Span. J. Psychol.* **16**:E21. [6]

Carrión, R. E., B. A. Cornblatt, C. Z. Burton, et al. 2016. Personalized Prediction of Psychosis: External Validation of the NAPLS-2 Psychosis Risk Calculator with the Edippp Project. *Am. J. Psychiatry* **173**:989-996. [8, 11]

Casey, B. J., N. Craddock, B. N. Cuthbert, et al. 2013. DSM-5 and RDoC: Progress in Psychiatry Research? *Nat. Rev. Neurosci.* **14**:810–814. [2]

Casey, B. J., and R. M. Jones. 2010. Neurobiology of the Adolescent Brain and Behavior: Implications for Substance Use Disorders. *J. Am. Acad. Child Adolesc. Psychiatry* **49**:1189–1201. [9]

Casey, B. J., M. E. Oliveri, and T. Insel. 2014. A Neurodevelopmental Perspective on the Research Domain Criteria (RDoC) Framework. *Biol. Psychiatry* **76**:350–353. [9]

Caspi, A., R. M. Houts, D. W. Belsky, et al. 2014. The P Factor: One General Psychopathology Factor in the Structure of Psychiatric Disorders? *Clin. Psychol. Sci.* **2**:119–137. [1, 14]

Caspi, A., and T. E. Moffitt. 2018. All for One and One for All: Mental Disorders in One Dimension. *Am. J. Psychiatry* **175**:831–844. [1]

Castro-Nallar, E., M. L. Bendall, M. Perez-Losada, et al. 2015. Composition, Taxonomy and Functional Diversity of the Oropharynx Microbiome in Individuals with Schizophrenia and Controls. *PeerJ* **3**:e1140. [7]

Caudill, W. 1973. The Influence of Social Structure and Culture on Human Behavior in Modern Japan. *Ethos* **1**:343–382. [6]

Cecil, C. A. M., E. Walton, R. G. Smith, et al. 2016. DNA Methylation and Substance-Use Risk: A Prospective, Genome-Wide Study Spanning Gestation to Adolescence. *Transl. Psychiatry* **6**:e976–e976. [6]

Celec, P., D. Ostatnikova, and J. Hodosy. 2015. On the Effects of Testosterone on Brain Behavioral Functions. *Front. Neurosci.* **9**:12. [7]

Cesta, C. E., M. Månsson, C. Palm, et al. 2016. Polycystic Ovary Syndrome and Psychiatric Disorders: Co-Morbidity and Heritability in a Nationwide Swedish Cohort. *Psychoneuroendocrinol.* **73**:196–203. [6]

Chalmers, J. B., and M. A. R. Townshend. 1990. The Effects of Training in Social Perspective Taking on Socially Maladjusted Girls. *Child Dev.* **61**:178–190. [4]

Chambers, D. A., and W. E. Norton. 2016. The Adaptome. *Am. J. Prev. Med.* **51**:124–131. [12]

Chambers, R. A., J. R. Taylor, and M. N. Potenza. 2003. Developmental Neurocircuitry of Motivation in Adolescence: A Critical Period of Addiction Vulnerability. *Am. J. Psychiatry* **160**:1041–1052. [9]

Chan, S. K. W., E. Y. N. Ching, K. S. C. Lam, et al. 2017. Newspaper Coverage of Mental Illness in Hong Kong between 2002 and 2012: Impact of Introduction of a New Chinese Name of Psychosis. *Early Interv. Psychiatry* **11**:342–345. [11]

Chanen, A. M. 2015. Borderline Personality Disorder in Young People: Are We There Yet? *J. Clin. Psychol.* **71**:778–791. [14]

Chanen, A. M., and L. McCutcheon. 2013. Prevention and Early Intervention for Borderline Personality Disorder: Current Status and Recent Evidence. The British Journal of Psychiatry Supplement. *Br. J. Psychiatry Suppl.* **54**:24–29. [10, 14]

Chanen, A. M., C. Sharp, Hoffman, P., and Global Alliance for Prevention and Early Intervention for Borderline Personality Disorder. 2017. Prevention and Early Intervention for Borderline Personality Disorder: A Novel Public Health Priority. *World Psychiatry* **16**:215–216. [10]

Chang, W. C., V. W. Y. Kwong, E. S. K. Lau, et al. 2017. Sustainability of Treatment Effect of a 3-Year Early Intervention Programme for First-Episode Psychosis. *Br. J. Psychiatry* **211**:37–44. [11]

Charalampopoulos, D., A. McLoughlin, C. E. Elks, and K. K. Ong. 2014. Age at Menarche and Risks of All-Cause and Cardiovascular Death: A Systematic Review and Meta-Analysis. *Am. J. Epidemiol.* **180**:29–40. [6]

Chauhan, A., V. Chauhan, and T. Brown. 2010. Autism: Oxidative Stress, Inflammation, and Immune Abnormalities. Boca Raton: Taylor & Francis. [7]

Cheer, J. F., K. M. Wassum, M. L. Heien, P. E. Phillips, and R. M. Wightman. 2004. Cannabinoids Enhance Subsecond Dopamine Release in the Nucleus Accumbens of Awake Rats. *J. Neurosci.* **24**:4393–4400. [7]

Chen, C. S., and S. Farruggia. 2002. Culture and Adolescent Development. *Online Read. Psychol. Culture* **6**:1–12. [5]

Chen, E., and G. E. Miller. 2013. Socioeconomic Status and Health: Mediating and Moderating Factors. *Annu. Rev. Clin. Psych.* **9**:723–749. [4]

Chen, E. Y. H., J. Y. M. Tang, C. L. M. Hui, et al. 2011. Three-Year Outcome of Phase-Specific Early Intervention for First-Episode Psychosis: A Cohort Study in Hong Kong. *Early Interv. Psychiatry* **5**:315–323. [11]

Chen, H., Y. Liu, Z. Li, and D. Xue. 2017. Urbanization, Economic Development and Health: Evidence from China's Labor-Force Dynamic Survey. *Int. J. Equity Health* **16**:207. [6]

Cheng, J. T., J. L. Tracy, T. Foulsham, A. Kingstone, and J. Henrich. 2013. Two Ways to the Top: Evidence That Dominance and Prestige Are Distinct yet Viable Avenues to Social Rank and Influence. *J. Personality Soc. Psychol.* **104**:103–125. [4]

Cherskov, A., A. Pohl, C. Allison, et al. 2018. Polycystic Ovary Syndrome and Autism: A Test of the Prenatal Sex Steroid Theory. *Transl. Psychiatry* **8**:136. [6]

Chiao, J. Y., and K. D. Blizinsky. 2013. Population Disparities in Mental Health: Insights from Cultural Neuroscience. *Am. J. Public Health* **103**:122–132. [5]

Chiao, J. Y., T. Iidaka, H. L. Gordon, et al. 2008. Cultural Specificity in Amygdala Response to Fear Faces. *J. Cog. Neurosci.* **20**:2167–2174. [6]

Chiu, C. P. Y., M. M. L. Lam, S. K. W. Chan, et al. 2010. Naming Psychosis: The Hong Kong Experience. *Early Interv. Psychiatry* **4**:270–274. [11]

Cho, Y., S.-H. Ryu, B. R. Lee, et al. 2015. Effects of Artificial Light at Night on Human Health: A Literature Review of Observational and Experimental Studies Applied to Exposure Assessment. *Chronobiol. Int.* **32**:1294–1310. [6]

Choe, A. S., C. K. Jones, S. E. Joel, et al. 2015. Reproducibility and Temporal Structure in Weekly Resting-State fMRI over a Period of 3.5 Years. *PLoS ONE* **10**:e0140134. [4]

Choi, E. Y., B. T. Yeo, and R. L. Buckner. 2012. The Organization of the Human Striatum Estimated by Intrinsic Functional Connectivity. *J. Neurophysiol.* **108**:2242–2263. [9]

Christoffel, D. J., S. A. Golden, and S. J. Russo. 2011. Structural and Synaptic Plasticity in Stress-Related Disorders. *Rev. Neurosci.* **22**:535–549. [7]

Clark, S. R., B. T. Baune, K. O. Schubert, et al. 2016. Prediction of Transition from Ultra-High Risk to First-Episode Psychosis Using a Probabilistic Model Combining History, Clinical Assessment and Fatty-Acid Biomarkers. *Transl. Psychiatry* **6**:e897. [14]

Clarke, G., S. Grenham, P. Scully, et al. 2013. The Microbiome-Gut-Brain Axis During Early Life Regulates the Hippocampal Serotonergic System in a Sex-Dependent Manner. *Mol. Psychiatr.* **18**:666–673. [7]

Clarke, G. N., W. Hawkins, M. Murphy, et al. 1995. Targeted Prevention of Unipolar Depressive Disorder in an At-Risk Sample of High School Adolescents: A Randomized Trial of a Group Cognitive Intervention. *J. Am. Acad. Child Adolesc. Psychiatry* **34**:312–321. [14]

Clarke, G. N., M. Hornbrook, F. Lynch, et al. 2001. A Randomized Trial of a Group Cognitive Intervention for Preventing Depression in Adolescent Offspring of Depressed Parents. *Arch. Gen. Psychiatry* **58**:1127–1134. [14]

Claxton, M., J. Onwumere, and M. Fornells-Ambrojo. 2017. Do Family Interventions Improve Outcomes in Early Psychosis? A Systematic Review and Meta-Analysis. *Front. Psychol.* **8**:371. [10]

Clementz, B. A., J. A. Sweeney, J. P. Hamm, et al. 2016. Identification of Distinct Psychosis Biotypes Using Brain-Based Biomarkers. *Am. J. Psychiatry* **173**:373–384. [6]

Cloutier, M., M. S. Aigbogun, A. Guerin, et al. 2016. The Economic Burden of Schizophrenia in the United States in 2013. *J. Clin. Psychiatry* **77**:764–771. [12]

Cocchi, A., V. Mapellli, A. Meneghelli, and A. Preti. 2011. Cost-Effectiveness of Treating First-Episode Psychosis: Five-Year Follow-up Results from an Italian Early Intervention Programme. *Early Interv. Psychiatry* **5**:203–211. [11]

Cohen, P., and J. Cohen. 1984. The Clinician's Illusion. *Arch. Gen. Psychiatry* **41**:1178–1182. [1, 14]

Colantuoni, C., B. K. Lipska, T. Ye, et al. 2011. Temporal Dynamics and Genetic Control of Transcription in the Human Prefrontal Cortex. *Nature* **478**:519–523. [8]

Collin, G., and M. Keshavan. 2018. Connectome Development and a Novel Extension to the Neurodevelopmental Model of Schizophrenia. *Dialogues Clin. Neurosci.* **20**:37–46. [9]

Collins, F. S., and H. Varmus. 2015. A New Initiative on Precision Medicine. *New England Journal of Medicine* **372**:793–795. [4]

Collins, W. A., D. P. Welsh, and W. Furman. 2009. Adolescent Romantic Relationships. *Annu. Rev. Psychol.* **60**:631–652. [5]

Collishaw, S. 2015. Annual Research Review: Secular Trends in Child and Adolescent Mental Health. *J. Child Psychol. Psychiatry* **56**:370–393. [9]

Collishaw, S., B. Maughan, R. Goodman, and A. Pickles. 2004. Time Trends in Adolescent Mental Health. *J. Child Psychol. Psychiatry* **45**:1350–1362. [1]

Colodro-Conde, L., B. Couvy-Duchesne, J. B. Whitfield, et al. 2018. Association between Population Density and Genetic Risk for Schizophrenia. *JAMA Psychiatry* **75**:901–910. [6]

Colombo, E., and C. Farina. 2016. Astrocytes: Key Regulators of Neuroinflammation. *Trends Immunol.* **37**:608–620. [9]

Colonnesi, C., E. M. Draijer, G. Jan J. M. Stams, et al. 2011. The Relation between Insecure Attachment and Child Anxiety: A Meta-Analytic Review. *J. Clin. Child Adolesc. Psychol.* **40**:630–645. [6]

Colon-Ramos, D. A. 2009. Synapse Formation in Developing Neural Circuits. *Curr. Top. Dev. Biol.* **87**:53–79. [7]

Compton, M. T., S. M. Goulding, C. E. Ramsay, et al. 2008. Early Detection and Intervention for Psychosis: Perspectives from North America. *Clin. Neuropsychiatry* **5**:263. [11]

Cook, J. A., M. E. Copeland, J. A. Jonikas, et al. 2012. Results of a Randomized Controlled Trial of Mental Illness Self-Management Using Wellness Recovery Action Planning. *Schizophr. Bull.* **38**:881-891. [13]

Cooley, L., and R. Kohl. 2006. Scaling Up: From Vision to Large-Scale Change: A Management Framework for Practitioners. Arlington, VA: Management Systems Intl. [14]

Copeland, W., L. Shanahan, E. J. Costello, and A. Angold. 2011. Cumulative Prevalence of Psychiatric Disorders by Young Adulthood: A Prospective Cohort Analysis from the Great Smoky Mountains Study. *J. Am. Acad. Child Adolesc. Psychiatry* **50**:252–261. [1]

Copeland, W. E., C. E. Adair, P. Smetanin, et al. 2013. Diagnostic Transitions from Childhood to Adolescence to Early Adulthood. *J. Child Psychol. Psychiatry* **54**:791–799. [2]

Copeland, W. E., L. Shanahan, S. Miller, et al. 2010. Outcomes of Early Pubertal Timing in Young Women: A Prospective Population-Based Study. *Am. J. Psychiatry* **167**:1218–1225. [6]

Corbetta, M., and G. L. Shulman. 2002. Control of Goal-Directed and Stimulus-Driven Attention in the Brain. *Nature reviews. Neuroscience* **3**:201–215. [9]

Cornblatt, B. A., R. E. Carrión, A. Auther, et al. 2015. Psychosis Prevention: A Modified Clinical High Risk Perspective from the Recognition and Prevention (RAP) Program. *Am. J. Psychiatry* **172**:986–994. [11]

Cornet, V. P., and R. J. Holden. 2018. Systematic Review of Smartphone-Based Passive Sensing for Health and Wellbeing. Journal of Biomedical Informatics. *J. Biomed. Inform.* **77**:120–132. [10]

Correll, C. U., B. Galling, A. Pawar, et al. 2018. Comparison of Early Intervention Services vs. Treatment as Usual for Early-Phase Psychosis: A Systematic Review, Meta-Analysis, and Meta-Regression. *JAMA Psychiatry* **75**:555–565. [12, 14]

Costello, E. J. 2016. Early Detection and Prevention of Mental Health Problems: Developmental Epidemiology and Systems of Support. *J. Clin. Child Adolesc. Psychol.* **45**:710–717. [7]

Costello, E. J., and A. Angold. 2016. Developmental Epidemiology. In: Developmental Psychopathology, Theory and Method, ed. D. Cicchetti, pp. 41–75, vol. 1. Hoboken: John Wiley & Sons. [4]

Costello, E. J., W. Copeland, and A. Angold. 2011. Trends in Psychopathology across the Adolescent Years: What Changes When Children Become Adolescents, and When Adolescents Become Adults? *J. Child Psychol. Psychiatry* **52**:1015–1025. [1]

Cousineau, T. M., D. L. Franko, M. Trant, et al. 2010. Teaching Adolescents About Changing Bodies: Randomized Controlled Trial of an Internet Puberty Education and Body Dissatisfaction Prevention Program. *Body Image* **7**:296–300. [4]

Craig, T. K., P. Garety, P. Power, et al. 2004. The Lambeth Early Onset (Leo) Team: Randomised Controlled Trial of the Effectiveness of Specialised Care for Early Psychosis. *BMJ* **329**:1067. [10]

Crone, E. A., and R. E. Dahl. 2012. Understanding Adolescence as a Period of Social–Affective Engagement and Goal Flexibility. *Nat. Rev. Neurosci.* **13**:636–650. [4, 5, 7]

Crone, E. A., and N. Steinbeis. 2017. Neural Perspectives on Cognitive Control Development During Childhood and Adolescence. *Trends Cogn. Sci.* **21**:205–215. [4]

Cross, S. P. M., D. F. Hermens, and I. B. Hickie. 2016. Treatment Patterns and Short-Term Outcomes in an Early Intervention Youth Mental Health Service. *Early Interv. Psychiatry* **10**:88–97. [2]

Cross, S. P. M., D. F. Hermens, E. M. Scott, et al. 2014. A Clinical Staging Model for Early Intervention Youth Mental Health Services. *Psychiatric Serv.* **65**:939–943. [3]

Cross, S. P. M., D. F. Hermens, J. Scott, L. Salvador-Carulla, and I. B. Hickie. 2017. Differential Impact of Current Diagnosis and Clinical Stage on Attendance at a Youth Mental Health Service. *Early Interv. Psychiatry* **11**:255–262. [2]

Cross, S. P. M., J. Scott, and I. B. Hickie. 2018a. Predicting Early Transition from Sub-Syndromal Presentations to Major Mental Disorders. *Br. J. Psychiatry Open* **3**:223–227. [2, 14]

Cross, S. P. M., J. L. Scott, D. F. Hermens, and I. B. Hickie. 2018b. Variability in Clinical Outcomes for Youths Treated for Subthreshold Severe Mental Disorders at an Early Intervention Service. *Psychiatric Serv.* **69**:555–561. [2]

Cross-Disorder Group of the Psychiatric Genomics Consortium. 2013. Identification of Risk Loci with Shared Effects on Five Major Psychiatric Disorders: A Genome-Wide Analysis. *Lancet* **381**:1371–1379. [8]

Crutchfield, J. P., J. D. Farmer, N. H. Packard, and R. S. Shaw. 1986. Chaos. *Sci. American* **255**:46–57. [6]

Cruz, D. A., S. M. Eggan, and D. A. Lewis. 2003. Postnatal Development of Pre- and Postsynaptic GABA Markers at Chandelier Cell Connections with Pyramidal Neurons in Monkey Prefrontal Cortex. *J. Comput. Neurol.* **465**:385–400. [7, 9]

Csillag, C., M. Nordentoft, M. Mizuno, et al. 2017. Early Intervention in Psychosis: From Clinical Intervention to Health System Implementation. *Early Interv. Psychiatry* **356**:i6681. [11]

Cuthbert, B. N., and T. R. Insel. 2010. Toward New Approaches to Psychotic Disorders: The NIMH Research Domain Criteria Project. *Schizophr. Bull.* **36**:1061–1062. [1, 3]

Cuthbert, B. N., and T. R. Insel. 2013. Toward the Future of Psychiatric Diagnosis: The Seven Pillars of RDoC. *BMC Med.* **11**:126. [1–3]

Dagani, J., G. Signorini, O. Nielssen, et al. 2017. Meta-Analysis of the Interval between the Onset and Management of Bipolar Disorder. *Can. J. of Psychiatry* **62**:247–258. [14]

Dahl, R. E., N. B. Allen, L. Wilbrecht, and A. B. Suleiman. 2018. Importance of Investing in Adolescence from a Developmental Science Perspective. *Nature* **554**:441–450. [3, 4, 7]

D'Alfonso, S., O. Santesteban-Echarri, S. Rice, et al. 2017. Artificial Intelligence-Assisted Online Social Therapy for Youth Mental Health. *Front. Psychol.* **8**:796. [10]

Damon, W. 1989. Child Development Today and Tomorrow. The Jossey-Bass Social and Behavioral Science Series. San Francisco: Jossey-Bass Publ. [6]

Dannlowski, U., A. Stuhrmann, V. Beutelmann, et al. 2012. Limbic Scars: Long-Term Consequences of Childhood Maltreatment Revealed by Functional and Structural Magnetic Resonance Imaging. *Biol. Psychiatry* **71**:286–293. [9]

Darling, N., and L. Steinberg. 1993. Parenting Style as Context: An Integrative Model. *Psychol. Bull.* **113**:487–496. [6]

Datta, D., D. Arion, and D. A. Lewis. 2015. Developmental Expression Patterns of GABAA Receptor Subunits in Layer 3 and 5 Pyramidal Cells of Monkey Prefrontal Cortex. *Cereb. Cortex* **25**:2295–2305. [9]

Daugherty, A. M., A. R. Bender, N. Raz, and N. Ofen. 2016. Age Differences in Hippocampal Subfield Volumes from Childhood to Late Adulthood. *Hippocampus* **26**:220–228. [9]

Davey, C. G., M. Yücel, and N. B. Allen. 2008. The Emergence of Depression in Adolescence: Development of the Prefrontal Cortex and the Representation of Reward. *Neurosci. Biobehav. Rev.* **32**:1–19. [4, 9]

Davydov, D. M., R. Stewart, K. Ritchie, and I. Chaudieu. 2010. Resilience and Mental Health. *Clin. Psychol. Rev.* **30**:479–495. [5]

Day, F. R., C. E. Elks, A. Murray, K. K. Ong, and J. R. B. Perry. 2015. Puberty Timing Associated with Diabetes, Cardiovascular Disease and Also Diverse Health Outcomes in Men and Women: The UK Biobank Study. *Scientific Rep.* **5**: [6]

Dean, D., A. D. Bryan, R. Newberry, et al. 2017. A Supervised Exercise Intervention for Youth at Risk for Psychosis: An Open-Label Pilot Study. *J. Clin. Psychiatry* **78**:e1167–e1173. [11]

De Angelis, M., R. Francavilla, M. Piccolo, A. De Giacomo, and M. Gobbetti. 2015. Autism Spectrum Disorders and Intestinal Microbiota. *Gut Microbes* **6**:207–213. [7]

de Faria, O., Jr., E. A. C. Pama, K. Evans, A. Luzhynskaya, and R. T. Karadottir. 2018. Neuroglial Interactions Underpinning Myelin Plasticity. *Dev. Neurobiol.* **78**:93–107. [7]

de Girolamo, G., J. Dagani, R. Purcell, A. Cocchi, and P. D. McGorry. 2012. Age of Onset of Mental Disorders and Use of Mental Health Services: Needs, Opportunities and Obstacles. *Epidemiol. Psychiatr. Sci.* **21**:47–57. [5, 14]

Deighton, S., and J. Addington. 2015. Exercise Practices in Individuals at Clinical High Risk of Developing Psychosis. *Early Interv. Psychiatry* **9**:284-291. [11]

Dekker, J., J. Peen, J. Koelen, F. Smit, and R. Schoevers. 2008. Psychiatric Disorders and Urbanization in Germany. *BMC Public Health* **8**:1–9. [6]

de Klepper, M., S. E. Sleebo, G. van de Bunt, and F. Agneessens. 2010. Similarity in Friendship Networks: Selection or Influence? The Effect of Constraining Contexts and Non-Visible Individual Attributes. *Social NetworksSocial Networks* **32**:82–90. [5]

Del Giudice, M., R. Angeleri, and V. Manera. 2009. The Juvenile Transition: A Developmental Switch Point in Human Life History. *Dev. Rev.* **29**:1–31. [6]

DeMaster, D., T. Pathman, J. K. Lee, and S. Ghetti. 2014. Structural Development of the Hippocampus and Episodic Memory: Developmental Differences Along the Anterior/Posterior Axis. *Cereb. Cortex* **24**:3036–3045. [9]

Desbonnet, L., G. Clarke, F. Shanahan, T. G. Dinan, and J. F. Cryan. 2014. Microbiota Is Essential for Social Development in the Mouse. *Mol. Psychiatr.* **19**:146–148. [7]

de Vries, E., C. J. Rincon, N. Tamayo Martínez, et al. 2018. Housing Index, Urbanisation Level and Lifetime Prevalence of Depressive and Anxiety Disorders: A Cross-Sectional Analysis of the Colombian National Mental Health Survey. *BMJ Open* **8**:e019065. [6]

Dickerson, F., E. Severance, and R. Yolken. 2017. The Microbiome, Immunity, and Schizophrenia and Bipolar Disorder. *Brain Behav. Immun.* **62**:46–52. [7]

Di Cristo, G. 2007. Development of Cortical GABAergic Circuits and Its Implications for Neurodevelopmental Disorders. *Clin. Genet.* **72**:1–8. [7]

Dimaggio, G., P. H. Lysaker, A. Carcione, G. Nicolo, and A. Semerari. 2008. Know Yourself and You Shall Know the Other... To a Certain Extent: Multiple Paths of Influence of Self-Reflection on Mindreading. *Conscious. Cogn.* **17**:778–789. [6]

Dixon, L. B., F. Dickerson, A. S. Bellack, et al. 2010. The 2009 Schizophrenia Port Psychosocial Treatment Recommendations and Summary Statements. *Schizophr. Bull.* **36**:48–70. [12]

Do, K. Q., J. H. Cabungcal, A. Frank, P. Steullet, and M. Cuenod. 2009. Redox Dysregulation, Neurodevelopment, and Schizophrenia. *Curr Opin. Neurobiol.* **19**:220–230. [7]

Do, K. Q., M. Cuenod, and T. K. Hensch. 2015. Targeting Oxidative Stress and Aberrant Critical Period Plasticity in the Developmental Trajectory to Schizophrenia. *Schizophr. Bull.* **41**:835–846. [7, 9]

Do, K. Q., A. H. Trabesinger, M. Kirsten-Kruger, et al. 2000. Schizophrenia: Glutathione Deficit in Cerebrospinal Fluid and Prefrontal Cortex *in Vivo*. *Eur. J. Neurosci.* **12**:3721–3728. [13]

Dobbyn, A., L. M. Huckins, J. Boocock, et al. 2018. Landscape of Conditional Eqtl in Dorsolateral Prefrontal Cortex and Co-Localization with Schizophrenia GWAS. *Am. J. Hum. Genet.* **102**:1169–1184. [8]

Dolsen, M. R., L. D. Asarnow, and A. G. Harvey. 2014. Insomnia as a Transdiagnostic Process in Psychiatric Disorders. *Curr. Psychiatry Rep.* **16**:471. [2]

Donato, F., S. B. Rompani, and P. Caroni. 2013. Parvalbumin-Expressing Basket-Cell Network Plasticity Induced by Experience Regulates Adult Learning. *Nature* **504**:272–276. [7]

Dorn, L. D. 2015. Moving Research on Puberty Forward: Measures Are the Key Component. *J. Adolesc. Health* **56**:580–581. [6]

Dosenbach, N. U. F., D. A. Fair, A. L. Cohen, B. L. Schlaggar, and S. E. Petersen. 2008. A Dual-Networks Architecture of Top-Down Control. *Trends Cogn. Sci.* **12**:99–105. [4]

Dosenbach, N. U. F., B. Nardos, A. L. Cohen, et al. 2010. Prediction of Individual Brain Maturity Using fMRI. *Science* **329**:1358–1361. [4, 9]

Dosenbach, N. U. F., K. M. Visscher, E. D. Palmer, et al. 2006. A Core System for the Implementation of Task Sets. *Neuron* **50**:99–812. [4]

Doucet, G., M. Naveau, L. Petit, et al. 2011. Brain Activity at Rest: A Multiscale Hierarchical Functional Organization. *J. Neurophysiol.* **105**:2753–2763. [9]

Dougherty, D., and P. H. Conway. 2008. The "3T's" Road Map to Transform Us Health Care: The "How" of High-Quality Care. *JAMA* **299**:2319–2321. [12]

Doupe, A. J., and P. K. Kuhl. 1999. Birdsong and Human Speech: Common Themes and Mechanisms. *Annu. Rev. Neurosci.* **22**:567–631. [3, 4]

Dray, J., J. Bowman, E. Campbell, et al. 2017. Systematic Review of Universal Resilience-Focused Interventions Targeting Child and Adolescent Mental Health in the School Setting. *J. Am. Acad. Child Adolesc. Psychiatry* **56**:813–824. [5]

Drysdale, A. T., L. Grosenick, J. Downar, et al. 2017. Resting-State Connectivity Biomarkers Define Neurophysiological Subtypes of Depression. *Nat. Med.* **23**:28–38. [6]

Drysdale, A. T., C. A. Hartley, S. S. Pattwell, et al. 2014. Fear and Anxiety from Principle to Practice: Implications for When to Treat Youth with Anxiety Disorders. *Biol. Psychiatry* **75**:e19–20. [9]

Duffy, A. 2014. Toward a Comprehensive Clinical Staging Model for Bipolar Disorder: Integrating the Evidence. *Can. J. of Psychiatry* **59**:659–666. [2]

———. 2018. Early Intervention in Bipolar Disorders: Where We Are Now and Need to Go Next. *Bipolar Disord.* **20**:490–491. [14]

Dumontheil, I. 2014. Development of Abstract Thinking During Childhood and Adolescence: The Role of Rostrolateral Prefrontal Cortex. *Dev. Cogn. Neurosci.* **10**:57–76. [4]

Dumontheil, I., I. A. Apperly, and S. J. Blakemore. 2010. Online Usage of Theory of Mind Continues to Develop in Late Adolescence. *Dev. Sci.* **12**:331–338. [4]

Dunaif, A. 2012. Genes, Aging and Sleep Apnea in Polycystic Ovary Syndrome: Polycystic Ovary Syndrome in 2011. *Nat. Rev. Endocrinol.* **8**:72–74. [6]

Duncan, C. E., M. J. Webster, D. A. Rothmond, et al. 2010. Prefrontal GABA(A) Receptor Alpha-Subunit Expression in Normal Postnatal Human Development and Schizophrenia. *J. Psychiatr. Res.* **44**:673–681. [9]

Dunn, E. C., T. W. Soare, M. R. Raffeld, et al. 2018. What Life Course Theoretical Models Best Explain the Relationship between Exposure to Childhood Adversity and Psychopathology Symptoms: Recency, Accumulation, or Sensitive Periods? *Psychol. Med.* **48**:2562–2572. [6]

Dunn, E. C., Y. Wang, J. Tse, et al. 2017. Sensitive Periods for the Effect of Childhood Interpersonal Violence on Psychiatric Disorder Onset among Adolescents. *Br. J. Psychiatry* **211**:365–372. [6]

Durstewitz, D., and T. Gabriel. 2007. Dynamical Basis of Irregular Spiking in NMDA-Driven Prefrontal Cortex Neurons. *Cereb. Cortex* **17**:894–908. [7]

Dwir, D., J.-H. Cabungcal, L. Tenenbaum, et al. 2017. Matrix Metalloproteinase Inhibition Prevents the Adult Excitatory-Inhibitory Imbalance Induced by the Reciprocal Interaction between Neuroinflammation and Oxidative Stress During Development. *Schizophr. Bull.* **43**:S32. [7]

Dwir, D., J. H. Cabungcal, L. Tenenbaum, et al. 2016. Interaction between Redox Dysregulation and Neuroinflammation During Early Development Could Lead to PVI Circuitry Impairments an Adulthood: Relevance for Schizophrenia. *Biol Psychiat* **79**:344s–344s. [13]

Dye, C. 2008. Health and Urban Living. *Science* **319**:766–769. [6]

Eagle, N., A. Pentland, and D. Lazer. 2009. Inferring Friendship Network Structure by Using Mobile Phone Data. *PNAS* **106**:15274–15278. [5]

Eaton, W. W. 2001. The Sociology of Mental Disorders. 3rd Ed. Westport, CT: Praeger. [14]

Ebner-Priemer, U. W., and J. F. Trull. 2009. Ecological Momentary Assessment of Mood Disorders and Mood Dysregulation. *Psychol. Assess.* **21**:463–475. [5]

Eccles, J. S., C. Midgley, A. Wigfield, et al. 1993. Development During Adolescence: The Impact of Stage-Environment Fit on Young Adolescents' Experiences in Schools and in Families. *Am. Psychol.* **48**:90. [11]

Edlow, A. G. 2017. Maternal Obesity and Neurodevelopmental and Psychiatric Disorders in Offspring. *Prenatal Diagn.* **37**:95–110. [7]

Edwards, J., J. Cocks, P. Burnett, et al. 2011. Randomized Controlled Trial of Clozapine and CBT for First-Episode Psychosis with Enduring Positive Symptoms: A Pilot Study. *Schizophr. Res. Treat.* **2011**:394896. [14]

Eggan, S. M., T. Hashimoto, and D. A. Lewis. 2008. Reduced Cortical Cannabinoid 1 Receptor Messenger RNA and Protein Expression in Schizophrenia. *Arch. Gen. Psychiatry* **65**:772–784. [7]

Eggan, S. M., Y. Mizoguchi, S. R. Stoyak, and D. A. Lewis. 2010a. Development of Cannabinoid 1 Receptor Protein and Messenger RNA in Monkey Dorsolateral Prefrontal Cortex. *Cereb. Cortex* **20**:1164–1174. [9]

Eggan, S. M., S. R. Stoyak, C. D. Verrico, and D. A. Lewis. 2010b. Cannabinoid CB1 Receptor Immunoreactivity in the Prefrontal Cortex: Comparison of Schizophrenia and Major Depressive Disorder. *Neuropsychopharmacology* **35**:2060–2071. [7]

Ehrlichman, R. S., M. J. Gandal, C. R. Maxwell, et al. 2009. N-Methyl-D-Aspartic Acid Receptor Antagonist-Induced Frequency Oscillations in Mice Recreate Pattern of Electrophysiological Deficits in Schizophrenia. *Neuroscience* **158**:705–712. [8]

Eisenberg, D. P., and K. F. Berman. 2010. Executive Function, Neural Circuitry, and Genetic Mechanisms in Schizophrenia. *Neuropsychopharmacology* **35**:258–277. [9]

Eissler, K. R. 1958. Notes on Problems of Technique in the Psychoanalytic Treatment of Adolescents. *Psychoanalytic Study Child* **13**:223–254. [5]

Elfenbein, H. A. 2002. On the Universality and Cultural Specificity of Emotion Recognition: A Meta-Analysis. *Psychol. Bull.* **128**:203–235. [6]

Ellis, B. J. 2004. Timing of Pubertal Maturation in Girls: An Integrated Life History Approach. *Psychol. Bull.* **130**:920–958. [4]

Ellison, N. B., C. Steinfield, and C. Lampe. 2007. The Benefits of Facebook "Friends:" Social Capital and College Students' Use of Online Social Network Sites. *J. Comp.-Mediat. Commun.* **12**:1143–1168. [6]

Eloe-Fadrosh, E. A., and D. A. Rasko. 2013. The Human Microbiome: From Symbiosis to Pathogenesis. *Annu. Rev. Med.* **64**:145–163. [7]

Enwright, J. F., S. Sanapala, A. Foglio, et al. 2016. Reduced Labeling of Parvalbumin Neurons and Perineuronal Nets in the Dorsolateral Prefrontal Cortex of Subjects with Schizophrenia. *Neuropsychopharmacology* **41**:2206–2214. [9]

Erskine, H. E., T. E. Moffitt, W. E. Copeland, et al. 2015. A Heavy Burden on Young Minds: The Global Burden of Mental and Substance Use Disorders in Children and Youth. *Psychol. Med.* **45**:1511–1563. [2, 5, 6]

Essex, M. J., W. Thomas Boyce, C. Hertzman, et al. 2013. Epigenetic Vestiges of Early Developmental Adversity: Childhood Stress Exposure and DNA Methylation in Adolescence. *Child Dev.* **84**:58–75. [6]

Fagiolini, M., J. M. Fritschy, K. Low, et al. 2004. Specific GABAA Circuits for Visual Cortical Plasticity. *Science* **303**:1681–1683. [7]

Fair, D. A., A. L. Cohen, J. D. Power, et al. 2009. Functional Brain Networks Develop from a "Local to Distributed" Organization. *PLoS Comput. Biol.* **5**:e1000381. [9]

Fair, D. A., J. T. Nigg, S. Iyer, et al. 2013. Distinct Neural Signatures Detected for ADHD Subtypes after Controlling for Micro-Movements in Resting State Functional Connectivity MRI Data. *Front. Syst. Neurosci.* **6**:80. [4, 9]

Falloon, I. R. 1988. Handbook of Behavioral Family Therapy. London: Routledge. [10]

Fareri, D. S., L. Gabard-Durnam, B. Goff, et al. 2015. Normative Development of Ventral Striatal Resting State Connectivity in Humans. *Neuroimage* **118**:422–437. [9]

Fawcett, T. W., and W. E. Frankenhuis. 2015. Adaptive Explanations for Sensitive Windows in Development. *Front. Zool.* **12**:S3. [3, 4]

Feinberg, I. 1982. Schizophrenia: Caused by a Fault in Programmed Synaptic Elimination During Adolescence? *J. Psychiatr. Res.* **17**:319–334. [7, 8]

Feldstein Ewing, S. W., J. M. Bjork, and M. Luciana. 2018. Implications of the ABCD Study for Developmental Neuroscience. *Dev. Cogn. Neurosci.* **32**:161–164. [9]

Finne, E., J. Bucksch, T. Lampert, and P. Kolip. 2013. Physical Activity and Screen-Based Media Use: Cross-Sectional Associations with Health-Related Quality of Life and the Role of Body Satisfaction in a Representative Sample of German Adolescents. *Health Psychol. Behav. Med.* **1**:15–30. [5]

Firth, J., J. Cotter, R. Elliott, P. French, and A. R. Yung. 2015. A Systematic Review and Meta-Analysis of Exercise Interventions in Schizophrenia Patients. *Psychol. Med.* **45**:1343-1361. [11]

Firth, J., S. Rosenbaum, P. B. Ward, et al. 2018. Adjunctive Nutrients in First-Episode Psychosis: A Systematic Review of Efficacy, Tolerability and Neurobiological Mechanisms. *Early Interv. Psychiatry* **1**:S44. [11]

Fisher, A. J., J. D. Medaglia, and B. F. Jeronimus. 2018. Lack of Group-to-Individual Generalizability Is a Threat to Human Subjects Research. *PNAS* **115**:6106–6115. [3]

Föcking, M., P. Dicker, L. M. Lopez, et al. 2016. Differential Expression of the Inflammation Marker IL12p40 in the At-Risk Mental State for Psychosis: A Predictor of Transition to Psychotic Disorder? *BMC Psychiat.* **16**:326. [13]

Fonareva, I., and B. S. Oken. 2014. Physiological and Functional Consequences of Caregiving for Relatives with Dementia. *Int. Psychogeriatr.* **26**:725–747. [10]

Forbes, E. E., and R. E. Dahl. 2011. Research Review: Altered Reward Function in Adolescent Depression: What, When and How? *J. Child Psychol. Psychiatry Allied Discipl.* **53**:3–15. [9]

Forbes, M. K., A. G. C. Wright, K. E. Markon, and R. F. Krueger. 2017. Evidence That Psychopathology Symptom Networks Have Limited Replicability. *J. Abnorm. Psycholog.* **126**:969. [14]

Forrest, M. P., E. Parnell, and P. Penzes. 2018. Dendritic Structural Plasticity and Neuropsychiatric Disease. *Nature reviews. Neuroscience* **19**:215–234. [7]

Foulkes, L., and S. J. Blakemore. 2016. Is There Heightened Sensitivity to Social Reward in Adolescence? *Curr. Opin. Neurobiol.* **40**:81-85. [5]

Fraguas, D., J. Merchán-Naranjo, P. Laita, et al. 2008. Metabolic and Hormonal Side Effects in Children and Adolescents Treated with Second-Generation Antipsychotics. *J. Clin. Psychiatry* **69**:1166–1175. [11]

Frances, A. 2012. Predicting Psychosis Risk Is Pretty Risky. July 29, 2018. Huffington Post. https://www.huffingtonpost.com/allen-frances/psychosis-risk_b_1289022.html?guccounter=1. (accessed Nov. 23, 2018). [14]

———. 2013. Saving Normal: An Insider's Revolt against out-of-Control Psychiatric Diagnosis, DSM-5, Big Pharma, and the Medicalization of Ordinary Life. New York: William Morrow. [14]

Francis, T. C., R. Chandra, D. M. Friend, et al. 2015. Nucleus Accumbens Medium Spiny Neuron Subtypes Mediate Depression-Related Outcomes to Social Defeat Stress. *Biol. Psychiatry* **77**:212–222. [7]

Frangou, S. 2011. Brain Structural and Functional Correlates of Resilience to Bipolar Disorder. *Front. Hum. Neurosci.* **5**:184. [9]

Frantseva, M. V., P. B. Fitzgerald, and R. Chen. 2008. Evidence for Impaired Long-Term Potentiation in Schizophrenia and Its Relationship to Motor Skill Learning. *Cereb. Cortex* **18**:990–996. [8]

Freeman, M. P., J. R. Hibbeln, K. L. Wisner, et al. 2006. Omega-3 Fatty Acids: Evidence Basis for Treatment and Future Research in Psychiatry. *J. Clin. Psychiatry* **67**:1954–1967. [10]

Freund, T. F. 2003. Interneuron Diversity Series: Rhythm and Mood in Perisomatic Inhibition. *Trends Neurosci.* **26**:489–495. [9]

Fudge, J. L., M. A. Breitbart, and C. McClain. 2004. Amygdaloid Inputs Define a Caudal Component of the Ventral Striatum in Primates. *J. Comput. Neurol.* **476**:330–347. [9]

Fusar-Poli, P. 2019. Integrated Mental Health Services for the Developmental Period (0 to 25 Years): A Critical Review of the Evidence. *Front. Psychiatry* **10**:355. [13]

Fusar-Poli, P., I. Bonoldi, A. R. Yung, et al. 2012. Predicting Psychosis: Meta-Analysis of Transition Outcomes in Individuals at High Clinical Risk. *Arch. Gen. Psychiatry* **69**:220–229. [11]

Fusar-Poli, P., S. Borgwardt, A. Bechdolf, et al. 2013a. The Psychosis High-Risk State: A Comprehensive State-of-the-Art Review. *JAMA Psychiatry* **70**:107–120. [1]

Fusar-Poli, P., M. Byrne, L. Valmaggia, et al. 2010. Social Dysfunction Predicts Two Years Clinical Outcome in People at Ultra High Risk for Psychosis. *J. Psychiatr. Res.* **44**:294–301. [2]

Fusar-Poli, P., M. Cappucciati, S. Borgwardt, et al. 2016. Heterogeneity of Psychosis Risk within Individuals at Clinical High Risk: A Meta-Analytical Stratification. *JAMA Psychiatry* **73**:113–120. [11]

Fusar-Poli, P., M. Cappucciati, G. Rutigliano, et al. 2015. At Risk or Not at Risk? A Meta-Analysis of the Prognostic Accuracy of Psychometric Interviews for Psychosis Prediction. *World Psychiatry* **14**:322–332. [1]

Fusar-Poli, P., M. Solmi, N. Brondino, et al. 2019. Transdiagnostic Psychiatry: A Systematic Review. *World Psychiatry* **18**:192–207. [1]

Fusar-Poli, P., A. R. Yung, P. McGorry, and J. Van Os. 2013b. Lessons Learned from the Psychosis High-Risk State: Towards a General Staging Model of Prodromal Intervention. *Psychol. Med.* **44**:17–24. [11]

Galea, S. 2005. Urban Built Environment and Depression: A Multilevel Analysis. *J. Epidemiol. Community Health* **59**:822–827. [6]

Galvan, A., T. A. Hare, M. Davidson, et al. 2005. The Role of Ventral Frontostriatal Circuitry in Reward-Based Learning in Humans. *J. Neurosci.* **25**:8650–8656. [9]

Gandal, M. J., J. R. Haney, N. N. Parikshak, et al. 2018. Shared Molecular Neuropathology across Major Psychiatric Disorders Parallels Polygenic Overlap. *Science* **359**:693–697. [8]

Gao, B., and J. M. Fritschy. 1994. Selective Allocation of GABAA Receptors Containing the Alpha 1 Subunit to Neurochemically Distinct Subpopulations of Rat Hippocampal Interneurons. *Eur. J. Neurosci.* **6**:837–853. [7]

Gao, B., J. M. Fritschy, D. Benke, and H. Mohler. 1993. Neuron-Specific Expression of GABAA-Receptor Subtypes: Differential Association of the Alpha 1- and Alpha 3-Subunits with Serotonergic and GABAergic Neurons. *Neuroscience* **54**:881–892. [7]

Garber, J., G. N. Clarke, V. R. Weersing, et al. 2009. Prevention of Depression in At-Risk Adolescents: A Randomized Controlled Trial. *JAMA* **301**:2215–2224. [14]

Garber, J., S. A. Frankel, and C. G. Herrington. 2016. Developmental Demands of Cognitive Behavioral Therapy for Depression in Children and Adolescents: Cognitive, Social, and Emotional Processes. *Annu. Rev. Clin. Psych.* **12**:181–216. [4]

Gardosi, J., A. Francis, S. Turner, and M. Williams. 2018. Customized Growth Charts: Rationale, Validation and Clinical Benefits. *Am. J. Obstet. Gynecol.* **218**:S609-S618. [3]

Garland, M. R., and B. Hallahan. 2006. Essential Fatty Acids and Their Role in Conditions Characterised by Impulsivity. *Int. Rev. Psychiatry* **18**:99–105. [10]

Garland, M. R., B. Hallahan, M. McNamara, et al. 2007. Lipids and Essential Fatty Acids in Patients Presenting with Self-Harm. *Br. J. Psychiatry* **190**:112–117. [10]

Garner, A. S., J. P. Shonkoff, Committee on Psychosocial Aspects of Child and Family Health, Committee on Early Childhood Adoption and Dependent Care, and Section on Developmental and Behavioral Pediatrics. 2012. Early Childhood Adversity, Toxic Stress, and the Role of the Pediatrician: Translating Developmental Science into Lifelong Health. *Pediatrics* **129**:e224–231. [6]

Gawande, A. 2017. Being Mortal: Medicine and What Matters in the End. New York: Metropolitan Books. [14]

Gebicke-Haerter, P. J. 2016. Systems Psychopharmacology: A Network Approach to Developing Novel Therapies. *World J. Psychiatry* **6**:66. [8]

Geddes, J. R., and S. M. Lawrie. 1995. Obstetric Complications and Schizophrenia: A Meta-Analysis. *Br. J. Psychiatry* **167**:786–793. [8]

Gee, D. G., and T. D. Cannon. 2011. Prediction of Conversion to Psychosis: Review and Future Directions. *Rev. Brasil. Psiquiatr.* **33**:s129–s142. [11]

Gee, D. G., K. L. Humphreys, J. Flannery, et al. 2013. A Developmental Shift from Positive to Negative Connectivity in Human Amygdala-Prefrontal Circuitry. *J. Neurosci.* **33**:4584-4593. [5, 9]

Geier, C. F., R. Terwilliger, T. Teslovich, K. Velanova, and B. Luna. 2010. Immaturities in Reward Processing and Its Influence on Inhibitory Control in Adolescence. *Cereb. Cortex* **20**:1613–1629. [9]

Gershon, E. S., and N. Alliey-Rodriguez. 2013. New Ethical Issues for Genetic Counseling in Common Mental Disorders. *Am. J. Psychiatry* **170**:968–976. [8]

Gervain, J., B. W. Vines, L. M. Chen, et al. 2013. Valproate Reopens Critical-Period Learning of Absolute Pitch. *Front. Syst. Neurosci.* **7**:102. [5]

Geyer, M. A., and D. L. Braff. 1987. Startle Habituation and Sensorimotor Gating in Schizophrenia and Related Animal Models. *Schizophr. Bull.* **13**:643–668. [8]

Geyer, M. A., K. Krebs-Thomson, D. L. Braff, and N. R. Swerdlow. 2001. Pharmacological Studies of Prepulse Inhibition Models of Sensorimotor Gating Deficits in Schizophrenia: A Decade in Review. *Psychopharmacology* **156**:117–154. [8]

Ghetti, S., and S. A. Bunge. 2012. Neural Changes Underlying the Development of Episodic Memory During Middle Childhood. *Dev. Cogn. Neurosci.* **2**:381–395. [9]

Gianfranceschi, L., R. Siciliano, J. Walls, et al. 2003. Visual Cortex Is Rescued from the Effects of Dark Rearing by Overexpression of BDNF. *PNAS* **100**:12486–12491. [7]

Gibb, S. J., D. M. Fergusson, and L. J. Horwood. 2010. Burden of Psychiatric Disorder in Young Adulthood and Life Outcomes at Age 30. *Br. J. Psychiatry* **197**:122–127. [1]

Giedd, J. N., J. Blumenthal, N. O. Jeffries, et al. 1999. Brain Development During Childhood and Adolescence: A Longitudinal MRI Study. *Nat. Neurosci.* **2**:861–863. [7, 9]

Giedd, J. N., J. W. Snell, N. Lange, et al. 1996a. Quantitative Magnetic Resonance Imaging of Human Brain Development: Ages 4–18. *Cereb. Cortex* **6**:551–560. [9]

Giedd, J. N., A. C. Vaituzis, S. D. Hamburger, et al. 1996b. Quantitative MRI of the Temporal Lobe, Amygdala, and Hippocampus in Normal Human Development: Ages 4–18 Years. *J. Comput. Neurol.* **366**:223–230. [9]

Gilbody, S., E. Littlewood, C. Hewitt, et al. 2015. Computerised Cognitive Behaviour Therapy (CCBT) as Treatment for Depression in Primary Care (REEACT Trial): Large Scale Pragmatic Randomised Controlled Trial. *BMJ* **351**:h5627. [10]

Giles, J. 2012. Computational Social Science: Making the Links. *Nature* **488**:448–450. [6]

Ginovart, N., B. B. Tournier, M. Moulin-Sallanon, et al. 2012. Chronic Delta(9)-Tetrahydrocannabinol Exposure Induces a Sensitization of Dopamine D(2)/(3) Receptors in the Mesoaccumbens and Nigrostriatal Systems. *Neuropsychopharmacology* **37**:2355–2367. [7]

Giovanoli, S., H. Engler, A. Engler, et al. 2013. Stress in Puberty Unmasks Latent Neuropathological Consequences of Prenatal Immune Activation in Mice. *Science* **339**:1095–1099. [7]

Giuffrida, A., L. H. Parsons, T. M. Kerr, et al. 1999. Dopamine Activation of Endogenous Cannabinoid Signaling in Dorsal Striatum. *Nat. Neurosci.* **2**:358–363. [7]

Glantz, L. A., and D. A. Lewis. 2000. Decreased Dendritic Spine Density on Prefrontal Cortical Pyramidal Neurons in Schizophrenia. *Arch. Gen. Psychiatry* **57**:65–73. [8]

Glasziou, P., and B. Haynes. 2005. The Paths from Research to Improved Health Outcomes. *ACP J. Club* **142**:8–10. [12]

Glasziou, P., G. Ogrinc, and S. Goodman. 2011. Can Evidence-Based Medicine and Clinical Quality Improvement Learn from Each Other? *BMJ Qual. Saf.* **20**:i13–i17. [12]

Glatt, S. J., S. V. Faraone, and M. T. Tsuang. 2007. Genetic Risk Factors for Mental Disorders: General Principles and State of the Science. In: Recognition and Prevention of Major Mental and Substance Abuse Disorders, ed. M. T. Tsuang et al., pp. 3–20. Washington, D.C.: American Psychiatric Publ. [8]

Gleeson, J., S. M. Cotton, M. Alvarez-Jimenez, et al. 2010. Family Outcomes from a Randomized Control Trial of Relapse Prevention Therapy in First-Episode Psychosis. *J. Clin. Psychiatry* **71**:475–483. [10]

Gleeson, J., R. Lederman, H. Herrman, et al. 2017a. Moderated Online Social Therapy for Carers of Young People Recovering from First-Episode Psychosis: Study Protocol for a Randomised Controlled Trial. *Trials* **18**:27. [10]

Gleeson, J., R. Lederman, P. Koval, et al. 2017b. Moderated Online Social Therapy: A Model for Reducing Stress in Carers of Young People Diagnosed with Mental Health Disorders. *Front. Psychol.* **8**:485. [10]

Global Mental Health Group. 2007. Global Mental Health. *Lancet* **370**:2241–2252. [1]

Glouberman, S., and B. Zimmerman. 2002. Complicated and Complex Systems: What Would Successful Reform of Medicare Look Like? pp. 1–30, vol. 2. Commission on the Future of Health Care in Canada. [12]

Godsil, B. P., J. P. Kiss, M. Spedding, and T. M. Jay. 2013. The Hippocampal-Prefrontal Pathway: The Weak Link in Psychiatric Disorders. *Eur. Neuropsychopharmacol.* **23**:1165–1181. [9]

Gogolla, N., P. Caroni, A. Luthi, and C. Herry. 2009. Perineuronal Nets Protect Fear Memories from Erasure. *Science* **325**:1258–1261. [7]

Gogtay, N., J. N. Giedd, L. Lusk, et al. 2004. Dynamic Mapping of Human Cortical Development During Childhood through Early Adulthood. *PNAS* **101**:8174–8179. [7, 9]

Gogtay, N., T. F. Nugent III, D. H. Herman, et al. 2006. Dynamic Mapping of Normal Human Hippocampal Development. *Hippocampus* **16**:664–672. [9]

Golden, S. A., D. J. Christoffel, M. Heshmati, et al. 2013. Epigenetic Regulation of RAC1 Induces Synaptic Remodeling in Stress Disorders and Depression. *Nat. Med.* **19**:337–344. [7]

Goldman-Rakic, P. S., J.-P. Bourgeois, and P. Rakic. 1997. Synaptic Substrate of Cognitive Development: Life-Span Analysis of Synaptogenesis in the Prefrontal Cortex of the Nonhuman Primate. In: Development of the Prefontal Cortex, ed. N. A. Krasnegor et al., pp. 27–48. Baltimore: Paul H. Brookes Publishing. [7]

Goldsmith, D. R., M. H. Rapaport, and B. J. Miller. 2016. A Meta-Analysis of Blood Cytokine Network Alterations in Psychiatric Patients: Comparisons between Schizophrenia, Bipolar Disorder and Depression. *Mol. Psychiatr.* **21**:1696–1709. [7]

Gore, F. M., P. J. N. Bloem, G. C. Patton, et al. 2011. Global Burden of Disease in Young People Aged 10–24 Years: A Systematic Analysis. *Lancet* **377**:2093–2102. [2, 9]

Gorriti, M. A., F. Rodríguez de Fonseca, M. Navarro, and T. Palomo. 1999. Chronic (-)-Delta9-Tetrahydrocannabinol Treatment Induces Sensitization to the Psychomotor Effects of Amphetamine in Rats. *Eur. J. Pharmacol.* **365**:133–142. [8]

Goto, Y., and A. A. Grace. 2007. The Dopamine System and the Pathophysiology of Schizophrenia: A Basic Science Perspective. *Int. Rev. Neurobiol.* **78**:41–68. [7]

Gottesman, I. I., and T. D. Gould. 2003. The Endophenotype Concept in Psychiatry: Etymology and Strategic Intentions. *Am. J. Psychiatry* **160**:636–645. [8]

Gould, L. F., J. K. Dariotis, T. Mendelson, and M. T. Greenberg. 2012. A School-Based Mindfulness Intervention for Urban Youth: Exploring Moderators of Intervention Effects. *J. Commun. Psychol.* **40**:968–982. [4]

Gould, T. D., and I. I. Gottesman. 2006. Psychiatric Endophenotypes and the Development of Valid Animal Models. *Genes Brain Behav.* **5**:113–119. [8]

Graber, J. A., J. R. Seeley, J. Brooks-Gunn, and P. M. Lewinsohn. 2004. Is Pubertal Timing Associated with Psychopathology in Young Adulthood. *J. Am. Acad. Child Adolesc. Psychiatry* **43**:718–726. [9]

Gradisar, M., G. Gardner, and H. Dohnt. 2011. Recent Worldwide Sleep Patterns and Problems During Adolescence: A Review and Meta-Analysis of Age, Region, and Sleep. *Sleep Med.* **12**:110–118. [2]

Gray, E., T. L. Thomas, S. Betmouni, N. Scolding, and S. Love. 2008. Elevated Matrix Metalloproteinase-9 and Degradation of Perineuronal Nets in Cerebrocortical Multiple Sclerosis Plaques. *J. Neuropathol. Exp. Neurol.* **67**:888–899. [7]

Gray, J. A. 1995. Dopamine Release in the Nucleus Accumbens: The Perspective from Aberrations of Consciousness in Schizophrenia. *Neuropsychologia* **33**:1143–1153. [8]

Gray, M. 2012. Value: Operations Research and the New Health Care Paradigm. *Operations Res. Health Care* **1**:20–21. [12]

Grayson, D. S., and D. A. Fair. 2017. Development of Large-Scale Functional Networks from Birth to Adulthood: A Guide to the Neuroimaging Literature. *Neuroimage* **160**:15–31. [9]

Green, M. F., W. P. Horan, and J. Lee. 2015. Social Cognition in Schizophrenia. *Nat. Rev. Neurosci.* **16**:620–631. [6]

Green, M. F., D. L. Penn, R. Bentall, et al. 2008. Social Cognition in Schizophrenia: An NIMH Workshop on Definitions, Assessment, and Research Opportunities. *Schizophr. Bull.* **34**:1211–1220. [6]

Green, P., H. Hermesh, A. Monselise, et al. 2006. Red Cell Membrane Omega-3 Fatty Acids Are Decreased in Nondepressed Patients with Social Anxiety Disorder. *Eur. Neuropsychopharmacol.* **16**:107–113. [10]

Greenberg, G. 2013. The Book of Woe: The DSM and the Unmaking of Psychiatry. New York: Blue Rider Press. [14]

Greenough, W. T., J. E. Black, and C. S. Wallace. 1987. Experience and Brain Development. *Child Dev.* **58**:539–559. [5]

Gregor, C., S. Davidson, and H. Hingley-Jones. 2016. The Experience of Gender Dysphoria for Pre-Pubescent Children and Their Families: A Review of the Literature. *Child Fam. Social Work* **21**:339–346. [10]

Greiff, S., S. Wustenberg, T. Goetz, et al. 2015. A Longitudinal Study of Higher-Order Thinking Skills: Working Memory and Fluid Reasoning in Childhood Enhance Complex Problem Solving in Adolescence. *Front. Psychol.* **6**:1060. [7]

Grist, R., J. Porter, and P. Stallard. 2017. Mental Health Mobile Apps for Preadolescents and Adolescents: A Systematic Review. *J. Med. Internet Res.* **19**:e176. [13]

Gronholm, P. C., G. Thornicroft, K. R. Laurens, and S. Evans-Lacko. 2017. Mental Health-Related Stigma and Pathways to Care for People at Risk of Psychotic Disorders or Experiencing First-Episode Psychosis: A Systematic Review. *Psychol. Med.* **47**:1867–1879. [11]

Gu, S., T. D. Satterthwaite, J. D. Medaglia, et al. 2015. Emergence of System Roles in Normative Neurodevelopment. *PNAS* **112**:13681–13686. [9]

Guloksuz, S., J. van Os, and B. P. F. Rutten. 2018. The Exposome Paradigm and the Complexities of Environmental Research in Psychiatry. *JAMA Psychiatry* **75**:985-986. [6]

Gunderson, J. G., A. Fruzzetti, B. Unruh, and L. Choi-Kain. 2018. Competing Theories of Borderline Personality Disorder. *J. Pers. Disord.* **32**:148–167. [10]

Gusev, A., N. Mancuso, H. Won, et al. 2018. Transcriptome-Wide Association Study of Schizophrenia and Chromatin Activity Yields Mechanistic Disease Insights. *Nat. Genet.* **50**:538–548. [8]

Gustavsson, A., M. Svensson, F. Jacobi, et al. 2011. Cost of Disorders of the Brain in Europe 2010. *Eur. Neuropsychopharmacol.* **21**:718–779. [2]

Gysin, R., R. Kraftsik, J. Sandell, et al. 2007. Impaired Glutathione Synthesis in Schizophrenia: Convergent Genetic and Functional Evidence. *PNAS* **104**:16621–16626. [13]

Haber, S. N., and B. Knutson. 2010. The Reward Circuit: Linking Primate Anatomy and Human Imaging. *Neuropsychopharmacology* **35**:4–26. [9]

Hadad, C. 2015. Why Some 13-Year-Olds Check Social Media 100 Times a Day. https://edition.cnn.com/2015/10/5/health/being-13-teens-social-media-study/index.html. (accessed July 22, 2019). [10]

Haddad, L., A. Schäfer, F. Streit, et al. 2015. Brain Structure Correlates of Urban Upbringing, an Environmental Risk Factor for Schizophrenia. *Schizophr. Bull.* **41**:115–122. [6]

Hafeman, D. M., J. Merranko, D. Axelson, et al. 2016. Toward the Definition of a Bipolar Prodrome: Dimensional Predictors of Bipolar Spectrum Disorders in At-Risk Youths. *Am. J. Psychiatry* **173**:695–704. [2]

Hafizi, S., T. Da Silva, C. Gerritsen, et al. 2017a. Imaging Microglial Activation in Individuals at Clinical High Risk for Psychosis: An *in Vivo* PET Study with [(18)F] Feppa. *Neuropsychopharmacology* **42**:2474–2481. [7]

Hafizi, S., H. H. Tseng, N. Rao, et al. 2017b. Imaging Microglial Activation in Untreated First-Episode Psychosis: A PET Study with [(18)F]Feppa. *Am. J. Psychiatry* **174**:118–124. [7]

Häfner, H., W. an der Heiden, and K. Maurer. 2008. Evidence for Separate Diseases? Stages of One Disease or Different Combinations of Symptom Dimensions? *Eur. Arch. Psychiatry Clin. Neurosci.* **258 Suppl 2**:85–96. [2]

Häfner, H., A. Riecher, K. Maurer, et al. 1989. How Does Gender Influence Age at First Hospitalization for Schizophrenia? A Transnational Case Register Study. *Psychol. Med.* **19**:903–918. [4]

Häfner, H., A. Riecher-Rössler, M. Hambrecht, et al. 1992. Iraos: An Instrument for the Assessment of Onset and Early Course of Schizophrenia. *Schizophr. Res.* **6**:209–223. [14]

Haggarty, S. J., M. C. Silva, A. Cross, N. J. Brandon, and R. H. Perlis. 2016. Advancing Drug Discovery for Neuropsychiatric Disorders Using Patient-Specific Stem Cell Models. *Mol. Cell. Neurosci.* **73**:104–115. [8]

Hallahan, B., T. Ryan, J. R. Hibbeln, et al. 2016. Efficacy of Omega-3 Highly Unsaturated Fatty Acids in the Treatment of Depression. *Br. J. Psychiatry* **209**:192–201. [10]

Halsall, T., I. Manion, S. N. Iyer, et al. 2019. Trends in Mental Health System Transformation: Integrating Youth Services within the Canadian Context. *Healthcare Management Forum* **32**:51–55. [13]

Hamilton, M. P., S. E. Hetrick, C. Mihalopoulos, et al. 2017. Identifying Attributes of Care That May Improve Cost-Effectiveness in the Youth Mental Health Service System. *Med. J. Austral.* **207**:S27–S37. [13, 14]

Hamm, M. P., A. S. Newton, A. Chisholm, et al. 2015. Prevalence and Effect of Cyberbullying on Children and Young People: A Scoping Review of Social Media Studies. *JAMA Pediatrics* **169**:770–777. [5]

Hanover, J. L., Z. J. Huang, S. Tonegawa, and M. P. Stryker. 1999. Brain-Derived Neurotrophic Factor Overexpression Induces Precocious Critical Period in Mouse Visual Cortex. *J. Neurosci.* **19**:RC40. [7]

Happel, M. F., H. Niekisch, L. L. Castiblanco Rivera, et al. 2014. Enhanced Cognitive Flexibility in Reversal Learning Induced by Removal of the Extracellular Matrix in Auditory Cortex. *PNAS* **111**:2800–2805. [7]

Haque, F. N., T. V. Lipina, J. C. Roder, and A. H. Wong. 2012. Social Defeat Interacts with Disc1 Mutations in the Mouse to Affect Behavior. *Behav. Brain Res.* **233**:337–344. [8]

Hardingham, G. E., and K. Q. Do. 2016. Linking Early-Life NMDAR Hypofunction and Oxidative Stress in Schizophrenia Pathogenesis. *Nat. Rev. Neurosci.* **17**:125–134. [13]

Harris, W. S. 2008. The Omega-3 Index as a Risk Factor for Coronary Heart Disease. *Am. J. Clin. Nutrition* **87**:1997S–2002S. [10]

Harris, W. S., and C. von Schacky. 2004. The Omega-3 Index: A New Risk Factor for Death from Coronary Heart Disease? *Prev. Med.* **39**:212–220. [10]

Hartley, C. A., and L. H. Somerville. 2015. The Neuroscience of Adolescent Decision-Making. *Curr. Opin. Behav. Sci.* **5**:108–115. [4]

Hartmann, J. A., B. Nelson, R. Spooner, et al. 2019. Broad Clinical High-Risk Mental State (CHARMS): Methodology of a Cohort Study Validating Criteria for Pluripotent Risk. *Early Interv. Psychiatry* [2, 14]

Harvey, A. G., G. Murray, R. A. Chandler, and A. Soehner. 2011. Sleep Disturbance as Transdiagnostic: Consideration of Neurobiological Mechanisms. *Clin. Psychol. Rev.* **31**:225–235. [2]

Hasan, S., Y. Alviany, C. Clarissa, and S. S. Kusuma. 2017. High Perceived Discrimination and No Family Support Increase Risk of Poor Quality of Life in Gender Dysphoria. *Universa Medicina* **36**:187–196. [10]

Hashimoto, T., Q. L. Nguyen, D. Rotaru, et al. 2009. Protracted Developmental Trajectories of GABAA Receptor Alpha1 and Alpha2 Subunit Expression in Primate Prefrontal Cortex. *Biol. Psychiatry* **65**:1015–1023. [7, 9]

Hasler, G., W. C. Drevets, T. D. Gould, I. I. Gottesman, and H. K. Manji. 2006. Toward Constructing an Endophenotype Strategy for Bipolar Disorders. *Biol Psychiat* **60**:93–105. [8]

Hastrup, L. H., C. Kronborg, M. Bertelsen, et al. 2013. Cost-Effectiveness of Early Intervention in First-Episode Psychosis: Economic Evaluation of a Randomised Controlled Trial (the OPUS Study). *Br. J. Psychiatry* **202**:35–41. [11]

Hawe, P., A. Shiell, and T. Riley. 2004. Complex Interventions: How "Out of Control" Can a Randomised Controlled Trial Be? *BMJ* **328**:1561–1563. [12]

Hedelin, M., M. Löf, M. Olsson, et al. 2010. Dietary Intake of Fish, Omega-3, Omega-6 Polyunsaturated Fatty Acids and Vitamin D and the Prevalence of Psychotic-Like Symptoms in a Cohort of 33,000 Women from the General Population. *BMC Psychiat.* **10**:38. [10]

Hegelstad, W. T. V., T. K. Larsen, B. Auestad, et al. 2012. Long-Term Follow-up of the TIPS Early Detection in Psychosis Study: Effects on 10-Year Outcome. *Am. J. Psychiatry* **169**:374–380. [14]

Helbich, M., D. de Beurs, M.-P. Kwan, R. C. O'Connor, and P. P. Groenewegen. 2018. Natural Environments and Suicide Mortality in the Netherlands: A Cross-Sectional, Ecological Study. *Lancet Planet. Health* **2**:e134–e139. [6]

Hensch, T. K. 2003. Controlling the Critical Period. *Neurosci. Res.* **47**:17–22. [7]

———. 2005a. Critical Period Plasticity in Local Cortical Circuits. *Nature reviews. Neuroscience* **6**:877–888. [4]

———. 2005b. Recovery in the Blink of an Eye. *Neuron* **48**:166–168. [3]

Hermens, D. F., S. L. Naismith, J. Lagopoulos, et al. 2013. Neuropsychological Profile According to the Clinical Stage of Young Persons Presenting for Mental Health Care. *BMC Psychol.* **1**:8. [2, 13]

Heron, K. E., and J. M. Smyth. 2010. Ecological Momentary Interventions: Incorporating Mobile Technology into Psychosocial and Health Behaviour Treatments. *Br. J. Health Psychol.* **15**:1–39. [10]

Herpertz-Dahlmann, B., K. Bühren, and H. Remschmidt. 2013. Growing up Is Hard: Mental Disorders in Adolescence. *Dtsch. Arztebl. Int.* **110**:432–439. [5]

Hertzman, C. 1999. The Biological Embedding of Early Experience and Its Effects on Health in Adulthood. *Ann. NY Acad. Sci.* **896**:85–95. [6]

———. 2012. Putting the Concept of Biological Embedding in Historical Perspective. *PNAS* **109**:17160–17167. [6]

Heshmati, M., H. Aleyasin, C. Menard, et al. 2018. Cell-Type-Specific Role for Nucleus Accumbens Neuroligin-2 in Depression and Stress Susceptibility. *PNAS* **115**:1111–1116. [7]

Hetrick, S. E., A. P. Bailey, K. E. Smith, et al. 2017. Integrated (One-Stop Shop) Youth Health Care: Best Available Evidence and Future Directions. *Med. J. Austral.* **207**:S5–S18. [13, 14]

Hetrick, S. E., J. E. McKenzie, and S. N. Merry. 2010. The Use of Ssris in Children and Adolescents. *Curr. Opin. Psychiatry* **23**:53–57. [10]

Hibbeln, J. R. 1998. Fish Consumption and Major Depression. *Lancet* **351**:1213. [10]

Hickie, I. B., D. F. Hermens, S. L. Naismith, et al. 2013a. Evaluating Differential Developmental Trajectories to Adolescent-Onset Mood and Psychotic Disorders. *BMC Psychiat.* **13**:303. [2]

Hickie, I. B., E. M. Scott, D. F. Hermens, et al. 2013b. Applying Clinical Staging to Young People Who Present for Mental Health Care. *Early Interv. Psychiatry* **7**:31–43. [2, 14]

Hickie, I. B., J. Scott, D. F. Hermens, et al. 2013c. Clinical Classification in Mental Health at the Cross-Roads: Which Direction Next? *BMC Med.* **11**:125. [2]

Hickie, I. B., J. Scott, and P. D. McGorry. 2013d. Clinical Staging for Mental Disorders: A New Development in Diagnostic Practice in Mental Health. *Med. J. Austral.* **198**:461–462. [2]

Hilferty, F., R. Cassells, K. Muir, et al. 2015. Is Headspace Making a Difference to Young People's Lives? Final Report of the Independent Evaluation of the Headspace Program. Sydney: Social Policy Research Centre. [13, 14]

Hill, A. B. 1965. The Environment and Disease: Association or Causation? *Proc. Med.* **58**:295–300. [8]

Hill, E. M., F. E. Griffiths, and T. House. 2015. Spreading of Healthy Mood in Adolescent Social Networks. *Proc. Biol. Sci.* **282**:20151180. [6]

Hinde, R. 1987. Interpersonal Relationships and Child Development. *Dev. Rev.* **7**:1–21. [6]

Hirayama, T., T. Kobayashi, T. Fujita, and O. Fujino. 2004. Two Cases of Adult Down Syndrome Treated with Selective Serotonin Re-Uptake Inhibitor for Behavior Disorders. [article in Japanese] *No To Hattatsu* **36**:391–394. [10]

Hjemdal, O., P. A. Vogel, S. Solem, K. Hagen, and T. C. Stiles. 2011. The Relationship between Resilience and Levels of Anxiety, Depression, and Obsessive–Compulsive Symptoms in Adolescents. *Clin. Psychol. Psychother.* **18**:314–321. [5]

Hockfield, S., R. G. Kalb, S. Zaremba, and H. Fryer. 1990. Expression of Neural Proteoglycans Correlates with the Acquisition of Mature Neuronal Properties in the Mammalian Brain. *Cold Spring Harb. Symp. Quant. Biol.* **55**:505–514. [7]

Hodes, G. E., M. L. Pfau, I. Purushothaman, et al. 2015. Sex Differences in Nucleus Accumbens Transcriptome Profiles Associated with Susceptibility Versus Resilience to Subchronic Variable Stress. *J. Neurosci.* **35**:16362–16376. [7]

Hoek, H. W., A. I. Bartelds, J. J. Bosveld, et al. 1995. Impact of Urbanization on Detection Rates of Eating Disorders. *Am. J. Psychiatry* **152**:1272–1278. [6]

Hofstede, G. 2015. Dimensionalizing Cultures: The Hofstede Model in Context. 2. https://scholarworks.gvsu.edu/orpc/vol2/iss1/8/. (accessed July 26, 2019). [5]

Hogan, B., J. R. Melville, G. L. Philips, et al. 2016. Evaluating the Paper-to-Screen Translation of Participant-Aided Sociograms with High-Risk Participants. *Proc. SIGCHI Conf. Hum. Factor Comput. Syst.* **2016**:5360–5371. [6]

Hokanson, J. E., and M. A. Austin. 1996. Plasma Triglyceride Level Is a Risk Factor for Cardiovascular Disease Independent of High-Density Lipoprotein Cholesterol Level: A Meta-Analysis of Population-Based Prospective Studies. *J. Cardiovasc. Risk* **3**:213–219. [10]

Holmes, S. E., R. Hinz, S. Conen, et al. 2018. Elevated Translocator Protein in Anterior Cingulate in Major Depression and a Role for Inflammation in Suicidal Thinking: A Positron Emission Tomography Study. *Biol. Psychiatry* **83**:61–69. [7]

Homan, P., and J. M. Kane. 2018. Clozapine as an Early-Stage Treatment. *Acta Psychiat. Scand.* **138**:279–280. [14]

Horan, W. P., K. L. Subotnik, K. S. Snyder, and K. H. Nuechterlein. 2006. Do Recent-Onset Schizophrenia Patients Experience a "Social Network Crisis"? *Psychiatry* **69**:115–129. [10]

Hoshiko, M., I. Arnoux, E. Avignone, N. Yamamoto, and E. Audinat. 2012. Deficiency of the Microglial Receptor CX3CR1 Impairs Postnatal Functional Development of Thalamocortical Synapses in the Barrel Cortex. *J. Neurosci.* **32**:15106–15111. [7]

Hostinar, C. E., A. E. Johnson, and M. R. Gunnar. 2015. Parent Support Is Less Effective in Buffering Cortisol Stress Reactivity for Adolescents Compared to Children. *Dev. Sci.* **18**:281–297. [5]

Houle, D., D. R. Govindaraju, and S. Omholt. 2010. Phenomics: The Next Challenge. *Nat. Rev. Genet.* **11**:855–866. [6]

Huang, D., L. H. Yang, and B. A. Pescosolido. 2019. Understanding the Public's Profile of Mental Health Literacy in China: A Nationwide Study. *BMC Psychiat.* **19**:20. [11]

Huang, Z. J., A. Kirkwood, T. Pizzorusso, et al. 1999. BDNF Regulates the Maturation of Inhibition and the Critical Period of Plasticity in Mouse Visual Cortex. *Cell* **98**:739–755. [7]

Huntley, G. W., D. L. Benson, E. G. Jones, and P. J. Isackson. 1992. Developmental Expression of Brain Derived Neurotrophic Factor mRNA by Neurons of Fetal and Adult Monkey Prefrontal Cortex. *Brain Res. Dev. Brain Res.* **70**:53–63. [7]

Hutsler, J. J., and H. Zhang. 2010. Increased Dendritic Spine Densities on Cortical Projection Neurons in Autism Spectrum Disorders. *Brain Res.* **1309**:83–94. [7]

Huttenlocher, P. R. 2002. Neural Plasticity: The Effects of Environment on the Development of the Cerebral Cortex. Cambridge, MA: Harvard Univ. Press. [7, 9]

Huys, Q. J. M., T. V. Maia, and M. J. Frank. 2016. Computational Psychiatry as a Bridge from Neuroscience to Clinical Applications. *Nat. Neurosci.* **19**:404–413. [6]

Hwang, K., M. N. Hallquist, and B. Luna. 2013. The Development of Hub Architecture in the Human Functional Brain Network. *Cereb. Cortex* **23**:2380–2393. [9]

Hyde, T. M., J. C. Ziegler, and D. R. Weinberger. 1992. Psychiatric Disturbances in Metachromatic Leukodystrophy: Insights into the Neurobiology of Psychosis. *Arch. Neurol.* **49**:401–406. [7]

Hyman, S. E. 2013. Psychiatric Drug Development: Diagnosing a Crisis. *Cerebrum* **2013**:5. [1]

Ibáñez, L., A. López-Bermejo, M. Díaz, M. V. Marcos, and F. de Zegher. 2011. Early Metformin Therapy (Age 8–12 Years) in Girls with Precocious Pubarche to Reduce Hirsutism, Androgen Excess, and Oligomenorrhea in Adolescence. *J. Clin. Endocrinol. Metab.* **96**:E1262–1267. [6]

Insel, T. R. 2007. The Arrival of Preemptive Psychiatry. *Early Interv. Psychiatry* **1**:5–6. [2]

———. 2009. Translating Scientific Opportunity into Public Health Impact: A Strategic Plan for Research on Mental Illness. *Arch. Gen. Psychiatry* **66**:128–133. [2]

———. 2017. Digital Phenotyping: Technology for a New Science of Behavior. *JAMA* **318**:1215–1216. [6, 10]

Insel, T. R., B. N. Cuthbert, M. Garvey, et al. 2010. Research Domain Criteria (RDoC): Toward a New Classification Framework for Research on Mental Disorders. *Am. J. Psychiatry* **167**:748–751. [2, 3, 9]

Insel, T. R., and W. S. Fenton. 2005. Psychiatric Epidemiology: It's Not Just About Counting Anymore. *Arch. Gen. Psychiatry* **62**:590–592. [1, 12]

Institute of Medicine. 2013. Observational Studies in a Learning Health System: Workshop Summary, C. Grossmann and J. Alper, series ed. Washington, D.C.: National Academies Press. [12]

Institute of Medicine's Quality of Health Care in America. 2001. Crossing the Quality Chasm: A New Health System for the 21st Century. Crossing the Quality Chasm: A New Health System for the 21st Century. Institute of Medicine Committee on Quality of Health Care in America. Washington, D.C.: National Academies Press. [12]

Ioannidis, J. P. A., E. Y. Loy, R. Poulton, and K. S. Chia. 2009. Researching Genetic Versus Nongenetic Determinants of Disease: A Comparison and Proposed Unification. *Sci. Transl. Med.* **1**:7ps8–7ps8. [6]

Iorfino, F., D. F. Hermens, S. P. M. Cross, et al. 2018. Prior Suicide Attempts Predict Worse Clinical and Functional Outcomes in Young People Attending a Mental Health Service. *J. Affective Disord.* **238**:563–569. [2]

Iossi Silva, M., B. Pereira, D. Mendonça, B. Nunes, and W. Oliveira. 2013. The Involvement of Girls and Boys with Bullying: An Analysis of Gender Differences. *Int. J. Environ. Res. Pub. Health* **10**:6820–6831. [6]

Itami, C., F. Kimura, and S. Nakamura. 2007. Brain-Derived Neurotrophic Factor Regulates the Maturation of Layer 4 Fast-Spiking Cells after the Second Postnatal Week in the Developing Barrel Cortex. *J. Neurosci.* **27**:2241–2252. [7]

Jablensky, A., J. McGrath, H. Herrman, et al. 1999. People Living with Psychotic Illness: An Australian Study 1997–1998, vol. 4. Canberra: Commonwealth of Australia Department of Health and Aging. [14]

Jacobson, D. M., and S. Teutsch. 2012. An Environmental Scan of Integrated Approaches for Defining and Measuring Total Population Health by the Clinical Care System, the Government Public Health System, and Stakeholder Organizations. Oakland, CA: Public Health Institute. [12]

Jalbrzikowski, M., B. Larsen, M. N. Hallquist, et al. 2017. Development of White Matter Microstructure and Intrinsic Functional Connectivity between the Amygdala and Ventromedial Prefrontal Cortex: Associations with Anxiety and Depression. *Biol Psychiat* **82**:511–521. [9]

James, M. J., T. R. Sullivan, R. G. Metcalf, and L. G. Cleland. 2014. Pitfalls in the Use of Randomised Controlled Trials for Fish Oil Studies with Cardiac Patients. *Br. J. Nutrition* **112**:812–820. [10]

Javitt, D. C., C. E. Schroeder, M. Steinschneider, et al. 1995. Cognitive Event-Related Potentials in Human and Non-Human Primates: Implications for the PCP/NMDA Model of Schizophrenia. *Electroencephalogr. Clin. Neurophysiol. Suppl.* **44**:161–175. [8]

Jensen, C. B. 2008. Sociology, Systems and (Patient) Safety: Knowledge Translations in Healthcare Policy. *Soc. Health Ill.* **30**:309–324. [12]

Jiang, B., Z. J. Huang, B. Morales, and A. Kirkwood. 2005. Maturation of GABAergic Transmission and the Timing of Plasticity in Visual Cortex. *Brain Res. Brain Res. Rev.* **50**:126–133. [7]

Joa, I., J. O. Johannessen, B. Auestad, et al. 2007. The Key to Reducing Duration of Untreated First Psychosis: Information Campaigns. *Schizophr. Bull.* **34**:466–472. [14]

Johnson, M. H., T. Grossmann, and K. C. Kadosh. 2009. Mapping Functional Brain Development: Building a Social Brain through Interactive Specialization. *Dev. Psychol.* **45**:151–159. [4]

Johnson, W., D. Kuh, and R. Hardy. 2015. A Life Course Perspective on Body Size and Cardio-Metabolic Health. In: A Life Course Perspective on Health Trajectories and Transitions, ed. C. Burton-Jeangros et al., pp. 61–83. Cham: Springer. [9]

Jolles, D. D., and E. A. Crone. 2012. Training the Developing Brain: A Neurocognitive Perspective. *Front. Hum. Neurosci.* **6**:76. [4]

Jones, P. B. 2013. Adult Mental Health Disorders and Their Age at Onset. *Br. J. Psychiatry* **202**:s5–s10. [4, 12]

Jones, S. G., and R. M. Benca. 2015. Circadian Disruption in Psychiatric Disorders. *Sleep Med. Clin.* **10**:481–493. [2]

Jung, Y., L. S. Hsieh, A. M. Lee, et al. 2016. An Epigenetic Mechanism Mediates Developmental Nicotine Effects on Neuronal Structure and Behavior. *Nat. Neurosci.* **19**:905–914. [6]

Kaiser, S., A. Roth, M. Rentrop, et al. 2008. Intra-Individual Reaction Time Variability in Schizophrenia, Depression and Borderline Personality Disorder. *Brain Cognition* **66**:73–82. [3]

Kamil, M. L., P. B. Mosenthal, P. D. Pearson, and R. Barr, eds. 2016. Handbook of Reading Research, vol. 3. New York: Routledge. [3]

Kane, J. M., D. G. Robinson, N. R. Schooler, et al. 2016. Comprehensive Versus Usual Community Care for First-Episode Psychosis: 2-Year Outcomes from the NIMH RAISE Early Treatment Program. *Am. J. Psychiatry* **173**:362–372. [13, 14]

Kapczinski, F., V. V. Dias, M. Kauer-Sant'Anna, et al. 2009. Clinical Implications of a Staging Model for Bipolar Disorders. *Expert Rev. Neurotherap.* **9**:957–966. [2]

Karatsoreos, I. N. 2014. Links between Circadian Rhythms and Psychiatric Disease. *Front. Behav. Neurosci.* **8**:162. [2]

Kass, N. E., R. R. Faden, S. N. Goodman, et al. 2013. The Research-Treatment Distinction: A Problematic Approach for Determining Which Activities Should Have Ethical Oversight *Hastings Cent. Rep.* **43(S1)**:S4–S15. [12]

Katagiri, H., M. Fagiolini, and T. K. Hensch. 2007. Optimization of Somatic Inhibition at Critical Period Onset in Mouse Visual Cortex. *Neuron* **53**:805–812. [7]

Kaufmann, T., D. Alnæs, N. T. Doan, et al. 2017. Delayed Stabilization and Individualization in Connectome Development Are Related to Psychiatric Disorders. *Nat. Neurosci.* **20**:513–515. [4]

Kauppi, K., S. B. Rosenthal, M. T. Lo, et al. 2018. Revisiting Antipsychotic Drug Actions through Gene Networks Associated with Schizophrenia. *Am. J. Psychiatry* **175**:674–682. [8]

Kelleher, I., H. Keeley, P. Corcoran, et al. 2012a. Clinicopathological Significance of Psychotic Experiences in Non-Psychotic Young People: Evidence from Four Population-Based Studies. *Br. J. Psychiatry* **201**:26–32. [2, 14]

Kennard, B. D., G. J. Emslie, T. L. Mayes, and J. L. Hughes. 2006. Relapse and Recurrence in Pediatric Depression. *Child Adolesc. Psychiatr. Clin. N. Am.* **15**:1057–1079. [10]

Kennard, B. D., T. Goldstein, A. A. Foxwell, et al. 2018. As Safe as Possible (ASAP): A Brief App-Supported Inpatient Intervention to Prevent Postdischarge Suicidal Behavior in Hospitalized, Suicidal Adolescents. *Am. J. Psychiatry* **175**:864–872. [3]

Kesek, A., P. D. Zelazo, and M. D. Lewis. 2008. The Development of Executive Function and Emotion Regulation in Adolescence. In: Adolescent Emotional Development and the Emergence of Depressive Disorders, ed. N. B. Allen and L. B. Sheeber, pp. 135–155. New York: Cambridge Univ. Press. [4]

Keshavan, M. S., S. Anderson, and J. W. Pettergrew. 1994. Is Schizophrenia Due to Excessive Synaptic Pruning in the Prefrontal Cortex? The Feinberg Hypothesis Revisited. *J. Psychiatr. Res.* **28**:239–265. [7, 8]

Keshavan, M. S., A. N. Lawler, H. A. Nasrallah, and R. Tandon. 2017. New Drug Developments in Psychosis: Challenges, Opportunities and Strategies. *Prog. Neurobiol.* **152**:3–20. [8]

Keshavan, M. S., U. M. Mehta, J. L. Padmanabhan, and J. L. Shah. 2015. Dysplasticity, Metaplasticity, and Schizophrenia: Implications for Risk, Illness, and Novel Interventions. *Dev. Psychopathol.* **27**:615–635. [8]

Kessler, R. C., G. P. Amminger, S. Aguilar-Gaxiola, et al. 2007. Age of Onset of Mental Disorders: A Review of Recent Literature. *Curr. Opin. Psychiatry* **20**:359–364. [9, 12, 13]

Kessler, R. C., S. Avenevoli, E. J. Costello, et al. 2012. Prevalence, Persistence, and Sociodemographic Correlates of DSM-IV Disorders in the National Comorbidity Survey Replication Adolescent Supplement. *Arch. Gen. Psychiatry* **69**:372–380. [1]

Kessler, R. C., P. Berglund, O. Demler, et al. 2005. Lifetime Prevalence and Age-of-Onset Distributions of DSM-IV Disorders in the National Comorbidity Survey Replication. *Arch. Gen. Psychiatry* **62**:593–602. [1–4, 7, 9]

Kessler, R. C., K. A. McLaughlin, J. G. Green, et al. 2010. Childhood Adversities and Adult Psychopathology in the Who World Mental Health Surveys. *Br. J. Psychiatry* **197**:378–385. [6]

Kessler, R. C., N. A. Sampson, P. Berglund, et al. 2015. Anxious and Non-Anxious Major Depressive Disorder in the World Health Organization World Mental Health Surveys. *Epidemiol. Psychiatr. Sci.* **24**:210–226. [9]

Kessler, R. C., and P. S. Wang. 2008. The Descriptive Epidemiology of Commonly Occurring Mental Disorders in the United States. *Annu. Rev. Public Health* **29**:115–129. [4]

Kettenmann, H., F. Kirchhoff, and A. Verkhratsky. 2013. Microglia: New Roles for the Synaptic Stripper. *Neuron* **77**:10–18. [7]

Kiecolt-Glaser, J. K., M. A. Belury, R. Andridge, W. B. Malarkey, and R. Glaser. 2011. Omega-3 Supplementation Lowers Inflammation and Anxiety in Medical Students: A Randomized Controlled Trial. *Brain Behav. Immun.* **25**:1725–1734. [10]

Kilford, E. J., E. Garrett, and S.-J. Blakemore. 2016. The Development of Social Cognition in Adolescence: An Integrated Perspective. *Neurosci. Biobehav. Rev.* **70**:106–120. [6]

Killackey, E., K. Allott, H. J. Jackson, et al. 2019. Individual Placement and Support for Vocational Recovery in First-Episode Psychosis: Randomised Controlled Trial. *Br. J. Psychiatry* **214(2)**:76–78. [14]

Killackey, E., H. J. Jackson, and P. D. McGorry. 2008. Vocational Intervention in First-Episode Psychosis: Individual Placement and Support Versus Treatment as Usual. *Br. J. Psychiatry* **193**:114–120. [14]

Killackey, E. J., H. J. Jackson, J. Gleeson, I. B. Hickie, and P. D. McGorry. 2006. Exciting Career Opportunity Beckons! Early Intervention and Vocational Rehabilitation in First Episode Psychosis: Employing Cautious Optimism. *Aust. N. Z. J. Psychiatry* **40**:951–962. [1]

Kim, H. H. 2017. The Impact of Online Social Networking on Adolescent Psychological Well-Being (WB): A Population-Level Analysis of Korean School-Aged Children. *Int. J. Adolesc. Youth* **22**:364–376. [6]

Kim, J. J., and M. S. Fanselow. 1992. Modality-Specific Retrograde Amnesia of Fear. *Science* **256**:675–677. [9]

Kim, S.-W., M. Jhon, J.-M. Kim, et al. 2016. Relationship between Erythrocyte Fatty Acid Composition and Psychopathology in the Vienna Omega-3 Study. *PLoS ONE* **11**:e0151417. [10]

Kim-Cohen, J., A. Caspi, T. E. Moffitt, et al. 2003. Prior Juvenile Diagnoses in Adults with Mental Disorder: Developmental Follow-Back of a Prospective-Longitudinal Cohort. *Arch. Gen. Psychiatry* **60**:709–717. [1–3, 5]

Kim-Spoon, J., D. Maciejewski, J. Lee, K. Deater-Deckard, and B. King-Casas. 2017. Longitudinal Associations among Family Environment, Neural Cognitive Control, and Social Competence among Adolescents. *Dev. Cogn. Neurosci.* **26**:69–76. [6]

Kindig, D., and G. Stoddart. 2003. What Is Population Health? *Am. J. Public Health* **93**:380–383. [12]

Kindig, D. A., Y. Asada, and B. Booske. 2008. A Population Health Framework for Setting National and State Health Goals. *JAMA* **299**:2081–2083. [12]

Kirch, W., ed. 2008. Encyclopedia of Public Health, vol. Dordrecht: Springer Netherlands. [6]

Kirkbride, J. B. 2015. Epidemiology on Demand: Population-Based Approaches to Mental Health Service Commissioning. *BJ Psych. Bull.* **39**:242–247. [6]

Kirkwood, A., H. K. Lee, and M. F. Bear. 1995. Co-Regulation of Long-Term Potentiation and Experience-Dependent Synaptic Plasticity in Visual Cortex by Age and Experience. *Nature* **375**:328–331. [7]

Klausberger, T., J. D. Roberts, and P. Somogyi. 2002. Cell Type- and Input-Specific Differences in the Number and Subtypes of Synaptic GABAA Receptors in the Hippocampus. *J. Neurosci.* **22**:2513–2521. [7]

Kleibeuker, S. W., C. K. W. De Dreu, and E. A. Crone. 2016. Creativity Development in Adolescence: Insight from Behavior, Brain, and Training Studies. *New Direct. Child and Adolesc. Dev.* **151**:73–84. [4]

Klein, R. S., and C. A. Hunter. 2017. Protective and Pathological Immunity During Central Nervous System Infections. *Immunity* **46**:891–909. [7]

Kleinman, A. 1999. Experience and Its Moral Modes: Culture, Human Conditions, and Disorder, vol. 20. The Tanner Lectures on Human Values. Salt Lake City: Univ. of Utah Press. [6]

———. 2004. Culture and Depression. *New England Journal of Medicine* **351**:951–953. [6]

Kleinman, A., and P. Benson. 2006. Anthropology in the Clinic: The Problem of Cultural Competency and How to Fix It. *PLoS Med.* **3**:e294. [6]

Knapp, M., A. Andrew, D. McDaid, et al. 2014. Investing in Recovery: Making the Business Case for Effective Interventions for People with Schizophrenia and Psychosis. PSSRU, The London School of Economics and Political Science, and Centre for Mental Health. [11]

Knox, P. L., and L. McCarthy. 2005. Urbanization: An Introduction to Urban Geography. Upper Saddle River: Pearson Prentice Hall. [6]

Kobayashi, C., G. H. Glover, and E. Temple. 2007. Cultural and Linguistic Effects on Neural Bases of "Theory of Mind" in American and Japanese Children. *Brain Res.* **1164**:95–107. [6]

Koenen, K. C., S. Rudenstine, E. Susser, and S. Galea, eds. 2013. A Life Course Approach to Mental Disorders, vol. Oxford: Oxford Univ. Press. [6]

Koike, H., P. A. Arguello, M. Kvajo, M. Karayiorgou, and J. A. Gogos. 2006. Disc1 Is Mutated in the 129S6/SvEv Strain and Modulates Working Memory in Mice. *PNAS* **103**:3693–2697. [8]

Koivukangas, J., T. Tammelin, M. Kaakinen, et al. 2010. Physical Activity and Fitness in Adolescents at Risk for Psychosis within the Northern Finland 1986 Birth Cohort. *Schizophr. Res.* **116**:152–158. [11]

Kong, A., G. Thorleifsson, M. L. Frigge, et al. 2018. The Nature of Nurture: Effects of Parental Genotypes. *Science* **359**:424–428. [5]

Koolschijn, P. C., J. S. Peper, and E. A. Crone. 2014. The Influence of Sex Steroids on Structural Brain Maturation in Adolescence. *PLoS ONE* **9**:e83929. [7]

Korotkova, T., E. C. Fuchs, A. Ponomarenko, J. von Engelhardt, and H. Monyer. 2010. NMDA Receptor Ablation on Parvalbumin-Positive Interneurons Impairs Hippocampal Synchrony, Spatial Representations, and Working Memory. *Neuron* **68**:557–569. [7]

Koshy, A. N., J. K. Sajeev, N. Nerlekar, et al. 2018. Smart Watches for Heart Rate Assessment in Atrial Arrhythmias. *Int. J. Cardiol.* **266**:124–127. [3]

Kotov, R., R. F. Krueger, and D. Watson. 2018. A Paradigm Shift in Psychiatric Classification: The Hierarchical Taxonomy of Psychopathology (HiTOP). *World Psychiatry* **17**:24–25. [1, 14]

Kouzarides, T., and S. L. Berger. 2007. Chromatin Modifications and Their Mechanism of Action. In: Epigenetics ed. C. D. Allis et al., pp. 191–210. Cold Spring Harbor: Cold Spring Harbor Laboratory Press. [8]

Kozak, M. J., and B. N. Cuthbert. 2016. The NIMH Research Domain Criteria Initiative: Background, Issues, and Pragmatics. *Psychophysiology* **53**:286–297. [2]

Krabbendam, L. 2005. Schizophrenia and Urbanicity: A Major Environmental Influence–Conditional on Genetic Risk. *Schizophr. Bull.* **31**:795–799. [6]

Kraemer, H. C. 2016. Messages for Clinicians: Moderators and Mediators of Treatment Outcome in Randomized Clinical Trials. *Am. J. Psychiatry* **173**:672–679. [10]

Kraemer, H. C., G. T. Wilson, C. G. Fairburn, and W. S. Agras. 2002. Mediators and Moderators of Treatment Effects in Randomized Clinical Trials. *Arch. Gen. Psychiatry* **59**:877–883. [4]

Kraepelin, E. 1909. Psychiatrie. Ein Lehrbuch Für Studierende Und Ärzte. Achte, Vollständig Umgearbeitete Auflage. I. Band. Allgemeine Psychiatrie. Leipzig: Barth. [14]

Kroken, R. A., E. M. Loberg, T. Dronen, et al. 2014. A Critical Review of Pro-Cognitive Drug Targets in Psychosis: Convergence on Myelination and Inflammation. *Front. Psychiatry* **5**:11. [7]

Kuh, D., Y. Ben-Shlomo, J. Lynch, J. Hallqvist, and C. Power. 2003. Life Course Epidemiology. *J. Epidemiol. Community Health* **57**:778–783. [9]

Kuhn, D. 2006. Do Cognitive Changes Accompany Developments in the Adolescent Brain? *Persp. Psychologic. Sci.* **1**:59–67. [4]

Kurvers, R. H. J. M., and F. Holker. 2015. Bright Nights and Social Interactions: A Neglected Issue. *Behav. Ecol.* **26**:334–339. [6]

Kuzawa, C. W., H. T. Chugani, L. I. Grossman, et al. 2014. Metabolic Costs and Evolutionary Implications of Human Brain Development. *PNAS* **111**:13010–13015. [7]

Kuzirian, M. S., and S. Paradis. 2011. Emerging Themes in GABAergic Synapse Development. *Prog. Neurobiol.* **95**:68–87. [7]

Lagopoulos, J., D. F. Hermens, S. N. Hatton, et al. 2013. Microstructural White Matter Changes Are Correlated with the Stage of Psychiatric Illness. *Transl. Psychiatry* **3**:e248. [2]

Lagopoulos, J., D. F. Hermens, S. L. Naismith, E. M. Scott, and I. B. Hickie. 2012. Frontal Lobe Changes Occur Early in the Course of Affective Disorders in Young People. *BMC Psychiat.* **12**:4. [2, 13]

Lambe, E. K., L. S. Krimer, and P. S. Goldman-Rakic. 2000. Differential Postnatal Development of Catecholamine and Serotonin Inputs to Identified Neurons in Prefrontal Cortex of Rhesus Monkey. *J. Neurosci.* **20**:8780–8787. [7]

Lamblin, M., C. Murawski, S. Whittle, and A. Fornito. 2017. Social Connectedness, Mental Health and the Adolescent Brain. *Neurosci. Biobehav. Rev.* **80**:57–68. [6]

Landstedt, E., K. Asplund, and G. K. Gillander. 2009. Understanding Adolescent Mental Health: The Influence of Social Processes, Doing Gender and Gendered Power Relations. *Soc. Health Ill.* **31**:962–978. [5]

Lane, J. P., and J. L. Flagg. 2010. Translating Three States of Knowledge—Discovery, Invention, and Innovation. *Implement. Sci.* **5**:9. [12]

Larsen, B., and B. Luna. 2018. Adolescence as a Neurobiological Critical Period for the Development of Higher-Order Cognition. *Neurosci. Biobehav. Rev.* **94**:179–195. [3, 9]

Larsen, B., T. D. Verstynen, F.-C. Yeh, and B. Luna. 2018. Developmental Changes in the Integration of Affective and Cognitive Corticostriatal Pathways Are Associated with Reward-Driven Behavior. *Cereb. Cortex* **28**:2834–2845. [9]

Lau, J. Y. F., and A. M. Waters. 2017. Annual Research Review: An Expanded Account of Information-Processing Mechanisms in Risk for Child and Adolescent Anxiety and Depression. *J. Child Psychol. Psychiatry* **58**:387–407. [5]

Lavin, A., H. M. Moore, and A. A. Grace. 2005. Prenatal Disruption of Neocortical Development Alters Prefrontal Cortical Neuron Responses to Dopamine in Adult Rats. *Neuropsychopharmacology* **30**:1426–1435. [8]

Lazer, D., A. Pentland, L. Adamic, et al. 2009. Social Science: Computational Social Science. *Science* **323**:721–723. [6]

Lebel, C., and C. Beaulieu. 2011. Longitudinal Development of Human Brain Wiring Continues from Childhood into Adulthood. *J. Neurosci.* **31**:10937–10947. [9]

Lebel, C., and S. Deoni. 2018. The Development of Brain White Matter Microstructure. *Neuroimage* **182**:207–218. [7]

Lebel, C., M. Gee, R. Camicioli, et al. 2012. Diffusion Tensor Imaging of White Matter Tract Evolution over the Lifespan. *Neuroimage* **60**:340–352. [9]

Lee, D. 2008. Game Theory and Neural Basis of Social Decision Making. *Nat. Neurosci.* **11**:404–409. [6]

Lee, F. S., H. Heimer, J. N. Giedd, et al. 2014a. Mental Health. Adolescent Mental Health: Opportunity and Obligation. *Science* **346**:547–549. [1]

Lee, H., D. Dvorak, H. Y. Kao, et al. 2012. Early Cognitive Experience Prevents Adult Deficits in a Neurodevelopmental Schizophrenia Model. *Neuron* **75**:714–724. [9]

Lee, H. H. C., C. Bernard, Z. Ye, et al. 2017. Genetic Otx2 Mis-Localization Delays Critical Period Plasticity across Brain Regions. *Mol. Psychiatr.* **22**:680–688. [7]

Lee, J. K., A. D. Ekstrom, and S. Ghetti. 2014b. Volume of Hippocampal Subfields and Episodic Memory in Childhood and Adolescence. *Neuroimage* **94**:162–171. [9]

Lee, R. S., D. F. Hermens, S. L. Naismith, et al. 2015. Neuropsychological and Functional Outcomes in Recent-Onset Major Depression, Bipolar Disorder and Schizophrenia-Spectrum Disorders: A Longitudinal Cohort Study. *Transl. Psychiatry* **5**:e555. [2]

Lee, R. S., D. F. Hermens, M. A. Redoblado-Hodge, et al. 2013. Neuropsychological and Socio-Occupational Functioning in Young Psychiatric Outpatients: A Longitudinal Investigation. *PLoS ONE* **8**:e58176. [2]

Lee, R. S. C., D. F. Hermens, J. Scott, et al. 2014c. A Meta-Analysis of Neuropsychological Functioning in First-Episode Bipolar Disorders. *J. Psychiatr. Res.* **57C**:1–11. [2]

Lee, T. H. 2010. Putting the Value Framework to Work. *New Engl. J. Med.* **363**:2481–2483. [12]

Lee, Y., and D. Styne. 2013. Influences on the Onset and Tempo of Puberty in Human Beings and Implications for Adolescent Psychological Development. *Horm. Behav.* **64**:250–261. [5]

LeGates, T. A., C. M. Altimus, H. Wang, et al. 2012. Aberrant Light Directly Impairs Mood and Learning through Melanopsin-Expressing Neurons. *Nature* **491**:594–598. [6]

Lencz, T., and A. K. Malhotra. 2015. Targeting the Schizophrenia Genome: A Fast Track Strategy from GWAS to Clinic. *Mol. Psychiatr.* **20**:820–826. [8]

Lenroot, R. K., N. Gogtay, D. K. Greenstein, et al. 2007. Sexual Dimorphism of Brain Developmental Trajectories During Childhood and Adolescence. *Neuroimage* **36**:1065–1073. [9]

Lensjo, K. K., M. E. Lepperod, G. Dick, T. Hafting, and M. Fyhn. 2017. Removal of Perineuronal Nets Unlocks Juvenile Plasticity through Network Mechanisms of Decreased Inhibition and Increased Gamma Activity. *J. Neurosci.* **37**:1269–1283. [7]

Lenzenweger, M. F. 2013. Thinking Clearly About the Endophenotype-Intermediate Phenotype-Biomarker Distinctions in Developmental Psychopathology Research. *Dev. Psychopathol.* **25**:1347–1357. [8]

Lepeta, K., and L. Kaczmarek. 2015. Matrix Metalloproteinase-9 as a Novel Player in Synaptic Plasticity and Schizophrenia. *Schizophr. Bull.* **41**:1003–1009. [7]

Leussis, M. P., K. Lawson, K. Stone, and S. L. Andersen. 2008. The Enduring Effects of an Adolescent Social Stressor on Synaptic Density, Part II: Poststress Reversal of Synaptic Loss in the Cortex by Adinazolam and MK-801. *Synapse* **62**:185–192. [5]

Levinson, D. F. 2003. Molecular Genetics of Schizophrenia: A Review of the Recent Literature. *Curr. Opin. Psychiatry* **16**:157–170. [8]

Lewinsohn, P. M., R. Zinbarg, J. R. Seeley, M. Lewinsohn, and W. H. Sack. 1997. Lifetime Comorbidity among Anxiety Disorders and between Anxiety Disorders and Other Mental Disorders in Adolescents. *J. Anxiety Disord.* **11**:377–394. [9]

Lewis, D. A., and J. A. Lieberman. 2000. Catching up on Schizophrenia: Natural History and Neurobiology. *Neuron* **28**:325–334. [7]

Li, Q., Y. Han, A. B. C. Dy, and R. J. Hagerman. 2017. The Gut Microbiota and Autism Spectrum Disorders. *Front. Cell. Neurosci.* **11**:120. [7]

Li, S.-C. 2003. Biocultural Orchestration of Developmental Plasticity across Levels: The Interplay of Biology and Culture in Shaping the Mind and Behavior across the Life Span. *Psychol. Bull.* **129**:171–194. [6]

Lichenstein, S. D., T. Verstynen, and E. E. Forbes. 2016. Adolescent Brain Development and Depression: A Case for the Importance of Connectivity of the Anterior Cingulate Cortex. *Neurosci. Biobehav. Rev.* **70**:271–287. [7]

Lichtenstein, P., B. H. Yip, C. Björk, et al. 2009. Common Genetic Determinants of Schizophrenia and Bipolar Disorder in Swedish Families: A Population-Based Study. *Lancet* **373**:234–239. [2]

Lidow, M. S., and P. Rakic. 1992. Scheduling of Monoaminergic Neurotransmitter Receptor Expression in the Primate Neocortex During Postnatal Development. *Cereb. Cortex* **2**:401–416. [7]

Lieberman, J. A., D. Perkins, A. Belger, et al. 2001. The Early Stages of Schizophrenia: Speculations on Pathogenesis, Pathophysiology, and Therapeutic Approaches. *Biol Psychiat* **50**:884–897. [2]

Lillard, A. 1998. Ethnopsychologies: Cultural Variations in Theories of Mind. *Psychol. Bull.* **123**:3–32. [6]

Lim, K., T. Lee, M. Kim, et al. 2016. Early Referral and Comorbidity as Possible Causes of the Declining Transition Rate in Subjects at Clinical High Risk for Psychosis. *Early Interv. Psychiatry* **74**:149. [11]

Lin, A., S. J. Wood, B. Nelson, et al. 2015. Outcomes of Nontransitioned Cases in a Sample at Ultra-High Risk for Psychosis. *Am. J. Psychiatry* **172**:249–258. [1, 14]

Lin, A., A. R. Yung, B. Nelson, et al. 2013. Neurocognitive Predictors of Transition to Psychosis: Medium- to Long-Term Findings from a Sample at Ultra-High Risk for Psychosis. *Psychol. Med.* **43**:2349–2360. [2]

Lin, P.-Y., C.-H. Chang, M. F.-F. Chong, H. Chen, and K.-P. Su. 2017. Polyunsaturated Fatty Acids in Perinatal Depression: A Systematic Review and Meta-Analysis. *Biol Psychiat* **82**:560–569. [10]

Lipska, B. K., G. E. Jaskiw, S. Chrapusta, F. Karoum, and D. R. Weinberger. 1992. Ibotenic Acid Lesion of the Ventral Hippocampus Differentially Affects Dopamine and Its Metabolites in the Nucleus Accumbens and Prefrontal Cortex in the Rat. *Brain Res.* **585**:1–6. [8]

Lipska, B. K., G. E. Jaskiw, and D. R. Weinberger. 1993. Postpubertal Emergence of Hyperresponsiveness to Stress and to Amphetamine after Neonatal Excitotoxic Hippocampal Damage: A Potential Animal Model of Schizophrenia. *Neuropsychopharmacology* **9**:67–75. [9]

Liu, G., B. S. Mühlhäusler, and R. A. Gibson. 2014a. A Method for Long Term Stabilisation of Long Chain Polyunsaturated Fatty Acids in Dried Blood Spots and Its Clinical Application. *PLEFA* **91**:251–260. [10]

Liu, H., P. F. Gao, H. W. Xu, et al. 2013a. Perineuronal Nets Increase Inhibitory GABAergic Currents During the Critical Period in Rats. *Int. J. Ophthalmol.* **6**:120–125. [7]

Liu, H., Y. Tang, F. Womer, et al. 2014b. Differentiating Patterns of Amygdala-Frontal Functional Connectivity in Schizophrenia and Bipolar Disorder. *Schizophr. Bull.* **40**:469–477. [9]

Liu, J. J., H. C. Galfalvy, T. B. Cooper, et al. 2013b. Omega-3 Polyunsaturated Fatty Acid (PUFA) Status in Major Depressive Disorder with Comorbid Anxiety Disorders. *J. Clin. Psychiatry* **74**:732–738. [10]

Liu, Y., W. C. Hsiao, and K. Eggleston. 1999. Equity in Health and Health Care: The Chinese Experience. *Soc. Sci. Med.* **49**:1349–1356. [6]

Lockhart, S., A. Sawa, and M. Niwa. 2018. Developmental Trajectories of Brain Maturation and Behavior: Relevance to Major Mental Illnesses. *J. Pharmacol. Sci.* **137**:1–4. [7]

Loebel, A. D., J. A. Lieberman, J. M. Alvir, et al. 1992. Duration of Psychosis and Outcome in First-Episode Schizophrenia. *Am. J. Psychiatry* **149**:1183–1188. [14]

Lopez, A. D., C. D. Mathers, M. Ezzati, D. T. Jamison, and C. J. L. Murray. 2006. Global and Regional Burden of Disease and Risk Factors, 2001: Systematic Analysis of Population Health Data. *Lancet* **367**:1747–1757. [2]

Lozano, R., M. Naghavi, K. Foreman, et al. 2012. Global and Regional Mortality from 235 Causes of Death for 20 Age Groups in 1990 and 2010: A Systematic Analysis for the Global Burden of Disease Study 2010. *Lancet* **380**:2095–2128. [6]

Lu, J., L. Lu, Y. Yu, et al. 2018. Effects of Intestinal Microbiota on Brain Development in Humanized Gnotobiotic Mice. *Scientific Rep.* **8**:5443. [7]

Luengo Kanacri, B. P., N. Eisenberg, E. Thartori, et al. 2017. Longitudinal Relations among Positivity, Perceived Positive School Climate, and Prosocial Behavior in Colombian Adolescents. *Child Dev.* **88**:1100–1114. [6]

Luna, B., S. Marek, B. Larsen, B. Tervo-Clemmens, and R. Chahal. 2015. An Integrative Model of the Maturation of Cognitive Control. *Annu. Rev. Neurosci.* **38**:151–170. [9]

Luna, B., D. J. Paulsen, A. Padmanabhan, and C. F. Geier. 2013. Cognitive Control and Motivation. *Curr. Dir. Psychol. Sci.* **22**:94–100. [9]

Lund, C., C. Brooke-Sumner, F. Baingana, et al. 2018. Social Determinants of Mental Disorders and the Sustainable Development Goals: A Systematic Review of Reviews. *Lancet Psychiatry* **5**:357–369. [5]

Luthar, S. S., and D. Cicchetti. 2000. The Construct of Resilience: Implications for Interventions and Social Policies. *Dev. Psychopathol.* **12**:857–885. [5]

Luthar, S. S., and L. B. Zelazo. 2003. An Integrative Review. In: Resilience and Vulnerability: Adaptation in the Context of Childhood Adversities, ed. S. S. Luthar, pp. 510–549. New York: Cambridge Univ. Press. [5]

MacCarron, P., K. Kaski, and R. Dunbar. 2016. Calling Dunbar's Numbers. *Social Networks* **47**:151–155. [6]

Mackenzie, M., C. O'Donnell, E. Halliday, S. Sridharan, and S. Platt. 2010. Do Health Improvement Programmes Fit with MRC Guidance on Evaluating Complex Interventions? *BMJ* **340**:c185. [12]

Mahadik, S. P., and R. E. Scheffer. 1996. Oxidative Injury and Potential Use of Antioxidants in Schizophrenia. *PLEFA* **55**:45–54. [7]

Maharana, A., and E. O. Nsoesie. 2018. Use of Deep Learning to Examine the Association of the Built Environment with Prevalence of Neighborhood Adult Obesity. *JAMA Network Open* **1**:e181535. [6]

Malenka, R. C., and M. F. Bear. 2004. LTP and LTD: An Embarrassment of Riches. *Neuron* **44**:5–21. [9]

Malhi, G. S., G. Morris, A. Hamilton, T. Outhred, and Z. Mannie. 2017. Is "Early Intervention" in Bipolar Disorder What It Claims to Be? *Bipolar Disord.* **19**:627–636. [14]

Malla, A., R. Joober, S. Iyer, et al. 2017. Comparing Three-Year Extension of Early Intervention Service to Regular Care Following Two Years of Early Intervention Service in First-Episode Psychosis: A Randomized Single Blind Clinical Trial. *World Psychiatry* **16**:278–286. [13, 14]

Mallya, A. P., H. D. Wang, H. N. R. Lee, and A. Y. Deutch. 2018. Microglial Pruning of Synapses in the Prefrontal Cortex During Adolescence. *Cereb. Cortex* **Apr 13**: doi: 10.1093/cercor/bhy1061. [7]

Manjunatha, N., C. N. Kumar, S. B. Math, and J. Thirthalli. 2018. Designing and Implementing an Innovative Digitally Driven Primary Care Psychiatry Program in India. *Indian J. Psychiatry* **60**:236–244. [6]

Marco, E. M., S. Macrì, and G. Laviola. 2011. Critical Age Windows for Neurodevelopmental Psychiatric Disorders: Evidence from Animal Models. *Neurotox. Res.* **19**:286–307. [5]

Marek, S., K. Hwang, W. Foran, M. N. Hallquist, and B. Luna. 2015. The Contribution of Network Organization and Integration to the Development of Cognitive Control. *PLoS Biol.* **13**:e1002328. [9]

Markham, J. A., S. E. Mullins, and J. I. Koenig. 2013. Periadolescent Maturation of the Prefrontal Cortex Is Sex-Specific and Is Disrupted by Prenatal Stress. *J. Comput. Neurol.* **521**:1828–1843. [8]

Markulev, C., P. D. McGorry, B. Nelson, et al. 2017. NEURAPRO-E Study Protocol: A Multicentre Randomized Controlled Trial of Omega-3 Fatty Acids and Cognitive-Behavioural Case Management for Patients at Ultra High Risk of Schizophrenia and Other Psychotic Disorders. *Early Interv. Psychiatry* **11**:418–428. [11]

Marler, P., S. Peters, G. F. Ball, A. M. Dufty Jr., and J. C. Wingfield. 1988. The Role of Sex Steroids in the Acquisition and Production of Birdsong. *Nature* **336**:770–772. [4]

Marlinge, E., F. Bellivier, and J. Houenou. 2014. White Matter Alterations in Bipolar Disorder: Potential for Drug Discovery and Development. *Bipolar Disord.* **16**:97–112. [7]

Marquand, A. F., S. M. Kia, M. Zabihi, et al. 2019. Conceptualizing Mental Disorders as Deviations from Normative Functioning. *Mol. Psychiatr.* **June 14**: doi: 10.1038/s41380–41019–40441–41381. [1]

Mars, R. B., F. X. Neubert, M. P. Noonan, et al. 2012. On the Relationship between the "Default Mode Network" and the "Social Brain." *Front. Hum. Neurosci.* **6**:189. [9]

Marshall, M., S. Lewis, A. Lockwood, et al. 2005. Association between Duration of Untreated Psychosis and Outcome in Cohorts of First-Episode Patients: A Systematic Review. *Arch. Gen. Psychiatry* **62**:975–983. [1, 14]

Masten, A. S., and D. Cicchetti. 2010. Developmental Cascades. *Dev. Psychopathol.* **22**:491–495. [6]

Matragrano, L. L., M. M. LeBlanc, A. Chitrapu, Z. E. Blanton, and D. L. Maney. 2013. Testosterone Alters Genomic Responses to Song and Monoaminergic Innervation of Auditory Areas in a Seasonally Breeding Songbird. *Dev. Neurobiol.* **73**:455–468. [4]

Mauney, S. A., K. M. Athanas, H. Pantazopoulos, et al. 2013. Developmental Pattern of Perineuronal Nets in the Human Prefrontal Cortex and Their Deficit in Schizophrenia. *Biol. Psychiatry* **74**:427–435. [7]

Mauney, S. A., C. Y. Pietersen, K. C. Sonntag, and T.-U. W. Woo. 2015. Differentiation of Oligodendrocyte Precursors Is Impaired in the Prefrontal Cortex in Schizophrenia. *Schizophr. Res.* **169**:374–380. [7]

Mayr, E. 1982. The Growth of Biological Thought: Diversity, Evolution and Intelligence. Cambridge, MA: Harvard Univ. Press. [4]

Maziade, M., N. Rouleau, C. Merette, et al. 2011. Verbal and Visual Memory Impairments among Young Offspring and Healthy Adult Relatives of Patients with Schizophrenia and Bipolar Disorder: Selective Generational Patterns Indicate Different Developmental Trajectories. *Schizophr. Bull.* **37**:1218–1228. [2]

McCormick, C. M., M. R. Green, and J. J. Simone. 2017. Translational Relevance of Rodent Models of Hypothalamic-Pituitary-Adrenal Function and Stressors in Adolescence. *Neurobiol. Stress* **6**:31–43. [5]

McCrone, P. 2011. Mental Health Economics: Current Methodological Issues. *Epidemiol. Psychiatr. Sci.* **20**:239–243. [12]

McCrone, P., T. K. Craig, P. Power, and P. A. Garety. 2010. Cost-Effectiveness of an Early Intervention Service for People with Psychosis. *Br. J. Psychiatry* **196**:377–382. [11]

McCrone, P., S. Dhanasiri, A. Patel, M. Knapp, and S. Lawton-Smith. 2008. Paying the Price: The Cost of Mental Health Care in England to 2026. London: The King's Fund. [1]

McDonald, A. J., P. G. Hamilton, and C. J. Barnstable. 2018. Perineuronal Nets Labeled by Monoclonal Antibody VC1.1 Ensheath Interneurons Expressing Parvalbumin and Calbindin in the Rat Amygdala. *Brain Struct. Funct.* **223**:1133–1148. [7]

McFarland, L. A., and R. E. Ployhart. 2015. Social Media: A Contextual Framework to Guide Research and Practice. *J. Appl. Psychol.* **100**:1653–1677. [6]

McFarlane, W. R., W. L. Cook, D. Downing, et al. 2010. Portland Identification and Early Referral: A Community-Based System for Identifying and Treating Youths at High Risk of Psychosis. *Psychiatric Serv.* **61**:512–515. [11]

McFarlane, W. R., E. Susser, R. McCleary, et al. 2014. Reduction in Incidence of Hospitalizations for Psychotic Episodes through Early Identification and Intervention. *Psychiatric Serv.* **65**:1194–1200. [11]

McGlashan, T. H., J. Addington, T. Cannon, et al. 2007. Recruitment and Treatment Practices for Help-Seeking "Prodromal" Patients. *Schizophr. Bull.* **33**:715–726. [11]

McGlashan, T. H., and R. E. Hoffman. 2000. Schizophrenia as a Disorder of Developmentally Reduced Synaptic Connectivity. *Arch. Gen. Psychiatry* **57**:637–648. [7]

McGlashan, T. H., B. Walsh, and S. W. Woods. 2010. The Psychosis-Risk Syndrome. London: Oxford Univ. Press. [11]

McGorry, P. D. 1985. The Aubrey Lewis Unit: The Origins, Development and First Year of Operation of the Clinical Research Unit and Royal Park Psychiatric Hospital. Dissertation, Royal Australian and New Zealand College of Psychiatrists, Melbourne. [14]

McGorry, P. D.. 1993. Early Psychosis Prevention and Intervention Centre. *Australas. Psychiatry* **1**:32–34. [11]

———. 1995. A Treatment-Relevant Classification of Psychotic Disorders. *Aust. N. Z. J. Psychiatry* **29**:555–558. [2]

———. 2007. Issues for DSM-V: Clinical Staging: A Heuristic Pathway to Valid Nosology and Safer, More Effective Treatment in Psychiatry. *Am. J. Psychiatry* **164**:859–860. [1, 2]

———. 2010. Risk Syndromes, Clinical Staging and DSM V: New Diagnostic Infrastructure for Early Intervention in Psychiatry. *Schizophr. Res.* **120**:49–53. [2]

———. 2015. Early Intervention in Psychosis: Obvious, Effective, Overdue. *J. Nervous Mental Dis.* **203**:310–318. [13, 14]

McGorry, P. D., J. Cocks, P. Power, et al. 2011. Very Low-Dose Risperidone in First-Episode Psychosis: A Safe and Effective Way to Initiate Treatment. *Schizophr. Res. Treat.* **2011**:631690. [14]

McGorry, P. D., J. Edwards, C. Mihalopoulos, S. M. Harrigan, and H. J. Jackson. 1996. EPPIC: An Evolving System of Early Detection and Optimal Management. *Schizophr. Bull.* **22**:305–326. [14]

McGorry, P. D., S. D. Goldstone, A. G. Parker, D. J. Rickwood, and I. B. Hickie. 2014a. Cultures for Mental Health Care of Young People: An Australian Blueprint for Reform. *Lancet Psychiatry* **1**:559–568. [2, 13, 14]

McGorry, P. D., J. A. Hartmann, R. Spooner, and B. Nelson. 2018a. Beyond the "At-Risk Mental State" Concept: Transitioning to Transdiagnostic Psychiatry. *World Psychiatry* **17**:133–142. [1, 3, 14]

McGorry, P. D., and I. B. Hickie. 2019. Clinical Staging in Psychiatry: Making Diagnosis Work for Research and Treatment. Cambridge: Cambridge Univ. Press. [13]

McGorry, P. D., I. B. Hickie, A. R. Yung, C. Pantelis, and H. J. Jackson. 2006. Clinical Staging of Psychiatric Disorders: A Heuristic Framework for Choosing Earlier, Safer and More Effective Interventions. *Aust. N. Z. J. Psychiatry* **40**:616–622. [1, 2, 13, 14]

McGorry, P. D., M. Keshavan, S. D. Goldstone, et al. 2014b. Biomarkers and Clinical Staging in Psychiatry. *World Psychiatry* **13**:211–223. [13, 14]

McGorry, P. D., E. Killackey, and A. R. Yung. 2008a. Early Intervention in Psychosis: Concepts, Evidence and Future Directions. *World Psychiatry* **7**:148–156. [1, 10, 11, 14]

McGorry, P. D., and C. Mei. 2018. Early Intervention in Youth Mental Health: Progress and Future Directions. *Evid. Based Mental Health* **21**:182–184. [13]

McGorry, P. D., B. Nelson, C. Markulev, et al. 2017. Effect of Ω-3 Polyunsaturated Fatty Acids in Young People at Ultrahigh Risk for Psychotic Disorders: The Neurapro Randomized Clinical Trial. *JAMA Psychiatry* **74**:19–27. [10, 11]

McGorry, P. D., R. Purcell, I. B. Hickie, et al. 2007a. Clinical Staging: A Heuristic Model for Psychiatry and Youth Mental Health. *Med. J. Austral.* **187**:S40–S42. [2]

McGorry, P. D., A. Ratheesh, M. Berk, and P. Conus. 2018b. Is "Early Intervention" in Bipolar Disorder What It Claims to Be? Malhi et al. *Bipolar Disord.* **20**:181–183. [14]

McGorry, P. D., A. Ratheesh, and B. O'Donoghue. 2018c. Early Intervention: An Implementation Challenge for 21st Century Mental Health Care. *JAMA Psychiatry* **75**:545–546. [2, 12, 14]

McGorry, P. D., and B. S. Singh. 1995. Schizophrenia: Risk and Possibility. Handbook of Preventive Psychiatry, B. Raphael and G. D. Burrows, series ed. New York: Elsevier. [14]

McGorry, P. D., C. Tanti, R. Stokes, et al. 2007b. Headspace: Australia's National Youth Mental Health Foundation: Where Young Minds Come First. *Med. J. Austral.* **187**:S68. [11, 14]

McGorry, P. D., J. Trethowan, and D. Rickwood. 2019. Creating Headspace for Integrated Youth Mental Health Care. *World Psychiatry* **18**:140. [13]

McGorry, P. D., and J. van Os. 2013. Redeeming Diagnosis in Psychiatry: Timing Versus Specifi City. *Lancet* **381**:343–345. [14]

McGorry, P. D., A. R. Yung, A. Bechdolf, and P. Amminger. 2008b. Back to the Future: Predicting and Reshaping the Course of Psychotic Disorder. *Arch. Gen. Psychiatry* **65**:25–26. [2]

McGorry, P. D., A. R. Yung, and L. J. Phillips. 2003. The "Close-in" or Ultra High-Risk Model: A Safe and Effective Strategy for Research and Clinical Intervention in Prepsychotic Mental Disorder. *Schizophr. Bull.*771–790. [3]

McHugh, S. B., M. Fillenz, J. P. Lowry, J. N. Rawlins, and D. M. Bannerman. 2011. Brain Tissue Oxygen Amperometry in Behaving Rats Demonstrates Functional Dissociation of Dorsal and Ventral Hippocampus During Spatial Processing and Anxiety. *Eur. J. Neurosci.* **33**:322–337. [9]

McLaughlin, K. A., J. Greif Green, M. J. Gruber, et al. 2012. Childhood Adversities and First Onset of Psychiatric Disorders in a National Sample of Us Adolescents. *Arch. Gen. Psychiatry* **69**:1151. [6]

McLaughlin, K. A., M. A. Sheridan, F. Tibu, et al. 2015. Causal Effects of the Early Caregiving Environment on Development of Stress Response Systems in Children. *PNAS* **112**:5637–5642. [6]

McPherson, M., L. Smith-Lovin, and J. M. Cook. 2001. Birds of a Feather: Homophily in Social Networks. *Annu. Rev. Sociol.* **27**:415–444. [5]

McVey Neufeld, K. A., P. Luczynski, C. Seira Oriach, T. G. Dinan, and J. F. Cryan. 2016. What's Bugging Your Teen? The Microbiota and Adolescent Mental Health. *Neurosci. Biobehav. Rev.* **70**:300–312. [7]

Meares, A. 1959. The Diagnosis of Prepsychotic Schizophrenia. *Lancet* **273**:55–58. [14]

Mehta, U. M., J. Thirthalli, D. K. Subbakrishna, et al. 2013. Social and Neuro-Cognition as Distinct Cognitive Factors in Schizophrenia: A Systematic Review. *Schizophr. Res.* **148**:3–11. [6]

Meissner, A., T. S. Mikkelsen, H. Gu, et al. 2008. Genome-Scale DNA Methylation Maps of Pluripotent and Differentiated Cells. *Nature* **454**:766–770. [8]

Melle, I., T. K. Larsen, U. Haahr, et al. 2004. Reducing the Duration of Untreated First-Episode Psychosis: Effects on Clinical Presentation. *Arch. Gen. Psychiatry* **61**:143–150. [10]

Mercken, L., T. A. B. Snijders, C. Steglich, E. Vartiainen, and H. de Vries. 2010. Smoking-Based Selection and Influence in Gender-Segregated Friendship Networks: A Social Network Analysis of Adolescent Smoking. *Addiction* **105**:1280–1289. [5]

Merikangas, K. R., L. Cui, G. Kattan, et al. 2012. Mania with and without Depression in a Community Sample of Us Adolescents. *Arch. Gen. Psychiatry* **69**:943–951. [2]

Merikangas, K. R., J.-P. He, M. Burstein, et al. 2010. Lifetime Prevalence of Mental Disorders in U.S. Adolescents: Results from the National Comorbidity Survey Replication–Adolescent Supplement (NCS-A). *J. Am. Acad. Child Adolesc. Psychiatry* **49**:980–989. [2]

———. 2011. Service Utilization for Lifetime Mental Disorders in U.S. Adolescents: Results of the National Comorbidity Survey-Adolescent Supplement (NCS-A). *J. Am. Acad. Child Adolesc. Psychiatry* **50**:32–45. [1]

Merikangas, K. R., R. Herrell, J. Swendsen, et al. 2008. Specificity of Bipolar Spectrum Conditions in the Comorbidity of Mood and Substance Use Disorders: Results from the Zurich Cohort Study. *Arch. Gen. Psychiatry* **65**:47–52. [2]

Merikangas, K. R., E. F. Nakamura, and R. C. Kessler. 2009. Epidemiology of Mental Disorders in Children and Adolescents. *Dialogues Clin. Neurosci.* **11**:7–20. [5, 7, 13]

Merlo, M. C., H. Hofer, W. Gekle, et al. 2002. Risperidone, 2 mg/day vs. 4 mg/day, in First-Episode, Acutely Psychotic Patients: Treatment Efficacy and Effects on Fine Motor Functioning. *J. Clin. Psychiatry* **63**:885–891. [14]

Meshi, D., D. I. Tamir, and H. R. Heekeren. 2015. The Emerging Neuroscience of Social Media. *Trends Cogn. Sci.* **19**:771–782. [6]

Meyer, U. 2014. Prenatal Poly(I:C) Exposure and Other Developmental Immune Activation Models in Rodent Systems. *Biol. Psychiatry* **75**:307–315. [7]

Michie, S., L. Yardley, R. West, K. Patrick, and F. Greaves. 2017. Developing and Evaluating Digital Interventions to Promote Behavior Change in Health and Health Care: Recommendations Resulting from an International Workshop. *J. Med. Internet Res.* **19**:e232. [10]

Mighdoll, M. I., R. Tao, J. E. Kleinman, and T. M. Hyde. 2015. Myelin, Myelin-Related Disorders, and Psychosis. *Schizophr. Res.* **161**:85–93. [7]

Mihalopoulos, C., M. Harris, L. Henry, S. M. Harrigan, and P. D. McGorry. 2009. Is Early Intervention in Psychosis Cost-Effective over the Long Term? *Schizophr. Bull.* **35**:909–918. [11]

Millan, M. J., Y. Agid, M. Brüne, et al. 2012. Cognitive Dysfunction in Psychiatric Disorders: Characteristics, Causes and the Quest for Improved Therapy. *Nation. Rev. Drug Discov.* **11**:141–168. [3]

Miller, B., E. Messias, J. Miettunen, et al. 2011. Meta-Analysis of Paternal Age and Schizophrenia Risk in Male Versus Female Offspring. *Schizophr. Bull.* **37**:1039–1047. [8]

Miller, D. J., T. Duka, C. D. Stimpson, et al. 2012. Prolonged Myelination in Human Neocortical Evolution. *PNAS* **109**:16480–16485. [7]

Miller, T. J., T. H. McGlashan, J. L. Rosen, et al. 2003. Prodromal Assessment with the Structured Interview for Prodromal Syndromes and the Scale of Prodromal Symptoms: Predictive Validity, Interrater Reliability, and Training to Reliability. *Schizophr. Bull.* **29**:703–715. [11]

Mirsu-Paun, A., and J. A. Oliver. 2017. How Much Does Love Really Hurt? A Meta-Analysis of the Association between Romantic Relationship Quality, Breakups and Mental Health Outcomes in Adolescents and Young Adults. *J. Reationships Res.* **8**:e5. [3]

Mirwald, R. L., A. D. G. Baxter-Jones, D. A. Bailey, and G. P. Beunen. 2002. An Assessment of Maturity from Anthropometric Measurements. *Med. Sci. Sports Exerc.* **34**:689-694. [4]

Miyamoto, A., H. Wake, A. W. Ishikawa, et al. 2016. Microglia Contact Induces Synapse Formation in Developing Somatosensory Cortex. *Nat. Commun.* **7**:12540. [7]

Miyata, S., Y. Komatsu, Y. Yoshimura, C. Taya, and H. Kitagawa. 2012. Persistent Cortical Plasticity by Upregulation of Chondroitin 6-Sulfation. *Nat. Neurosci.* **15**:414–422, S411–412. [7]

Miyata, S., M. Taniguchi, Y. Koyama, et al. 2016. Association between Chronic Stress-Induced Structural Abnormalities in Ranvier Nodes and Reduced Oligodendrocyte Activity in Major Depression. *Scientific Rep.* **6**:23084. [7]

Mohr, D. C., H. Riper, and S. M. Schueller. 2018. A Solution-Focused Research Approach to Achieve an Implementable Revolution in Digital Mental Health. *JAMA Psychiatry* **75**:113–114. [10]

Mohr, D. C., S. M. Schueller, W. T. Riley, et al. 2015. Trials of Intervention Principles: Evaluation Methods for Evolving Behavioral Intervention Technologies. *J. Med. Internet Res.* **17**:e166. [10]

Mohr, D. C., M. Zhang, and S. M. Schueller. 2017. Personal Sensing: Understanding Mental Health Using Ubiquitous Sensors and Machine Learning. *Annu. Rev. Clin. Psych.* **13**:23–47. [3]

Moloney, R. D., L. Desbonnet, G. Clarke, T. G. Dinan, and J. F. Cryan. 2014. The Microbiome: Stress, Health and Disease. *Mammalian Genome* **25**:49–74. [7]

Monji, A., T. Kato, and S. Kanba. 2009. Cytokines and Schizophrenia: Microglia Hypothesis of Schizophrenia. *Psychiatry Clin. Neurosci.* **63**:257–265. [7]

Montez, D. F., F. J. Calabro, and B. Luna. 2017. The Expression of Established Cognitive Brain States Stabilizes with Working Memory Development. *eLife* **6**:e25606. [3, 9]

Morawski, M., T. Reinert, W. Meyer-Klaucke, et al. 2015. Ion Exchanger in the Brain: Quantitative Analysis of Perineuronally Fixed Anionic Binding Sites Suggests Diffusion Barriers with Ion Sorting Properties. *Scientific Rep.* **5**:16471. [7]

Moretti, M. M., and M. Peled. 2004. Adolescent-Parent Attachment: Bonds That Support Healthy Development. *Paediatr. Child Health* **9**:551–555. [6]

Morgan, C., and H. Fisher. 2007. Environment and Schizophrenia: Environmental Factors in Schizophrenia: Childhood Trauma: A Critical Review. *Schizophr. Bull.* **33**:3–10. [8]

Morgan, J. T., G. Chana, C. A. Pardo, et al. 2010. Microglial Activation and Increased Microglial Density Observed in the Dorsolateral Prefrontal Cortex in Autism. *Biol. Psychiatry* **68**:368–376. [7]

Morgan-Trimmer, S., and F. Wood. 2016. Ethnographic Methods for Process Evaluations of Complex Health Behaviour Interventions. *Trials* **17**:232. [6]

Moser, E., M. B. Moser, and P. Andersen. 1993. Spatial Learning Impairment Parallels the Magnitude of Dorsal Hippocampal Lesions, but Is Hardly Present Following Ventral Lesions. *J. Neurosci.* **13**:3916–3925. [9]

Moser, M. B., and E. I. Moser. 1998. Functional Differentiation in the Hippocampus. *Hippocampus* **8**:608–619. [9]

Moses, T. 2009. Self-Labeling and Its Effects among Adolescents Diagnosed with Mental Disorders. *Soc. Sci. Med.* **68**:570–578. [11]

Mossaheb, N., K. Papageorgiou, M. R. Schäfer, et al. 2015. Changes in Triglyceride Levels in Ultra-High Risk for Psychosis Individuals Treated with Omega-3 Fatty Acids. *Early Interv. Psychiatry* **12**:30–36. [10]

Mossaheb, N., M. Schloegelhofer, M. R. Schaefer, et al. 2012. Polyunsaturated Fatty Acids in Emerging Psychosis. *Curr. Pharmaceut. Design* **18**:576–591. [10]

Mottahedin, A., M. Ardalan, T. Chumak, et al. 2017. Effect of Neuroinflammation on Synaptic Organization and Function in the Developing Brain: Implications for Neurodevelopmental and Neurodegenerative Disorders. *Front. Cell. Neurosci.* **11**:190. [9]

MRC Strategic Review Group. 2010. Report of the Strategic Review Group. https://mrc.ukri.org/documents/pdf/mrc-mental-health-research-report-2010/. (accessed July 1, 2019). [1]

Muly, E. C., 3rd, K. Szigeti, and P. S. Goldman-Rakic. 1998. D1 Receptor in Interneurons of Macaque Prefrontal Cortex: Distribution and Subcellular Localization. *J. Neurosci.* **18**:10553–10565. [7]

Munoz, D. P., I. T. Armstrong, K. A. Hampton, and K. D. Moore. 2003. Altered Control of Visual Fixation and Saccadic Eye Movements in Attention-Deficit Hyperactivity Disorder. *J. Neurophysiol.* **90**:503–514. [3]

Murase, S., C. L. Lantz, and E. M. Quinlan. 2017. Light Reintroduction after Dark Exposure Reactivates Plasticity in Adults Via Perisynaptic Activation of MMP-9. *eLife* **6**:e27345. [7]

Murphy, S. M., S. Kucukgoncu, Y. Bao, et al. 2018. An Economic Evaluation of Coordinated Specialty Care (Csc) Services for First-Episode Psychosis in the U.S. Public Sector. *J. Ment. Health Policy Econ.* **21**:123–130. [12]

Murray, G. K., and P. B. Jones. 2012. Psychotic Symptoms in Young People without Psychotic Illness: Mechanisms and Meaning. *Br. J. Psychiatry* **201**:4–6. [2]

Murray, R. M., V. Bhavsar, G. Tripoli, and O. Howes. 2017a. 30 Years On: How the Neurodevelopmental Hypothesis of Schizophrenia Morphed into the Developmental Risk Factor Model of Psychosis. *Schizophr. Bull.* **43**:1190–1196. [7]

Murray, R. M., A. Englund, A. Abi-Dargham, et al. 2017b. Cannabis-Associated Psychosis: Neural Substrate and Clinical Impact. *Neuropharmacology* **124**:89–104. [7]

Murty, V. P., H. Shah, D. F. Montez, et al. 2018. Age-Related Trajectories of Functional Coupling between the VTA and Nucleus Accumbens Depend on Motivational State. *J. Neurosci.* **38**:7420–7427. [9]

Musci, R. J., C. P. Bradshaw, B. Maher, et al. 2014. Reducing Aggression and Impulsivity through School-Based Prevention Programs: A Gene by Intervention Interaction. *Prev. Sci.* **15**:831–840. [4]

Myin-Germeys, I., Z. Kasanova, T. Vaessen, et al. 2018. Experience Sampling Methodology in Mental Health Research: New Insights and Technical Developments. *World Psychiatry* **17**:123–132. [6]

Myin-Germeys, I., A. Klippel, H. Steinhart, and U. Reininghaus. 2016. Ecological Momentary Interventions in Psychiatry. *Curr. Opin. Psychiatry* **29**:258–263. [10]

Myin-Germeys, I., M. Oorschot, D. Collip, et al. 2009. Experience Sampling Research in Psychopathology: Opening the Black Box of Daily Life. *Psychol. Med.* **39**:1533–1547. [10]

Naismith, S. L., D. F. Hermens, T. K. Ip, et al. 2012. Circadian Profiles in Young People During the Early Stages of Affective Disorder. *Transl. Psychiatry* **2**:e123. [2, 13]

Naismith, S. L., J. Lagopoulos, D. F. Hermens, et al. 2014. Delayed Circadian Phase Is Linked to Glutamatergic Functions in Young People with Affective Disorders: A Proton Magnetic Resonance Spectroscopy Study. *BMC Psychiat.* **14**:345. [2]

Najjar, S., D. M. Pearlman, S. Hirsch, et al. 2014. Brain Biopsy Findings Link Major Depressive Disorder to Neuroinflammation, Oxidative Stress, and Neurovascular Dysfunction: A Case Report. *Biol. Psychiatry* **75**:e23–26. [7]

NCCMH. 2013. Psychosis and Schizophrenia in Children and Young People: Recognition and Management. London: National Collaborating Centre for Mental Health. [11]

Neier, K., E. H. Marchlewicz, D. C. Dolinoy, and V. Padmanabhan. 2015. Assessing Human Health Risk to Endocrine Disrupting Chemicals: A Focus on Prenatal Exposures and Oxidative Stress. *Endocr. Disruptors (Austin)* **3**:e1069916. [7]

Nelson, B., P. D. McGorry, M. Wichers, J. T. W. Wigman, and J. A. Hartmann. 2017. Moving from Static to Dynamic Models of the Onset of Mental Disorder: A Review. *JAMA Psychiatry* **74**:528–534. [7, 14]

Nelson, B., H. P. Yuen, S. J. Wood, et al. 2013. Long-Term Follow-up of a Group at Ultra High Risk ("Prodromal") for Psychosis: The PACE 400 Study. *JAMA Psychiatry* **70**:793–802. [11]

Nelson, C. A. 2017. Hazards to Early Development: The Biological Embedding of Early Life Adversity. *Neuron* **96**:262–266. [6]

Nelson, E. E., J. M. Jarcho, and A. E. Guyer. 2016. Social Re-Orientation and Brain Development: An Expanded and Updated View. *Dev. Cogn. Neurosci.* **17**:118–127. [5]

Neniskyte, U., and C. T. Gross. 2017. Errant Gardeners: Glial-Cell-Dependent Synaptic Pruning and Neurodevelopmental Disorders. *Nature reviews. Neuroscience* **18**:658–670. [7]

Neubauer, K., A. Weigel, A. Daubmann, et al. 2014. Paths to First Treatment and Duration of Untreated Illness in Anorexia Nervosa: Are There Differences According to Age of Onset? *Eur. Eat. Disord. Rev.* **22**:292–298. [14]

Neufang, S., K. Specht, M. Hausmann, et al. 2009. Sex Differences and the Impact of Steroid Hormones on the Developing Human Brain. *Cereb. Cortex* **19**:464–473. [9]

Neufeld, K. M., N. Kang, J. Bienenstock, and J. A. Foster. 2011. Reduced Anxiety-Like Behavior and Central Neurochemical Change in Germ-Free Mice. *Neurogastroenterol. Motility* **23**:255–264, e119. [7]

Niendam, T. A., M. Jalbrzikowski, and C. E. Bearden. 2009. Exploring Predictors of Outcome in the Psychosis Prodrome: Implications for Early Identification and Intervention. *Neuropsychol. Rev.* **19**:280–293. [11]

Nissen, J. B., C. S. Hansen, A. Starnawska, et al. 2016. DNA Methylation at the Neonatal State and at the Time of Diagnosis: Preliminary Support for an Association with the Estrogen Receptor 1, Gamma-Aminobutyric Acid B Receptor 1, and Myelin Oligodendrocyte Glycoprotein in Female Adolescent Patients with Ocd. *Front. Psychiatry* **7**:35. [7]

Niwa, M., H. Jaaro-Peled, S. Tankou, et al. 2013. Adolescent Stress-Induced Epigenetic Control of Dopaminergic Neurons Via Glucocorticoids. *Science* **339**:335–339. [9]

Noaghiul, S., and J. R. Hibbeln. 2003. Cross-National Comparisons of Seafood Consumption and Rates of Bipolar Disorders. *Am. J. Psychiatry* **160**:2222–2227. [10]

Numata, S., T. Ye, T. M. Hyde, et al. 2012. DNA Methylation Signatures in Development and Aging of the Human Prefrontal Cortex. *Am. J. Hum. Genet.* **90**:260–272. [8]

Nyffeler, M., U. Meyer, B. K. Yee, J. Feldon, and I. Knuesel. 2006. Maternal Immune Activation During Pregnancy Increases Limbic GABAA Receptor Immunoreactivity in the Adult Offspring: Implications for Schizophrenia. *Neuroscience* **143**:51–62. [8]

Nymberg, C., T. Jia, B. Ruggeri, and G. Schumann. 2013. Analytical Strategies for Large Imaging Genetic Datasets: Experiences from the Imagen Study. *Ann. NY Acad. Sci.* **1282**:92–106. [9]

O'Brien, S. F., and K. L. Bierman. 1988. Conceptions and Perceived Influence of Peer Groups: Interviews with Preadolescents and Adolescents. *Child Dev.* **59**:1360–1365. [5]

Ochsner, K. N., and J. J. Gross. 2005. The Cognitive Control of Emotion. *Trends Cogn. Sci.* **9**:242–249. [4]

O'Dea, B., N. Glozier, R. Purcell, et al. 2014. A Cross-Sectional Exploration of the Clinical Characteristics of Disengaged (NEET) Young People in Primary Mental Healthcare. *BMJ Open* **4**:e006378. [14]

O'Donnell, P. 2010. Adolescent Maturation of Cortical Dopamine. *Neurotox. Res.* **18**:306–312. [9]

O'Donoghue, B., S. M. Francey, B. Nelson, et al. 2019. Staged Treatment and Acceptability Guidelines in Early Psychosis Study (STAGES): A Randomized Placebo Controlled Trial of Intensive Psychosocial Treatment Plus or Minus Antipsychotic Medication for First-Episode Psychosis with Low-Risk of Self-Harm or Aggression. Study Protocol and Baseline Characteristics of Participants. *Early Interv. Psychiatry* **13**:953–960. [14]

Ogundele, O. M., A. O. Omoaghe, D. C. Ajonijebu, et al. 2014. Glia Activation and Its Role in Oxidative Stress. *Metab. Brain. Dis.* **29**:483–493. [9]

Okhuijsen-Pfeifer, C., E. A. H. Huijsman, A. Hasan, et al. 2018. Clozapine as a First- or Second-Line Treatment in Schizophrenia: A Systematic Review and Meta-Analysis. *Acta Psychiat. Scand.* **138**:281–288. [14]

Olde Loohuis, L. M., S. Mangul, A. P. S. Ori, et al. 2018. Transcriptome Analysis in Whole Blood Reveals Increased Microbial Diversity in Schizophrenia. *Translational psychiatry* **8**:96. [7]

Olsavsky, A. K., E. H. Telzer, M. Shapiro, et al. 2013. Indiscriminate Amygdala Response to Mothers and Strangers after Early Maternal Deprivation. *Biol Psychiat* **74**:853–860. [5]

O'Malley, A., C. O'Connell, K. J. Murphy, and C. M. Regan. 2000. Transient Spine Density Increases in the Mid-Molecular Layer of Hippocampal Dentate Gyrus Accompany Consolidation of a Spatial Learning Task in the Rodent. *Neuroscience* **99**:229–232. [8]

Onwumere, J., P. Bebbington, and E. Kuipers. 2011. Family Interventions in Early Psychosis: Specificity and Effectiveness. *Epidemiol. Psychiatr. Sci.* **20**:113–119. [10]

Onwumere, J., S. Grice, P. Garety, et al. 2014. Caregiver Reports of Patient-Initiated Violence in Psychosis. *Can. J. of Psychiatry* **59**:376–384. [10]

Onwumere, J., S. Sirykaite, J. Schulz, et al. 2018. Understanding the Experience of "Burnout" in First-Episode Psychosis Carers. *Compr. Psychiatry* **83**:19–24. [10]

Ordaz, S. J., W. Foran, K. Velanova, and B. Luna. 2013. Longitudinal Growth Curves of Brain Function Underlying Inhibitory Control through Adolescence. *J. Neurosci.* **33**:18109–18124. [9]

Oreskes, N., and E. Conway. 2010. Merchants of Doubt. London: Bloomsbury. [14]

Ormel, J., D. Raven, F. van Oort, et al. 2015. Mental Health in Dutch Adolescents: A Trails Report on Prevalence, Severity, Age of Onset, Continuity and Co-Morbidity of DSM Disorders. *Psychol. Med.* **45**:345–360. [2]

O'Sullivan, T., R. Batra, M. Nolan, and A. Scott. 2007. Goldberg and Huxley's Model 27 Years On. *Psychiatric Bulletin* **31**:316. [12]

Owen, M. J. 2014. New Approaches to Psychiatric Diagnostic Classification. *Neuron* **84**:564–571. [1]

Padmanabhan, J. L., J. L. Shah, N. Tandon, and M. S. Keshavan. 2017. The "Polyenviromic Risk Score": Aggregating Environmental Risk Factors Predicts Conversion to Psychosis in Familial High-Risk Subjects. *Schizophr. Res.* **181**:17–22. [6, 8]

Paksarian, D., B. B. Trabjerg, K. R. Merikangas, et al. 2018. The Role of Genetic Liability in the Association of Urbanicity at Birth and During Upbringing with Schizophrenia in Denmark. *Psychol. Med.* **48**:305–314. [6]

Pantazopoulos, H., T.-U. W. Woo, M. P. Lim, N. Lange, and S. Berretta. 2010. Extracellular Matrix-Glial Abnormalities in the Amygdala and Entorhinal Cortex of Subjects Diagnosed with Schizophrenia. *Arch. Gen. Psychiatry* **67**:155–166. [7]

Paolicelli, R. C., and M. T. Ferretti. 2017. Function and Dysfunction of Microglia During Brain Development: Consequences for Synapses and Neural Circuits. *Front. Synaptic Neurosci.* **9**:9. [7]

Papachristou, E., S. Frangou, and A. Reichenberg. 2013. Expanding Conceptual Frameworks: Life Course Risk Modelling for Mental Disorders. *Psychiatry Res.* **206**:140–145. [9]

Pardinas, A. F., P. Holmans, A. J. Pocklington, et al. 2018. Common Schizophrenia Alleles Are Enriched in Mutation-Intolerant Genes and in Regions under Strong Background Selection. *Nat. Genet.* **50**:381–389. [8]

Parker, L., L. Bero, D. Gillies, et al. 2018. Mental Health Messages in Prominent Mental Health Apps. *Ann. Fam. Med.* **16**:338–342. [13]

Parletta, N., T. Niyonsenga, and J. Duff. 2016a. Omega-3 and Omega-6 Polyunsaturated Fatty Acid Levels and Correlations with Symptoms in Children with Attention Deficit Hyperactivity Disorder, Autistic Spectrum Disorder and Typically Developing Controls. *PLoS ONE* **11**:e0156432. [10]

Parletta, N., D. Zarnowiecki, J. Cho, et al. 2016b. People with Schizophrenia and Depression Have a Low Omega-3 Index. *PLEFA* **110**:42–47. [10]

Patel, A. A., and M. J. Budoff. 2016. Effects of Eicosapentaenoic Acid and Docosahexaenoic Acid on Lipoproteins in Hypertriglyceridemia. *Curr. Opin. Endocrinol. Diabetes Obes.* **23**:145–149. [10]

Patel, V., A. J. Flisher, S. Hetrick, and P. D. McGorry. 2007. Mental Health of Young People: A Global Public-Health Challenge. *Lancet* **369**:1302–1313. [5, 6]

Patterson, G. R., B. D. DeBaryshe, and E. Ramsey. 1989. A Developmental Perspective on Antisocial Behavior. *Am. Psychol.* **44**:329–335. [6]

Patterson, P., M. Birchwood, and R. Cochrane. 2005. Expressed Emotion as an Adaptation to Loss: Prospective Study in First-Episode Psychosis. *Br. J. Psychiatry Suppl.* **48**:s59–64. [10]

Patton, G. C., and R. Viner. 2007. Pubertal Transitions in Health. *Lancet* **369**:1130–1139. [4, 6]

Pattwell, S. S., K. G. Bath, B. J. Casey, I. Ninan, and F. S. Lee. 2011. Selective Early-Acquired Fear Memories Undergo Temporary Suppression During Adolescence. *PNAS* **108**:1182–1187. [1, 9]

Pattwell, S. S., S. Duhoux, C. A. Hartley, et al. 2012. Altered Fear Learning across Development in Both Mouse and Human. *PNAS* **109**:16318–16323. [9]

Pattwell, S. S., C. Liston, D. Jing, et al. 2016. Dynamic Changes in Neural Circuitry During Adolescence Are Associated with Persistent Attenuation of Fear Memories. *Nat. Commun.* **7**:11475. [9]

Paus, T. 2010. Population Neuroscience: Why and How. *Hum. Brain Mapp.* **31**:891–903. [6]

Paus, T., M. Keshavan, and J. N. Giedd. 2008. Why Do Many Psychiatric Disorders Emerge During Adolescence? *Nat. Rev. Neurosci.* **9**:947–957. [2, 4, 5, 7, 9]

Paylor, J. W., B. R. Lins, Q. Greba, et al. 2016. Developmental Disruption of Perineuronal Nets in the Medial Prefrontal Cortex after Maternal Immune Activation. *Scientific Rep.* **6**:37580. [7]

Paylor, R., K. L. McIlwain, R. McAninch, et al. 2001. Mice Deleted for the Digeorge/Velocardiofacial Syndrome Region Show Abnormal Sensorimotor Gating and Learning and Memory Impairments. *Hum. Mol. Genet.* **10**:2645–2650. [8]

Pearce, J., M. Jovev, C. Hulbert, et al. 2017. Evaluation of a Psychoeducational Group Intervention for Family and Friends of Youth with Borderline Personality Disorder. *Borderline Personal. Disord. Emot. Dysreg.* **4**:5. [10]

Pearlson, G. D., B. A. Clementz, J. A. Sweeney, M. S. Keshavan, and C. A. Tamminga. 2016. Does Biology Transcend the Symptom-Based Boundaries of Psychosis? *Psychiatry Clin. North Am.* **39**:165–174. [8]

Pedersen, C. B., and P. B. Mortensen. 2001. Evidence of a Dose-Response Relationship between Urbanicity During Upbringing and Schizophrenia Risk. *Arch. Gen. Psychiatry* **58**:1039–1046. [8]

Pena, C. J., H. G. Kronman, D. M. Walker, et al. 2017. Early Life Stress Confers Lifelong Stress Susceptibility in Mice Via Ventral Tegmental Area OTX2. *Science* **356**:1185–1188. [7]

Penn, D. L., L. J. Sanna, and D. L. Roberts. 2008. Social Cognition in Schizophrenia: An Overview. *Schizophr. Bull.* **34**:408–411. [6]

Peper, J. S., and R. E. Dahl. 2013. Surging Hormones: Brain-Behavior Interactions During Puberty. *Curr. Dir. Psychol. Sci.* **22**:134–139. [7]

Perkins, D. O., H. Gu, K. Boteva, and J. A. Lieberman. 2005. Relationship between Duration of Untreated Psychosis and Outcome in First-Episode Schizophrenia: A Critical Review and Meta-Analysis. *Am. J. Psychiatry* **162**:1785–1804. [14]

Perlman, W. R., M. J. Webster, M. M. Herman, J. E. Kleinman, and C. S. Weickert. 2007. Age-Related Differences in Glucocorticoid Receptor mRNA Levels in the Human Brain. *Neurobiol. Aging* **28**:447–458. [5]

Petanjek, Z., M. Judaš, G. Šimić, et al. 2011. Extraordinary Neoteny of Synaptic Spines in the Human Prefrontal Cortex. *PNAS* **108**:13281–13286. [7, 9]

Petersen, L., P. Jeppesen, A. Thorup, et al. 2005. A Randomised Multicentre Trial of Integrated Versus Standard Treatment for Patients with a First Episode of Psychotic Illness. *BMJ* **331**:602. [10]

Phillips, L. J., S. B. Leicester, L. E. O'dwyer, et al. 2002a. The PACE Clinic: Identification and Management of Young People at "Ultra" High Risk of Psychosis. *J. Psychiatr. Pract.* **8**:255–269. [14]

Phillips, L. J., A. R. Yung, and P. D. McGorry. 2000. Identification of Young People at Risk of Psychosis: Validation of Personal Assessment and Crisis Evaluation Clinic Intake Criteria. *Aust. N. Z. J. Psychiatry* **34**:S164–169. [11]

Phillips, M. R., V. Pearson, F. Li, M. Xu, and L. Yang. 2002b. Stigma and Expressed Emotion: A Study of People with Schizophrenia and Their Family Members in China. *Br. J. Psychiatry* **181**:488–493. [11]

Picton, T. W., and M. J. Taylor. 2007. Electrophysiological Evaluation of Human Brain Development. *Dev. Neuropsychol.* **31**:249–278. [7]

Piekarski, D. J., J. R. Boivin, and L. Wilbrecht. 2017a. Ovarian Hormones Organize the Maturation of Inhibitory Neurotransmission in the Frontal Cortex at Puberty Onset in Female Mice. *Curr. Biol.* **27**:1735–1745. [4, 7]

Piekarski, D. J., C. M. Johnson, J. R. Boivin, et al. 2017b. Does Puberty Mark a Transition in Sensitive Periods for Plasticity in the Associative Neocortex? *Brain Res.* **1654**:123–144. [4]

Pilowsky, I. 1969. Abnormal Illness Behaviour. *Br. J. Med. Psychol.* **42**:347–351. [14]

———. 1978. A General Classification of Abnormal Illness Behaviours. *Br. J. Med. Psychol.* **51**:131–137. [14]

Piomelli, D., G. Astarita, and R. Rapaka. 2007. A Neuroscientist's Guide to Lipidomics. *Nat. Rev. Neurosci.* **8**:743–754. [10]

Pizzorusso, T., P. Medini, N. Berardi, et al. 2002. Reactivation of Ocular Dominance Plasticity in the Adult Visual Cortex. *Science* **298**:1248–1251. [7]

Plana-Ripoll, O., C. B. Pedersen, Y. Holtz, et al. 2019. Exploring Comorbidity within Mental Disorders among a Danish National Population. *JAMA Psychiatry* **76**:259–270. [1]

Plomin, R., and D. Daniels. 1987. Why Are Children in the Same Family So Different from One Another? *Behav. Brain Sci.* **10**:1. [6]

Plsek, P. E., and T. Greenhalgh. 2001. Complexity Science: The Challenge of Complexity in Health Care. *BMJ* **323**:625–628. [12]

Polderman, T. J. C., B. Benyamin, C. A. de Leeuw, et al. 2015. Meta-Analysis of the Heritability of Human Traits Based on Fifty Years of Twin Studies. *Nat. Genet.* **47**:702–709. [6]

Pollard, J. M., J. D. Cahill, and V. H. Srihari. 2016. Building Early Intervention Services for Psychotic Disorders: A Primer for Early Adopters in the U.S. *Curr. Psychiatry Rev.* **12**:350–356. [12]

Poon, A. W. C., J. Curtis, P. Ward, C. Loneragan, and J. Lappin. 2018. Physical and Psychological Health of Carers of Young People with First Episode Psychosis. *Australas. Psychiatry* **26**:184–188. [10]

Porter, J. N., A. K. Roy, B. Benson, et al. 2015. Age-Related Changes in the Intrinsic Functional Connectivity of the Human Ventral vs. Dorsal Striatum from Childhood to Middle Age. *Dev. Cogn. Neurosci.* **11**:83–95. [9]

Porter, L. L., E. Rizzo, and J. P. Hornung. 1999. Dopamine Affects Parvalbumin Expression During Cortical Development *in Vitro*. *J. Neurosci.* **19**:8990–9003. [9]

Porter, M. E. 2010. What Is Value in Health Care? *New Engl. J. Med.* **363**:2477–2481. [12]

Porter, M. E., and R. S. Kaplan. 2015. How Should We Pay for Health Care? *HBS Working Paper Series* **15-041**:1–25. [12]

Porter, M. E., S. Larsson, and T. H. Lee. 2016. Standardizing Patient Outcomes Measurement. *New Engl. J. Med.* **374**:504–506. [12]

Porter, M. E., and T. H. Lee. 2013. The Strategy That Will Fix Health Care. *Harvard Bus. Rev.* **91(10)**:50–70. [14]

Powell, A., P. Singh, and J. Torous. 2018. The Complexity of Mental Health App Privacy Policies: A Potential Barrier to Privacy. *JMIR Mental Health* **6**:e158. [13]

Power, J. D., K. A. Barnes, A. Z. Snyder, B. L. Schlaggar, and S. E. Petersen. 2012. Spurious but Systematic Correlations in Functional Connectivity MRI Networks Arise from Subject Motion. *Neuroimage* **59**:2142–2154. [9]

Power, J. D., A. L. Cohen, S. M. Nelson, et al. 2011. Functional Network Organization of the Human Brain. *Neuron* **72**:665–678. [9]

Prasad, K. M., K. V. Chowdari, L. A. D'Aiuto, et al. 2018. Neuropil Contraction in Relation to Complement C4 Gene Copy Numbers in Independent Cohorts of Adolescent-Onset and Young Adult-Onset Schizophrenia Patients: A Pilot Study. *Transl. Psychiatry* **8**:134. [8]

Prasad, K. M., and M. S. Keshavan. 2007. Structural Cerebral Variations as Useful Endophenotypes in Schizophrenia: Do They Help Construct "Extended Endophenotypes"? *Schizophr. Bull.* **34**:774–790. [8]

Przybylski, A. K., and L. Bowes. 2017. Cyberbullying and Adolescent Well-Being in England: A Population-Based Cross-Sectional Study. *Lancet Child Adolesc. Health* **1**:19–26. [5]

Puetz, V. B., N. Kohn, B. Dahmen, et al. 2014. Neural Response to Social Rejection in Children with Early Separation Experiences. *J. Am. Acad. Child Adolesc. Psychiatry* **53**:1328–1337. [5]

Purcell, R., A. F. Jorm, I. B. Hickie, et al. 2015. Demographic and Clinical Characteristics of Young People Seeking Help at Youth Mental Health Services: Baseline Findings of the Transitions Study. *Early Interv. Psychiatry* **9**:487–497. [3, 14]

Quinn, S., and J. Oldmeadow. 2012. The Martini Effect and Social Networking Sites: Early Adolescents, Mobile Social Networking and Connectedness to Friends. *Mobile Media Commun.* **1**:237–247. [5]

Radua, J., V. Ramella-Cravaro, J. P. A. Ioannidis, et al. 2018. What Causes Psychosis? An Umbrella Review of Risk and Protective Factors. *World Psychiatry* **17**:49–66. [8]

Raichle, M. E., A. M. MacLeod, A. Z. Snyder, et al. 2001. A Default Mode of Brain Function. *PNAS* **98**:676–682. [9]

Rapaport, M. H., A. A. Nierenberg, P. J. Schettler, et al. 2015. Inflammation as a Predictive Biomarker for Response to Omega-3 Fatty Acids in Major Depressive Disorder: A Proof-of-Concept Study. *Mol. Psychiatr.* **21**:71–79. [10]

Ratheesh, A., C. Davey, S. Hetrick, et al. 2017. A Systematic Review and Meta-Analysis of Prospective Transition from Major Depression to Bipolar Disorder. *Acta Psychiat. Scand.* **135**:273–284. [2]

Raznahan, A., P. W. Shaw, J. P. Lerch, et al. 2014. Longitudinal Four-Dimensional Mapping of Subcortical Anatomy in Human Development. *PNAS* **111**:1592–1597. [9]

Reavley, N. J., S. Cvetkovski, A. F. Jorm, and D. I. Lubman. 2010. Help-Seeking for Substance Use, Anxiety and Affective Disorders among Young People: Results from the 2007 Australian National Survey of Mental Health and Wellbeing. *Aust. N. Z. J. Psychiatry* **44**:729–735. [10]

Reddy, R. D., M. S. Keshavan, and J. K. Yao. 2004. Reduced Red Blood Cell Membrane Essential Polyunsaturated Fatty Acids in First Episode Schizophrenia at Neuroleptic-Naive Baseline. *Schizophr. Bull.* **30**:901–911. [10]

Reemst, K., S. C. Noctor, P. J. Lucassen, and E. M. Hol. 2016. The Indispensable Roles of Microglia and Astrocytes During Brain Development. *Front. Hum. Neurosci.* **10**:566. [7]

Rees, E., M. C. O'Donovan, and M. J. Owen. 2015. Genetics of Schizophrenia. *Curr. Opin. Behav. Sci.* **2**:8–14. [8]

Reininghaus, U., M. J. Kempton, L. Valmaggia, et al. 2016. Stress Sensitivity, Aberrant Salience, and Threat Anticipation in Early Psychosis: An Experience Sampling Study. *Schizophr. Bull.* **42**:712–722. [3]

Reiter, A., A. Heinz, and L. Deserno. 2017. Linking Social Context and Addiction Neuroscience: A Computational Psychiatry Approach. *Nat. Rev. Neurosci.* **18**:450–450. [6]

Renard, J., H. J. Szkudlarek, C. P. Kramar, et al. 2017. Adolescent THC Exposure Causes Enduring Prefrontal Cortical Disruption of GABAergic Inhibition and Dysregulation of Sub-Cortical Dopamine Function. *Scientific Rep.* **7**:11420. [9]

Rice, S. M., S. Halperin, S. Cahill, et al. 2017. The Youth Mood Clinic: An Innovative Service for the Treatment of Severe and Complex Depression. *Australas. Psychiatry* **25**:112–116. [10]

Rice, S. M., M. R. Schäfer, C. Klier, et al. 2015. Erythrocyte Polyunsaturated Fatty Acid Levels in Young People at Ultra-High Risk for Psychotic Disorder and Healthy Adolescent Controls. *Psychiatry Res.* **228**: [10]

Richards, D., and T. Richardson. 2012. Computer-Based Psychological Treatments for Depression: A Systematic Review and Meta-Analysis. *Clin. Psychol. Rev.* **32**:329–342. [10]

Rickwood, D. J., F. P. Deane, and C. J. Wilson. 2007. When and How Do Young People Seek Professional Help for Mental Health Problems. *Med. J. Austral.* **187**:S35–39. [1]

Rickwood, D. J., K. R. Mazzer, N. R. Telford, et al. 2015. Changes in Psychological Distress and Psychosocial Functioning in Young People Visiting Headspace Centres for Mental Health Problems. *Med. J. Austral.* **202**:537–542. [13]

Rickwood, D. J., M. Paraskakis, Q. Quin, et al. 2019. Australia's Innovation in Youth Mental Health Care: The Headspace Centre Model. *Early Interv. Psychiatry* **13**:159–166. [13]

Rickwood, D. J., N. R. Telford, A. G. Parker, C. J. Tanti, and P. D. McGorry. 2014. Headspace: Australia's Innovation in Youth Mental Health: Who Are the Clients and Why Are They Presenting. *Med. J. Austral.* **200**:108–111. [13, 14]

Rickwood, D. J., M. Webb, V. Kennedy, and N. Telford. 2016. Who Are the Young People Choosing Web-Based Mental Health Support? Findings from the Implementation of Australia's National Web-Based Youth Mental Health Service, Eheadspace. *JMIR Mental Health* **3**:e40. [13]

Rideout, V. J. 2015. The Common Sense Census: Media Use by Tweens and Teens. Common Sense Media Inc. https://www.commonsensemedia.org/sites/default/files/uploads/research/census_researchreport.pdf. (accessed July 22, 2019). [10]

Rittel, H. W. J., and M. M. Webber. 1973. Dilemmas in a General Theory of Planning. *Policy Sci.* **4**:155–169. [12]

Robbe, D., S. M. Montgomery, A. Thome, et al. 2006. Cannabinoids Reveal Importance of Spike Timing Coordination in Hippocampal Function. *Nat. Neurosci.* **9**:1526–1533. [9]

Robillard, R., J. S. Carpenter, N. L. Rogers, et al. 2018. Circadian Rhythms and Psychiatric Profiles in Young Adults with Unipolar Depressive Disorders. *Translational psychiatry* **8**:213. [2]

Robillard, R., D. F. Hermens, R. S. Lee, et al. 2016a. Sleep-Wake Profiles Predict Longitudinal Changes in Manic Symptoms and Memory in Young People with Mood Disorders. *J. Sleep Res.* **25**:549–555. [2]

Robillard, R., D. F. Hermens, S. L. Naismith, et al. 2015. Ambulatory Sleep-Wake Patterns and Variability in Young People with Emerging Mental Disorders. *J. Psychiatr. Neurosci.* **40**:28–37. [2]

Robillard, R., J. Lagopoulos, D. F. Hermens, et al. 2017. Lower *in Vivo* Myo-Inositol in the Anterior Cingulate Cortex Correlates with Delayed Melatonin Rhythms in Young Persons with Depression. *Front. Neurosci.* **11**:336. [2]

Robillard, R., S. L. Naismith, N. L. Rogers, et al. 2013a. Delayed Sleep Phase in Young People with Unipolar or Bipolar Affective Disorders. *J. Affective Disord.* **145**:260–263. [2]

———. 2013b. Sleep-Wake Cycle and Melatonin Rhythms in Adolescents and Young Adults with Mood Disorders: Comparison of Unipolar and Bipolar Phenotypes. *Eur. Psychiatry* **28**:412–416. [2]

Robillard, R., S. L. Naismith, K. L. Smith, et al. 2014. Sleep-Wake Cycle in Young and Older Persons with a Lifetime History of Mood Disorders. *PLoS ONE* **9**:e87763. [2]

Robillard, R., C. Oxley, D. F. Hermens, et al. 2016b. The Relative Contributions of Psychiatric Symptoms and Psychotropic Medications on the Sleep-Wake Profile of Young Persons with Anxiety, Depression and Bipolar Disorders *Psychiatry Res.* **243**:403–406. [2]

Rodriguez, J. M., K. Murphy, C. Stanton, et al. 2015. The Composition of the Gut Microbiota Throughout Life, with an Emphasis on Early Life. *Microb. Ecol. Health Dis.* **26**:26050. [7]

Rosenberg, D. R., and D. A. Lewis. 1995. Postnatal Maturation of the Dopaminergic Innervation of Monkey Prefrontal and Motor Cortices: A Tyrosine Hydroxylase Immunohistochemical Analysis. *J. Compar. Neurol.* **358**:383–400. [7, 9]

Rosenberg, M. D., B. J. Casey, and A. J. Holmes. 2018. Prediction Complements Explanation in Understanding the Developing Brain. *Nat. Commun.* **9**:589. [7]

Rosenheck, R., D. Leslie, K. Sint, et al. 2016. Cost-Effectiveness of Comprehensive, Integrated Care for First Episode Psychosis in the NIMH RAISE Early Treatment Program. *Schizophr. Bull.* **42**:896-906. [11]

Rosenquist, J. N., J. H. Fowler, and N. A. Christakis. 2011. Social Network Determinants of Depression. *Mol. Psychiatr.* **16**:273–281. [6]

Ross, B. M. 2009. Omega-3 Polyunsaturated Fatty Acids and Anxiety Disorders. *PLEFA* **81**:309–312. [10]

Roudi, Y., and E. I. Moser. 2014. Grid Cells in an Inhibitory Network. *Nat. Neurosci.* **17**:639–641. [7]

Rouse, W. 2008. Health Care as a Complex Adaptive System: Implications for Design and Management, vol. 38. Washington, D.C.: National Academy of Engineering. [12]

Rubio, J. M., and C. U. Correll. 2017a. Duration and Relevance of Untreated Psychiatric Disorders, 1: Psychotic Disorders. *J. Clin. Psychiatry* **78**:358–359. [3]

———. 2017b. Duration and Relevance of Untreated Psychiatric Disorders, 2: Nonpsychotic Psychiatric Disorders and Substance Use Disorders. *J. Clin. Psychiatry* **78**:464–465. [3]

Rudolph, K. D., M. E. Miernicki, W. Troop-Gordon, M. M. Davis, and E. H. Telzer. 2016. Adding Insult to Injury: Neural Sensitivity to Social Exclusion Is Associated with Internalizing Symptoms in Chronically Peer-Victimized Girls. *Soc. Cogn. Affect. Neurosci.* **11**:829–842. [6]

Ruhe, H. G., G. van Rooijen, J. Spijker, F. P. Peeters, and A. H. Schene. 2012. Staging Methods for Treatment Resistant Depression. A Systematic Review. *J. Affective Disord.* **137**:35–45. [2]

Russo, S. J., J. W. Murrough, M. H. Han, D. S. Charney, and E. J. Nestler. 2012. Neurobiology of Resilience. *Nat. Neurosci.* **15**:1475–1484. [7]

Russo, S. J., and E. J. Nestler. 2013. The Brain Reward Circuitry in Mood Disorders. *Nature reviews. Neuroscience* **14**:609–625. [7]

Rutter, M. 1999. Resilience Concepts and Findings: Implications for Family Therapy. *J. Fam. Ther.* **21**:119–144. [6]

Rutter, M., and D. J. Smith. 1995. Psychosocial Disorders in Young People: Time Trends and Their Causes. Chichester: John Wiley & Sons. [1]

Ryan, R. M., C. O'Farrelly, and P. Ramchandani. 2017. Parenting and Child Mental Health. *Lond. J. Primary Care* **9**:86–94. [6]

Ryff, C. D., and C. L. M. Keyes. 1995. The Structure of Psychological Well-Being Revisited. *J. Personality Soc. Psychol.* **69**:719–727. [10]

Saks, E. R. 2007. The Center Cannot Hold: My Journey through Madness. New York: Hyperion. [14]

Sami, M. B., and S. Bhattacharyya. 2018. Are Cannabis-Using and Non-Using Patients Different Groups? Towards Understanding the Neurobiology of Cannabis Use in Psychotic Disorders. *J. Psychopharmacol.* **32**:825–849. [7]

Sanislow, C. A. 2016. Updating the Research Domain Criteria. *World Psychiatry* **15**:222–223. [14]

Sawyer, M. G., F. M. Arney, P. A. Baghurst, et al. 2000. The Mental Health of Young People in Australia. Canberra: Commonwealth Department of Health and Aged and Care. Mental Health and Special Programs Branch. [1]

Sawyer, S. M., R. A. Afifi, L. H. Bearinger, et al. 2012. Adolescence: A Foundation for Future Health. *Lancet* **379**:1630–1640. [6]

Schafer, D. P., and B. Stevens. 2010. Synapse Elimination During Development and Disease: Immune Molecules Take Centre Stage. *Biochem. Soc. Trans.* **38**:476–481. [7]

Schifano, F. 2008. Is Urbanization a Risk Factor for Substance Misuse? *Curr. Opin. Psychiatry* **21**:391–397. [6]

Schizophrenia Working Group of the Psychiatric Genomics Consortium. 2014. Biological Insights from 108 Schizophrenia-Associated Genetic Loci. *Nature* **511**:421–427. [8]

Schlögelhofer, M., G. P. Amminger, M. R. Schaefer, et al. 2014. Polyunsaturated Fatty Acids in Emerging Psychosis: A Safer Alternative? *Early Interv. Psychiatry* **8**:199–208. [10]

Schlosser, D. A., S. Jacobson, Q. Chen, et al. 2012. Recovery from an At-Risk State: Clinical and Functional Outcomes of Putatively Prodromal Youth Who Do Not Develop Psychosis. *Schizophr. Bull.* **38**:1225–1233. [11]

Schmidt, S. J., F. Schultze-Lutter, B. G. Schimmelmann, et al. 2015. EPA Guidance on the Early Intervention in Clinical High Risk States of Psychoses. *Eur. Psychiatry* **30**:388–404. [14]

Schroeder, S. A. 2007. Shattuck Lecture. We Can Do Better—Improving the Health of the American People. *New Engl. J. Med.* **357**:1221–1228. [12]

Schultze-Lutter, F., M. Debbane, A. Theodoridou, et al. 2016. Revisiting the Basic Symptom Concept: Toward Translating Risk Symptoms for Psychosis into Neurobiological Targets. *Front. Psychiatry* **7**:9. [1]

Schultze-Lutter, F., C. Michel, S. J. Schmidt, et al. 2015. EPA Guidance on the Early Detection of Clinical High Risk States of Psychoses. *Eur. Psychiatry* **30**:405–416. [11]

Schulz, K. M., and C. L. Sisk. 2016. The Organizing Actions of Adolescent Gonadal Steroid Hormones on Brain and Behavioral Development. *Neurosci. Biobehav. Rev.* **70**:148–158. [4]

Schweitzer, L., and W. H. Su. 1977. Population Density and the Rate of Mental Illness. *Am. J. Public Health* **67**:1165–1172. [6]

Scott, A. J., T. H. Monk, and L. L. Brink. 1997. Shiftwork as a Risk Factor for Depression: A Pilot Study. *Int. J. Occupat. Environ. Health* **3**:S2–S9. [6]

Scott, E. M., D. F. Hermens, N. Glozier, et al. 2012a. Targeted Primary Care-Based Mental Health Services for Young Australians. *Med. J. Austral.* **196**:136–140. [2]

Scott, E. M., D. F. Hermens, S. L. Naismith, et al. 2012b. Thoughts of Death or Suicidal Ideation Are Common in Young People Aged 12 to 30 Years Presenting for Mental Health Care. *BMC Psychiat.* **12**:234. [13]

———. 2013a. Distinguishing Young People with Emerging Bipolar Disorders from Those with Unipolar Depression. *J. Affective Disord.* **144**:208–215. [2]

———. 2013b. Distress and Disability in Young Adults Presenting to Clinical Services with Mood Disorders. *Int. J. Bipolar Disord.* **1**:23. [2]

Scott, E. M., R. Robillard, D. F. Hermens, et al. 2014a. Dysregulated Sleep-Wake Cycles in Young People Are Associated with Emerging Stages of Major Mental Disorders. *Early Interv. Psychiatry* **10**:63–70. [2]

Scott, E. S., N. D. Reppucci, and J. L. Woolard. 1995. Evaluating Adolescent Decision Making in Legal Contexts. *Law and Human Behav.* **19**:221. [11]

Scott, J. 2011. Bipolar Disorder: From Early Identification to Personalized Treatment. *Early Interv. Psychiatry* **5**:89–90. [2]

Scott, J., G. Murray, C. Henry, et al. 2017. Activation in Bipolar Disorders: A Systematic Review. *JAMA Psychiatry* **74**:189–196. [2]

Scott, J., E. Paykel, R. Morriss, et al. 2006. Cognitive-Behavioural Therapy for Severe and Recurrent Bipolar Disorders: Randomised Controlled Trial. *Br. J. Psychiatry* **188**:313–320. [2]

Scott, J., E. M. Scott, D. F. Hermens, et al. 2014b. Functional Impairment in Adolescents and Young Adults with Emerging Mood Disorders. *Br. J. Psychiatry* **205**:362–368. [2]

Scott, R. D. 1973. The Treatment Barrier, Part 2: The Patient as an Unrecognized Agent. *Br. J. Med. Psychol.* **46**:57–67. [14]

Sebastian, C. L., G. C. Tan, J. P. Roiser, et al. 2011. Developmental Influences on the Neural Bases of Responses to Social Rejection: Implications of Social Neuroscience for Education. *Neuroimage* **57**:686–694. [5]

Seeley, W. W., V. Menon, A. F. Schatzberg, et al. 2007. Dissociable Intrinsic Connectivity Networks for Salience Processing and Executive Control. *J. Neurosci.* **27**:2349–2356. [9]

Sekar, A., A. R. Bialas, H. de Rivera, et al. 2016. Schizophrenia Risk from Complex Variation of Complement Component 4. *Nature* **530**:177–183. [7, 8]

Semple, D. M., A. M. McIntosh, and S. M. Lawrie. 2005. Cannabis as a Risk Factor for Psychosis: Systematic Review. *J. Psychopharmacol.* **19**:187–194. [8]

Serhan, C. N., G. Fredman, R. Yang, et al. 2011. Novel Proresolving Aspirin-Triggered DHA Pathway. *Chem. Biol.* **18**:976–987. [10]

Serretti, A., L. Mandelli, E. Bajo, et al. 2009. The Socio-Economical Burden of Schizophrenia: A Simulation of Cost-Offset of Early Intervention Program in Italy. *Eur. Psychiatry* **24**:11–16. [11]

Sesack, S. R., V. A. Hawrylak, D. S. Melchitzky, and D. A. Lewis. 1998. Dopamine Innervation of a Subclass of Local Circuit Neurons in Monkey Prefrontal Cortex: Ultrastructural Analysis of Tyrosine Hydroxylase and Parvalbumin Immunoreactive Structures. *Cereb. Cortex* **8**:614–622. [7]

Shaikh, A., and C. Kauppi. 2010. Deconstructing Resilience: Myriad Conceptualizations and Interpretations. *Int. J. Arts Sci.* **3**:155–176. [5]

Shanafelt, T. D., L. N. Dyrbye, C. Sinsky, et al. 2016. Relationship between Clerical Burden and Characteristics of the Electronic Environment with Physician Burnout and Professional Satisfaction. *Mayo Clin. Proc.* **91**:836–848. [12]

Shaw, P., N. J. Kabani, J. P. Lerch, et al. 2008. Neurodevelopmental Trajectories of the Human Cerebral Cortex. *J. Neurosci.* **28**:3586–3594. [7]

Shelton, R. C., J. Claiborne, M. Sidoryk-Wegrzynowicz, et al. 2011. Altered Expression of Genes Involved in Inflammation and Apoptosis in Frontal Cortex in Major Depression. *Mol. Psychiatr.* **16**:751–762. [7]

Sheridan, M. A., and K. A. McLaughlin. 2014. Dimensions of Early Experience and Neural Development: Deprivation and Threat. *Trends Cogn. Sci.* **18**:580–585. [6]

Shiell, A., P. Hawe, and L. Gold. 2008. Complex Interventions or Complex Systems? Implications for Health Economic Evaluation. *BMJ* **336**:1281–1283. [12]

Shiffman, S. 2009. Ecological Momentary Assessment (EMA) in Studies of Substance Use. *Psychol. Assess.* **21**:486–497. [6]

Shiffman, S., A. A. Stone, and M. R. Hufford. 2008. Ecological Momentary Assessment. *Annu. Rev. Clin. Psych.* **4**:1–32. [10]

Shiina, A., N. Kanahara, T. Sasaki, et al. 2015. An Open Study of Sulforaphane-Rich Broccoli Sprout Extract in Patients with Schizophrenia. *Clin. Psychopharmacol. Neurosci.* **13**:62–67. [9]

Shinde, S., B. Pereira, P. Khandeparkar, et al. 2017. The Development and Pilot Testing of a Multicomponent Health Promotion Intervention (Seher) for Secondary Schools in Bihar, India. *Glob. Health Action* **10**:1385284. [6]

Shonkoff, J. P. 2010. Building a New Biodevelopmental Framework to Guide the Future of Early Childhood Policy. *Child Dev.* **81**:357–367. [6]

Shreiner, A. B., J. Y. Kao, and V. B. Young. 2015. The Gut Microbiome in Health and in Disease. *Curr. Opin. Gastroenterol.* **31**:69–75. [7]

Shrivastava, A., M. Johnston, K. Terpstra, and Y. Bureau. 2014. Cannabis and Psychosis: Neurobiology. *Indian J. Psychiatry* **56**:8–16. [7]

Simmonds, D. J., M. N. Hallquist, M. Asato, and B. Luna. 2014. Developmental Stages and Sex Differences of White Matter and Behavioral Development through Adolescence: A Longitudinal Diffusion Tensor Imaging (DTI) Study. *Neuroimage* **92**:356–368. [9]

Simmonds, D. J., M. N. Hallquist, and B. Luna. 2017. Protracted Development of Executive and Mnemonic Brain Systems Underlying Working Memory in Adolescence: A Longitudinal fMRI Study. *Neuroimage* **157**:695–704. [9]

Simon, A. E., S. Borgwardt, A. Riecher-Rössler, et al. 2013. Moving Beyond Transition Outcomes: Meta-Analysis of Remission Rates in Individuals at High Clinical Risk for Psychosis. *Psychiatry Res.* **209**:266–272. [11]

Simon, A. E., D. Umbricht, U. E. Lang, and S. Borgwardt. 2014. Declining Transition Rates to Psychosis: The Role of Diagnostic Spectra and Symptom Overlaps in Individuals with Attenuated Psychosis Syndrome. *Schizophr. Res.* **159**:292–298. [11]

Simon, A. E., E. Velthorst, D. H. Nieman, et al. 2011. Ultra High-Risk State for Psychosis and Non-Transition: A Systematic Review. *Schizophr. Res.* **132**:8–17. [11]

Simopoulos, A. P. 2011. Evolutionary Aspects of Diet: The Omega-6/Omega-3 Ratio and the Brain. *Mol. Neurobiol.* **44**:203–215. [10]

Singh, S. P. 2009. Transition of Care from Child to Adult Mental Health Services: The Great Divide. *Curr. Opin. Psychiatry* **22**:386. [1]

Sisk, C. L., and D. L. Foster. 2004. The Neural Basis of Puberty and Adolescence. *Nat. Neurosci.* **7**:1040–1047. [7]

Sisk, C. L., and J. L. Zehr. 2005. Pubertal Hormones Organize the Adolescent Brain and Behavior. *Front. Neuroendocrin.* **26**:163–174. [7]

Skene, N. G., J. Bryois, T. E. Bakken, et al. 2018. Genetic Identification of Brain Cell Types Underlying Schizophrenia. *Nat. Genet.* **50**:825–833. [8]

Skosnik, P. D., D. C. D'Souza, A. B. Steinmetz, et al. 2012. The Effect of Chronic Cannabinoids on Broadband EEG Neural Oscillations in Humans. *Neuropsychopharmacology* **37**:2184–2193. [9]

Sliwinski, M. J., J. A. Mogle, J. Hyun, et al. 2018. Reliability and Validity of Ambulatory Cognitive Assessments. *Assessment* **25**:14–30. [5]

Smith, E. A., L.-A. Palen, L. L. Caldwell, et al. 2008. Substance Use and Sexual Risk Prevention in Cape Town, South Africa: An Evaluation of the Healthwise Program. *Prev. Sci.* **9**:311–321. [6]

Smith, K. 2016. 47 Incredible Facebook Statistics and Facts for 2016. Brandwatch. https://www.brandwatch.com/?s=47+Incredible+Facebook+Statistics+and+Facts+for+2016%3A+Brandwatch. (accessed July 22, 2019). [10]

Snijders, T. A. B., G. G. van de Bunt, and C. E. G. Steglich. 2010. Introduction to Stochastic Actor-Based Models for Network Dynamics. *Social Networks* **32**:44–60. [5]

Sohal, V. S., F. Zhang, O. Yizhar, and K. Deisseroth. 2009. Parvalbumin Neurons and Gamma Rhythms Enhance Cortical Circuit Performance. *Nature* **459**:698–702. [9]

Soltesz, E. G., S. Kim, R. G. Laurence, et al. 2005a. Intraoperative Sentinel Lymph Node Mapping of the Lung Using near-Infrared Fluorescent Quantum Dots. *Ann. Thorac. Surg.* **79**:269–277; discussion 269–277. [9]

Soltesz, I. 2005b. Diversity in the Neuronal Machine. New York: Oxford Univ. Press. [7]

Sorg, B. A., S. Berretta, J. M. Blacktop, et al. 2016. Casting a Wide Net: Role of Perineuronal Nets in Neural Plasticity. *J. Neurosci.* **36**:11459–11468. [7]

Sousa, S. S., E. Amaro, Jr., A. Crego, O. F. Goncalves, and A. Sampaio. 2017. Developmental Trajectory of the Prefrontal Cortex: A Systematic Review of Diffusion Tensor Imaging Studies. *Brain Imaging Behav.* **12**:1197–1210. [7]

Sowell, E. R., P. M. Thompson, K. D. Tessner, and A. W. Toga. 2001. Mapping Continued Brain Growth and Gray Matter Density Reduction in Dorsal Frontal Cortex: Inverse Relationships During Postadolescent Brain Maturation. *J. Neurosci.* **21**:8819–8829. [7]

Spadaro, P. A., and T. W. Bredy. 2012. Emerging Role of Non-Coding RNA in Neural Plasticity, Cognitive Function, and Neuropsychiatric Disorders. *Front. Genet.* **3**:132. [8]

Spatazza, J., E. Di Lullo, A. Joliot, et al. 2013a. Homeoprotein Signaling in Development, Health, and Disease: A Shaking of Dogmas Offers Challenges and Promises from Bench to Bed. *Pharmacol. Rev.* **65**:90–104. [7]

Spatazza, J., H. H. Lee, A. A. Di Nardo, et al. 2013b. Choroid-Plexus-Derived Otx2 Homeoprotein Constrains Adult Cortical Plasticity. *Cell Rep.* **3**:1815–1823. [7]

Spear, L. P. 2000. The Adolescent Brain and Age-Related Behavioral Manifestations. *Neurosci. Biobehav. Rev.* **24**:417–463. [9]

Spielberg, J. M., T. M. Olino, E. E. Forbes, and R. E. Dahl. 2014. Exciting Fear in Adolescence: Does Pubertal Development Alter Threat Processing? *Dev. Cogn. Neurosci.* **8**:86–95. [4]

Srihari, V. H., A. Jani, and M. Gray. 2016. Early Intervention for Psychotic Disorders: Building Population Health Systems. *JAMA Psychiatry* **73**:101–102. [12]

Srihari, V. H., J. Shah, and M. S. Keshavan. 2012. Is Early Intervention for Psychosis Feasible and Effective? *Psychiatry Clin. North Am.* **35**:613–631. [12]

Srihari, V. H., C. Tek, J. Pollard, et al. 2014. Reducing the Duration of Untreated Psychosis and Its Impact in the U.S.: The STEP-ED Study. *BMC Psychiat.* **14**:335. [12]

Sroufe, L. A., and M. Rutter. 1984. The Domain of Developmental Psychopathology. *Child Dev.* **55**:17–29. [4]

Stafford, M. R., H. Jackson, E. Mayo-Wilson, A. P. Morrison, and T. Kendall. 2013. Early Interventions to Prevent Psychosis: Systematic Review and Meta-Analysis. *BMJ* **346**:f185–f185. [11]

Stein, J. G. 2002. The Cult of Efficiency. Toronto: House of Anansi Press. [12]

Steinberg, L. 2005. Cognitive and Affective Development in Adolescence. *Trends Cogn. Sci.* **9**:69–74. [4, 9]

Stephan, A. H., B. A. Barres, and B. Stevens. 2012. The Complement System: An Unexpected Role in Synaptic Pruning During Development and Disease. *Annu. Rev. Neurosci.* **35**:369–389. [8]

Stephan, K. E., and C. Mathys. 2014. Computational Approaches to Psychiatry. *Curr Opin. Neurobiol.* **25**:85–92. [6]

Steullet, P., J. H. Cabungcal, S. A. Bukhari, et al. 2017. The Thalamic Reticular Nucleus in Schizophrenia and Bipolar Disorder: Role of Parvalbumin-Expressing Neuron Networks and Oxidative Stress. *Mol. Psychiatr.* **23**:2057–2065. [7]

Steullet, P., J. H. Cabungcal, A. Monin, et al. 2016. Redox Dysregulation, Neuroinflammation, and NMDA Receptor Hypofunction: A "Central Hub" in Schizophrenia Pathophysiology. *Schizophr. Res.* **176**:41–51. [9, 13]

Stice, E., and H. Shaw. 2004. Eating Disorder Prevention Programs: A Meta-Analytic Review. *Psychol. Bull.* **130**:206–227. [4]

Stice, E., H. Shaw, C. Bohon, C. N. Marti, and P. Rohde. 2009. A Meta-Analytic Review of Depression Prevention Programs for Children and Adolescents: Factors That Predict Magnitude of Intervention Effects. *J. Consult. Clin. Psychol.* **77**:486–503. [4]

Stiles, J., and T. L. Jernigan. 2010. The Basics of Brain Development. *Neuropsychol. Rev.* **20**:327–348. [7]

Stockings, E., W. D. Hall, M. Lynskey, et al. 2016. Prevention, Early Intervention, Harm Reduction, and Treatment of Substance Use in Young People. *Lancet Psychiatry* **3**:280–296. [14]

Stone, W. S., and L. J. Seidman. 2016. Neuropsychological and Structural Imaging Endophenotypes in Schizophrenia. In: Developmental Psychopathology, ed. D. Cicchetti, pp. 931–965, vol. 2. Hoboken: John Wiley & Sons, Inc. [8]

Su, K.-P., Y. Matsuoka, and C.-U. Pae. 2015. Omega-3 Polyunsaturated Fatty Acids in Prevention of Mood and Anxiety Disorders. *Clin. Psychopharmacol. Neurosci.* **13**:129–137. [10]

Sublette, M. E., S. P. Ellis, A. L. Geant, and J. J. Mann. 2011. Meta-Analysis of the Effects of Eicosapentaenoic Acid (EPA) in Clinical Trials in Depression. *J. Clin. Psychiatry* **72**:1577–1584. [10]

Sublette, M. E., H. C. Galfalvy, J. R. Hibbeln, et al. 2014. Polyunsaturated Fatty Acid Associations with Dopaminergic Indices in Major Depressive Disorder. *Int. J. Neuropsychopharmacol.* **17**:383–391. [10]

Sublette, M. E., M. J. Russ, and G. S. Smith. 2004. Evidence for a Role of the Arachidonic Acid Cascade in Affective Disorders: A Review. *Bipolar Disord.* **6**:95–105. [10]

Sugiyama, S., A. A. Di Nardo, S. Aizawa, et al. 2008. Experience-Dependent Transfer of Otx2 Homeoprotein into the Visual Cortex Activates Postnatal Plasticity. *Cell* **134**:508–520. [7]

Suleiman, A. B., A. Galván, K. P. Harden, and R. E. Dahl. 2017. Becoming a Sexual Being: The "Elephant in the Room" of Adolescent Brain Development. *Dev. Cogn. Neurosci.* **25**:209–220. [5]

Sullivan, H. S. 1927. The Onset of Schizophrenia. *Am. J. Psychiatry* **84**:105–134. [14]

Sullivan, P. F., M. J. Daly, and M. O'Donovan. 2012. Genetic Architectures of Psychiatric Disorders: The Emerging Picture and Its Implications. *Nat. Rev. Genet.* **13**:537–551. [2]

Sullivan, P. F., K. S. Kendler, and M. C. Neale. 2003. Schizophrenia as a Complex Trait: Evidence from a Meta-Analysis of Twin Studies. *Arch. Gen. Psychiatry* **60**:1187–1192. [8]

Sumiyoshi, T., T. Miyanishi, T. Seo, and Y. Higuchi. 2013. Electrophysiological and Neuropsychological Predictors of Conversion to Schizophrenia in At-Risk Subjects. *Front. Behav. Neurosci.* **7**:148. [2]

Sun, Y., F. K. Mensah, P. Azzopardi, G. C. Patton, and M. Wake. 2017. Childhood Social Disadvantage and Pubertal Timing: A National Birth Cohort from Australia. *Pediatrics* **139**:e20164099. [9]

Supekar, K., M. Musen, and V. Menon. 2009. Development of Large-Scale Functional Brain Networks in Children. *PLoS Biol.* **7**:e1000157. [9]

Swierk, M., P. G. Williams, J. Wilcox, K. G. Russell, and B. J. Meyer. 2011. Validation of an Australian Electronic Food Frequency Questionnaire to Measure Polyunsaturated Fatty Acid Intake. *Nutrition* **27**:641–646. [10]

Syed, S. A., and C. B. Nemeroff. 2017. Early Life Stress, Mood, and Anxiety Disorders. *Chronic Stress* **1**:10.1177/2470547017694461. [7]

Tadokoro, Y., H. Ema, M. Okano, E. Li, and H. Nakauchi. 2007. De Novo DNA Methyltransferase Is Essential for Self-Renewal, but Not for Differentiation, in Hematopoietic Stem Cells. *J. Exp. Med.* **204**:715–722. [8]

Takesian, A. E., and T. K. Hensch. 2013. Balancing Plasticity/Stability across Brain Development. *Prog. Brain Res.* **207**:3–34. [5, 7, 9]

Tamminga, C. A., G. Pearlson, M. Keshavan, et al. 2014. Bipolar and Schizophrenia Network for Intermediate Phenotypes: Outcomes across the Psychosis Continuum. *Schizophr. Bull.* **40 Suppl 2**:S131–137. [8]

Tamnes, C. K., K. B. Walhovd, A. Engvig, et al. 2014. Regional Hippocampal Volumes and Development Predict Learning and Memory. *Dev. Neurosci.* **36**:161–174. [9]

Tanda, G., F. E. Pontieri, and G. Di Chiara. 1997. Cannabinoid and Heroin Activation of Mesolimbic Dopamine Transmission by a Common μ1 Opioid Receptor Mechanism. *Science* **276**:2048–2050. [7]

Tandon, R., M. S. Keshavan, and H. A. Nasrallah. 2008. Schizophrenia, "Just the Facts" What We Know in 2008, 2: Epidemiology and Etiology. *Schizophr. Res.* **102**:1–18. [8]

Tang, J. Y. M., G. H. Y. Wong, C. L. M. Hui, et al. 2010. Early Intervention for Psychosis in Hong Kong: The EASY Programme. *Early Interv. Psychiatry* **4**:214–219. [11]

Tanskanen, A., J. R. Hibbeln, J. Hintikka, et al. 2001. Fish Consumption, Depression, and Suicidality in a General Population. *Arch. Gen. Psychiatry* **58**:512–513. [10]

Tau, G. Z., and B. S. Peterson. 2010. Normal Development of Brain Circuits. *Neuropsychopharmacology* **35**:147–168. [7]

Tay, T. L., C. Bechade, I. D'Andrea, et al. 2017. Microglia Gone Rogue: Impacts on Psychiatric Disorders across the Lifespan. *Front. Mol. Neurosci.* **10**:421. [7]

Tennakoon, L., D. Fannon, V. Doku, et al. 2000. Experience of Caregiving: Relatives of People Experiencing a First Episode of Psychosis. *Br. J. Psychiatry* **177**:529–533. [10]

Tervo-Clemmens, B., D. J. Simmonds, F. J. Calabro, et al. 2018. Early Cannabis Use and Neurocognitive Risk: A prospective Functional Neuroimaging Study. *Biol. Psychiatry Cogn. Neurosci. Neuroimaging* **3**:713–725. [9]

Thesing, C. S., M. Bot, Y. Milaneschi, E. J. Giltay, and B. W. J. H. Penninx. 2018. Omega-3 and Omega-6 Fatty Acid Levels in Depressive and Anxiety Disorders. *Psychoneuroendocrinol.* **87**:53–62. [10]

Thien, K., M. Bowtell, S. Eaton, et al. 2018. Clozapine Use in Early Psychosis. *Schizophr. Res.* **199**:374–379. [14]

Thirthalli, J., and S. Jain. 2009. Better Outcome of Schizophrenia in India: A Natural Selection against Severe Forms? *Schizophr. Bull.* **35**:655–657. [6]

Thornicroft, G. 2011. Physical Health Disparities and Mental Illness: The Scandal of Premature Mortality. *Br. J. Psychiatry* **199**:441–442. [10]

Tickell, A. M., R. S. C. Lee, I. B. Hickie, and D. F. Hermens. 2017. The Course of Neuropsychological Functioning in Young People with Attenuated vs. Discrete Mental Disorders. *Early Interv. Psychiatry* **13(3)**:425–433. [2]

Tienda, M. 1991. Poor People, Poor Places: Deciphering Neighborhood Effects on Poverty Outcomes. In: Macro-Micro Linkages in Sociology, ed. J. Huber, pp. 204–212. Newbury Park, CA: Sage Publ. [5]

Tognini, P. 2017. Gut Microbiota: A Potential Regulator of Neurodevelopment. *Front. Cell. Neurosci.* **11**:25. [7]

Tomlinson, L., C. V. Leiton, and H. Colognato. 2016. Behavioral Experiences as Drivers of Oligodendrocyte Lineage Dynamics and Myelin Plasticity. *Neuropharmacology* **110**:548–562. [7]

Torous, J., G. Andersson, A. Bertagnoli, et al. 2019. Towards a Consensus around Standards for Smartphone Apps and Digital Mental Health. *World Psychiatry* **18**:97. [13]

Torous, J., M. V. Kiang, J. Lorme, J. P. Onnela, and R. Boland. 2016. New Tools for New Research in Psychiatry: A Scalable and Customizable Platform to Empower Data Driven Smartphone Research. *JMIR Mental Health* **3**:e16. [13]

Torous, J., M. E. Larsen, C. Depp, et al. 2018. Smartphones, Sensors, and Machine Learning to Advance Real-Time Prediction and Interventions for Suicide Prevention: A Review of Current Progress and Next Steps. *Curr. Psychiatry Rep.* **20**:51. [3, 10]

Torrey, E. F., J. A. Miller, R. Rawlings, and R. H. Yolken. 1997. Seasonality of Births in Schizophrenia and Bipolar Disorder: A Review of the Literature. *Schizophr. Res.* **28**:1–38. [8]

Torrey, W. C., R. E. Drake, L. Dixon, et al. 2001. Implementing Evidence-Based Practices for Persons with Severe Mental Illnesses. *Psychiatric Serv.* **52**:45–50. [12]

Tosic, M., J. Ott, S. Barral, et al. 2006. Schizophrenia and Oxidative Stress: Glutamate Cysteine Ligase Modifier as a Susceptibility Gene. *Am. J. Hum. Genet.* **79**:586–592. [13]

Tost, H., F. A. Champagne, and A. Meyer-Lindenberg. 2015. Environmental Influence in the Brain, Human Welfare and Mental Health. *Nat. Neurosci.* **18**:1421–1431. [5]

Toyoizumi, T., H. Miyamoto, Y. Yazaki-Sugiyama, et al. 2013. A Theory of the Transition to Critical Period Plasticity: Inhibition Selectively Suppresses Spontaneous Activity. *Neuron* **80**:51–63. [9]

Tremblay, L., and J. Y. Frigon. 2005. Precocious Puberty in Adolescent Girls: A Biomarker of Later Psychosocial Adjustment Problems. *Child Psychiatry Hum. Dev.* **36**:73–94. [9]

Trepanier, M. O., K. E. Hopperton, R. Mizrahi, N. Mechawar, and R. P. Bazinet. 2016. Postmortem Evidence of Cerebral Inflammation in Schizophrenia: A Systematic Review. *Mol. Psychiatr.* **21**:1009–1026. [7]

Tropea, D., G. Kreiman, A. Lyckman, et al. 2006. Gene Expression Changes and Molecular Pathways Mediating Activity-Dependent Plasticity in Visual Cortex. *Nat. Neurosci.* **9**:660–668. [7]

Tseng, K. Y., and P. O'Donnell. 2005. Post-Pubertal Emergence of Prefrontal Cortical up States Induced by D1-NMDA Co-Activation. *Cereb. Cortex* **15**:49–57. [9]

———. 2007. Dopamine Modulation of Prefrontal Cortical Interneurons Changes During Adolescence. *Cereb. Cortex* **17**:1235–1240. [7, 9]

Tsuang, M. T. 1975. Heterogeneity of Schizophrenia. *Biol. Psychiatry* **10**:465–474. [8]

Tsuang, M. T., S. V. Faraone, and S. J. Glatt. 2011. Schizophrenia. Oxford: Oxford Univ. Press. [8]

Tukker, J. J., P. Fuentealba, K. Hartwich, P. Somogyi, and T. Klausberger. 2007. Cell Type-Specific Tuning of Hippocampal Interneuron Firing During Gamma Oscillations *in Vivo*. *J. Neurosci.* **27**:8184–8189. [9]

Uchida, Y., and S. Kitayama. 2009. Happiness and Unhappiness in East and West: Themes and Variations. *Emotion* **9**:441–456. [6]

Ueno, M., Y. Fujita, T. Tanaka, et al. 2013. Layer V Cortical Neurons Require Microglial Support for Survival During Postnatal Development. *Nat. Neurosci.* **16**:543–551. [7]

Uher, R., and A. Zwicker. 2017. Etiology in Psychiatry: Embracing the Reality of Poly-Gene-Environmental Causation of Mental Illness. *World Psychiatry* **16**:121–129. [6]

Uhlhaas, P. J. 2013. Dysconnectivity, Large-Scale Networks and Neuronal Dynamics in Schizophrenia. *Curr Opin. Neurobiol.* **23**:283–290. [7]

Uhlhaas, P. J., F. Roux, E. Rodriguez, A. Rotarska-Jagiela, and W. Singer. 2010. Neural Synchrony and the Development of Cortical Networks. *Trends Cogn. Sci.* **14**:72–80. [7]

Uhlhaas, P. J., F. Roux, W. Singer, et al. 2009. The Development of Neural Synchrony Reflects Late Maturation and Restructuring of Functional Networks in Humans. *PNAS* **106**:9866–9871. [7]

Uhlhaas, P. J., and W. Singer. 2015. Oscillations and Neuronal Dynamics in Schizophrenia: The Search for Basic Symptoms and Translational Opportunities. *Biol. Psychiatry* **77**:1001–1009. [7]

UN. 2003. World Youth Report, Chapter 7: Juvenile Delinquency. New York: United Nations. https://www.un.org/esa/socdev/unyin/documents/ch07.pdf. (accessed Sept. 26, 2018). [5]

Ungar, M., M. Ghazinour, and J. Richter. 2013. Annual Research Review: What Is Resilience within the Social Ecology of Human Development? *J. Child Psychol. Psychiatry* **54**:348–366. [5]

Unguru, Y. 2011. The Successful Integration of Research and Care: How Pediatric Oncology Became the Subspecialty in Which Research Defines the Standard of Care. *Pediatr. Blood Cancer* **56**:1019–1025. [12]

Vafadari, B., A. Salamian, and L. Kaczmarek. 2016. MMP-9 in Translation: From Molecule to Brain Physiology, Pathology, and Therapy. *J. Neurochem.* **139(Suppl 2)**:91–114. [7]

Valipour, G., P. Saneei, and A. Esmaillzadeh. 2014. Serum Vitamin D Levels in Relation to Schizophrenia: A Systematic Review and Meta-Analysis of Observational Studies. *J. Clin. Endocrinol. Metab.* **99**:3863–3872. [8]

Valmaggia, L. R., P. McCrone, M. Knapp, et al. 2009. Economic Impact of Early Intervention in People at High Risk of Psychosis. *Psychol. Med.* **39**:1617–1626. [11]

Valmaggia, L. R., D. Stahl, A. R. Yung, et al. 2013. Negative Psychotic Symptoms and Impaired Role Functioning Predict Transition Outcomes in the At-Risk Mental State: A Latent Class Cluster Analysis Study. *Psychol. Med.* **43**:2311–2325. [2]

van der Gaag, M., F. Smit, A. Bechdolf, et al. 2013. Preventing a First Episode of Psychosis: Meta-Analysis of Randomized Controlled Prevention Trials of 12 Month and Longer-Term Follow-Ups. *Schizophr. Res.* **149**:56–62. [14]

van der Gaag, M., D. van den Berg, and H. Ising. 2019. CBT in the Prevention of Psychosis and Other Severe Mental Disorders in Patients with an At-Risk Mental State: A Review and Proposed Next Steps. *Schizophr. Res.* **203**:88–93. [14]

van Diessen, E., J. Senders, F. E. Jansen, M. Boersma, and H. Bruining. 2015. Increased Power of Resting-State Gamma Oscillations in Autism Spectrum Disorder Detected by Routine Electroencephalography. *Eur. Arch. Psychiatry Clin. Neurosci.* **265**:537–540. [7]

van Harmelen, A.-L., R. A. Kievit, K. Ioannidis, et al. 2017. Adolescent Friendships Predict Later Resilient Functioning across Psychosocial Domains in a Healthy Community Cohort. *Psychol. Med.* **47**:2312–2322. [6]

Van Leijenhorst, L., K. Zanolie, C. S. Van Meel, et al. 2010. What Motivates the Adolescent? Brain Regions Mediating Reward Sensitivity across Adolescence. *Cereb. Cortex* **20**:61–69. [9]

van Os, J., and S. Guloksuz. 2017. A Critique of the "Ultra-High Risk" and "Transition" Paradigm. *World Psychiatry* **16**:200–206. [14]

van Os, J., R. J. Linscott, I. Myin-Germeys, P. Delespaul, and L. Krabbendam. 2009. A Systematic Review and Meta-Analysis of the Psychosis Continuum: Evidence for a Psychosis Proneness–Persistence–Impairment Model of Psychotic Disorder. *Psychol. Med.* **39**:179–195. [14]

van Os, J., B. P. Rutten, and R. Poulton. 2008. Gene-Environment Interactions in Schizophrenia: Review of Epidemiological Findings and Future Directions. *Schizophr. Bull.* **34**:1066–1082. [8]

Van Son, G. E., D. Van Hoeken, A. I. M. Bartelds, E. F. Van Furth, and H. W. Hoek. 2006. Urbanisation and the Incidence of Eating Disorders. *Br. J. Psychiatry* **189**:562–563. [6]

Vassos, E., C. B. Pedersen, R. M. Murray, D. A. Collier, and C. M. Lewis. 2012. Meta-Analysis of the Association of Urbanicity with Schizophrenia. *Schizophr. Bull.* **38**:1118–1123. [6]

Veling, W., H. W. Hoek, and J. P. Mackenbach. 2008. Perceived Discrimination and the Risk of Schizophrenia in Ethnic Minorities: A Case-Control Study. *Soc. Psychiatr. Psychiatric Epidemiol.* **43**:953–959. [8]

Venna, V. R., D. Deplanque, C. Allet, et al. 2009. PUFA Induce Antidepressant-Like Effects in Parallel to Structural and Molecular Changes in the Hippocampus. *Psychoneuroendocrinol.* **34**:199–211. [10]

Verduijn, J., Y. Milaneschi, A. M. van Hemert, et al. 2015. Clinical Staging of Major Depressive Disorder: An Empirical Exploration. *J. Clin. Psychiatry* **76**:1200–1208. [2]

Verrico, C. D., H. Gu, M. L. Peterson, A. R. Sampson, and D. A. Lewis. 2014. Repeated Δ9-Tetrahydrocannabinol Exposure in Adolescent Monkeys: Persistent Effects Selective for Spatial Working Memory. *Am. J. Psychiatry* **171**:416–425. [9]

Vertes, P. E., and E. T. Bullmore. 2015. Annual Research Review: Growth Connectomics: The Organization and Reorganization of Brain Networks During Normal and Abnormal Development. *J. Child Psychol. Psychiatry Allied Discipl.* **56**:299–320. [4]

Vigil, P., J. P. Del Rio, B. Carrera, et al. 2016. Influence of Sex Steroid Hormones on the Adolescent Brain and Behavior: An Update. *Linacre Q.* **83**:308–329. [7]

Vlahovic, T. A., S. Roberts, and R. Dunbar. 2012. Effects of Duration and Laughter on Subjective Happiness within Different Modes of Communication: Happiness and Mode of Communication. *J. Comp.-Mediat. Commun.* **17**:436–450. [6]

Vogeley, K., and A. Roepstorff. 2009. Contextualising Culture and Social Cognition. *Trends Cogn. Sci.* **13**:511–516. [6]

von Schacky, C. 2009. Cardiovascular Disease Prevention and Treatment. *PLEFA* **81**:193–198. [10]

Vos, T., A. D. Flaxman, M. Naghavi, et al. 2012. Years Lived with Disability (YLDS) for 1160 Sequelae of 289 Diseases and Injuries 1990–2010: A Systematic Analysis for the Global Burden of Disease Study 2010. *Lancet* **380**:2163–2196. [3]

Vuillermot, S., L. Weber, J. Feldon, and U. Meyer. 2010. A Longitudinal Examination of the Neurodevelopmental Impact of Prenatal Immune Activation in Mice Reveals Primary Defects in Dopaminergic Development Relevant to Schizophrenia. *J. Neurosci.* **30**:1270–1287. [7]

Wahlstrom, D., T. White, and M. Luciana. 2010. Neurobehavioral Evidence for Changes in Dopamine System Activity During Adolescence. *Neurosci. Biobehav. Rev.* **34**:631–648. [7]

Wamsley, E. J., M. A. Tucker, A. K. Shinn, et al. 2012. Reduced Sleep Spindles and Spindle Coherence in Schizophrenia: Mechanisms of Impaired Memory Consolidation? *Biol. Psychiatry* **71**:154–161. [8]

Wang, D., and J. Fawcett. 2012. The Perineuronal Net and the Control of CNS Plasticity. *Cell Tissue Res.* **349**:147–160. [7]

Wang, H. X., and W. J. Gao. 2009. Cell Type-Specific Development of NMDA Receptors in the Interneurons of Rat Prefrontal Cortex. *Neuropsychopharmacology* **34**:2028–2040. [7]

Wang, R., D. Xue, Y. Liu, H. Chen, and Y. Qiu. 2018. The Relationship between Urbanization and Depression in China: The Mediating Role of Neighborhood Social Capital. *Int. J. Equity Health* **17**:105. [6]

Wang, X. J. 1999. Synaptic Basis of Cortical Persistent Activity: The Importance of NMDA Receptors to Working Memory. *J. Neurosci.* **19**:9587–9603. [7]

———. 2001. Synaptic Reverberation Underlying Mnemonic Persistent Activity. *Trends Neurosci.* **24**:455–463. [7]

———. 2002. Probabilistic Decision Making by Slow Reverberation in Cortical Circuits. *Neuron* **36**:955–968. [7]

Wang, X. J., and G. Buzsáki. 1996. Gamma Oscillation by Synaptic Inhibition in a Hippocampal Interneuronal Network Model. *J. Neurosci.* **16**:6402–6413. [9]

Wasser, T., J. Pollard, D. Fisk, and V. Srihari. 2017. First-Episode Psychosis and the Criminal Justice System: Using a Sequential Intercept Framework to Highlight Risks and Opportunities. *Psychiatr. Serv.* **68**:994–996. [12]

Wasserman, S., and K. Faust. 1994. Social Network Analysis: Methods and Applications. Structural Analysis in the Social Sciences. Cambridge: Cambridge Univ. Press. [6]

Waszczuk, M. A., H. M. Zavos, A. M. Gregory, and T. C. Eley. 2014. The Phenotypic and Genetic Structure of Depression and Anxiety Disorder Symptoms in Childhood, Adolescence, and Young Adulthood. *JAMA Psychiatry* **71**:905–916. [2]

Webster, M. J., C. S. Weickert, M. M. Herman, and J. E. Kleinman. 2002. BDNF mRNA Expression During Postnatal Development, Maturation and Aging of the Human Prefrontal Cortex. *Brain Res. Dev. Brain Res.* **139**:139–150. [7]

Wegner, L., A. J. Flisher, L. L. Caldwell, T. Vergnani, and E. A. Smith. 2007. Healthwise South Africa: Cultural Adaptation of a School-Based Risk Prevention Programme. *Health Educ. Res.* **23**:1085–1096. [6]

Weich, S., and G. Lewis. 1998. Poverty, Unemployment, and Common Mental Disorders: Population Based Cohort Study. *BMJ* **317**:115–119. [6]

Weil, M. T., W. Mobius, A. Winkler, et al. 2016. Loss of Myelin Basic Protein Function Triggers Myelin Breakdown in Models of Demyelinating Diseases. *Cell Rep.* **16**:314–322. [7]

Weinberger, D. R. 1987. Implications of Normal Brain Development for the Pathogenesis of Schizophrenia. *Arch. Gen. Psychiatry* **44**:660–669. [7]

Weinstein, N., H. S. Hodgins, and R. M. Ryan. 2010. Autonomy and Control in Dyads: Effects on Interaction Quality and Joint Creative Performance. *Personal. Soc. Psychol. Bull.* **36**:1603–1617. [6]

Welsh, P., and S. Brown. 2013. "I'm Not Insane, My Mother Had Me Tested": The Risk and Benefits of Being Labelled "At-Risk" for Psychosis. *Health Risk Soc.* **15**:648–662. [11]

Wen, T. H., S. Afroz, S. M. Reinhard, et al. 2017. Genetic Reduction of Matrix Metalloproteinase-9 Promotes Formation of Perineuronal Nets around Parvalbumin-Expressing Interneurons and Normalizes Auditory Cortex Responses in Developing Fmr1 Knock-out Mice. *Cereb. Cortex* **28**:3951–3964. [7]

Werker, J. F., and T. K. Hensch. 2015. Critical Periods in Speech Perception: New Directions. *Annu. Rev. Psychol.* **66**:173–196. [3–5]

Whittle, S., N. Vijayakumar, J. G. Simmons, et al. 2017. Role of Positive Parenting in the Association between Neighborhood Social Disadvantage and Brain Development across Adolescence. *JAMA Psychiatry* **74**:824-832. [3]

WHO. 2012. Risks to Mental Health: An Overview of Vulnerabilities and Risk Factors. Background Paper by Who Secretariat for the Development of a Comprehensive Mental Health Action Plan, Aug. 27, 2012. Geneva: World Health Organization. [5]

———. 2014. Health for the World's Adolescents: A Second Chance in the Second Decade. Geneva: World Health Organization. [3]

Wicks, S., A. Hjern, D. Gunnell, G. Lewis, and C. Dalman. 2005. Social Adversity in Childhood and the Risk of Developing Psychosis: A National Cohort Study. *Am. J. Psychiatry* **162**:1652–1657. [8]

Wild, C. P. 2005. Complementing the Genome with an "Exposome": The Outstanding Challenge of Environmental Exposure Measurement in Molecular Epidemiology. *Cancer Epidemiol. Biomarkers Prev.* **14**:1847–1850. [6]

Will, G.-J., P. A. C. van Lier, E. A. Crone, and B. Güroğlu. 2016. Chronic Childhood Peer Rejection Is Associated with Heightened Neural Responses to Social Exclusion During Adolescence. *J. Abnorm. Child Psycholog.* **44**:43–55. [6]

Williams, B. L., M. Hornig, T. Parekh, and W. I. Lipkin. 2012. Application of Novel PCR-Based Methods for Detection, Quantitation, and Phylogenetic Characterization of Sutterella Species in Intestinal Biopsy Samples from Children with Autism and Gastrointestinal Disturbances. *MBio* **3**:e00261-00211. [7]

Williams, G. V., and S. A. Castner. 2006. Under the Curve: Critical Issues for Elucidating D1 Receptor Function in Working Memory. *Neuroscience* **139**:263–276. [7]

Williamson, L. L., P. W. Sholar, R. S. Mistry, S. H. Smith, and S. D. Bilbo. 2011. Microglia and Memory: Modulation by Early-Life Infection. *J. Neurosci.* **31**:15511–15521. [7]

Wisdom, J. P., and C. A. Green. 2004. "Being in a Funk": Teens' Efforts to Understand Their Depressive Experiences. *Qual. Health Res.* **14**:1227–1238. [11]

Woelbert, E., A. Kirtley, N. Balmer, and S. Dix. 2019. How Much Is Spent on Mental Health Research: Developing a System for Categorising Grant Funding in the UK. *Lancet Psychiatry* **6**:445–452. [1]

Wohlwill, J. F. 1970. The Age Variable in Psychological Research. *Psychol. Rev.* **77**:49–64. [4]

Wolfer, R., K. S. Cortina, and J. Baumert. 2012. Embeddedness and Empathy: How the Social Network Shapes Adolescents' Social Understanding. *J. Adolesc.* **35**:1295–1305. [5]

Wolke, D., and S. T. Lereya. 2015. Long-Term Effects of Bullying. *Arch. Dis. Child.* **100**:879–885. [6]

Wong, G. H. Y., C. L. M. Hui, C. P. Y. Chiu, et al. 2008. Early Detection and Intervention of Psychosis in Hong Kong: Experience of a Population-Based Intervention Programme. *Clin. Neuropsychiatry* **5**:286–289. [11]

Wong, K. K., S. K. W. Chan, M. M. L. Lam, et al. 2011. Cost-Effectiveness of an Early Assessment Service for Young People with Early Psychosis in Hong Kong. *Aust. N. Z. J. Psychiatry* **45**:673–680. [11]

Woo, T.-U. W., and A. L. Crowell. 2005. Targeting Synapses and Myelin in the Prevention of Schizophrenia. *Schizophr. Res.* **73**:193–207. [7]

Woo, T.-U. W., M. L. Pucak, C. H. Kye, C. V. Matus, and D. A. Lewis. 1997. Peripubertal Refinement of the Intrinsic and Associational Circuitry in Monkey Prefrontal Cortex. *Neuroscience* **80**:1149–1158. [7]

Woo, T.-U. W., K. Spencer, and R. W. McCarley. 2010. Gamma Oscillation Deficits and the Onset and Early Progression of Schizophrenia. *Harvard Rev. Psychiatry* **18**:173–189. [7]

Woo, T.-U. W., J. P. Walsh, and F. M. Benes. 2004. Density of Glutamic Acid Decarboxylase 67 Messenger RNA-Containing Neurons That Express the N-Methyl-D-Aspartate Receptor Subunit NR2A in the Anterior Cingulate Cortex in Schizophrenia and Bipolar Disorder. *Arch. Gen. Psychiatry* **61**:649–657. [7]

Woodberry, K. A., D. I. Shapiro, C. Bryant, and L. J. Seidman. 2016. Progress and Future Directions in Research on the Psychosis Prodrome: A Review for Clinicians. *Harvard Rev. Psychiatry* **24**:87–103. [11]

Wyatt, R. J. 1991. Neuroleptics and the Natural Course of Schizophrenia. *Schizophr. Bull.* **17**:325–351. [14]

Xanthos, D. N., and J. Sandkuhler. 2014. Neurogenic Neuroinflammation: Inflammatory CNS Reactions in Response to Neuronal Activity. *Nature reviews. Neuroscience* **15**:43–53. [7]

Xia, C. H., Z. Ma, R. Ciric, et al. 2018. Linked Dimensions of Psychopathology and Connectivity in Functional Brain Networks. *Nat. Commun.* **9**:3003. [9]

Xin, L., R. Mekle, M. Fournier, et al. 2016. Genetic Polymorphism Associated Prefrontal Glutathione and Its Coupling with Brain Glutamate and Peripheral Redox Status in Early Psychosis. *Schizophr. Bull.* **42**:1185–1196. [13]

Yakovlev, P. I., and A.-R. Lecours. 1967. The Myelogenetic Cycles of Regional Maturation of the Brain. In: Regional Development of the Brain in Early Life, ed. A. Minkowski, pp. 3–70. Oxford: Blackwell Scientific. [9]

Yamaguchi, S., M. Mizuno, Y. Ojio, et al. 2017. Associations between Renaming Schizophrenia and Stigma-Related Outcomes: A Systematic Review. *Psychiatry Clin. Neurosci.* **71**:347–362. [11]

Yang, L. H., D. A. Anglin, A. J. Wonpat-Borja, et al. 2013. Public Stigma of the Psychosis Risk Syndrome in a College Population: Implications for Peer Stigma Intervention. *Psychiatric Serv.* **64**:284–288. [11]

Yang, L. H., and A. Kleinman. 2008. "Face" and the Embodiment of Stigma in China: The Cases of Schizophrenia and Aids. *Soc. Sci. Med.* **67**:398–408. [11]

Yang, L. H., A. Kleinman, B. G. Link, et al. 2007. Culture and Stigma: Adding Moral Experience to Stigma Theory. *Soc. Sci. Med.* **64**:1524–1535. [11]

Yang, L. H., B. G. Link, S. Ben-David, et al. 2015. Stigma Related to Labels and Symptoms in Individuals at Clinical High-Risk for Psychosis. *Schizophr. Res.* **168**:9–15. [11]

Yang, L. H., K. A. Woodberry, B. G. Link, et al. In review. Impact of Psychosis Risk Identification: A Multisite Study. *Schizophr. Res.* [11]

Yolken, R. H., E. G. Severance, S. Sabunciyan, et al. 2015. Metagenomic Sequencing Indicates That the Oropharyngeal Phageome of Individuals with Schizophrenia Differs from That of Controls. *Schizophr. Bull.* **41**:1153–1161. [7]

Yung, A. R., and P. D. McGorry. 1996. The Prodromal Phase of First-Episode Psychosis: Past and Current Conceptualizations. *Schizophr. Bull.* **22**:353–370. [11, 14]

Yung, A. R., P. D. McGorry, C. A. McFarlane, et al. 2004. Monitoring and Care of Young People at Incipient Risk of Psychosis. *Focus* [11]

Yung, A. R., P. D. McGorry, C. A. McFarlane, and G. C. Patton. 1995. The PACE Clinic: Development of a Clinical Service for Young People at High Risk of Psychosis. *Australas. Psychiatry* **3**:345–349. [11, 14]

Yung, A. R., B. Nelson, C. Stanford, et al. 2008. Validation of "Prodromal" Criteria to Detect Individuals at Ultra High Risk of Psychosis: 2 Year Follow-Up. *Schizophr. Res.* **105**:10–17. [11]

Yung, A. R., S. W. Woods, S. Ruhrmann, et al. 2012. Whither the Attenuated Psychosis Syndrome? *Schizophr. Bull.* **38**:1130–1134. [1]

Yung, A. R., H. P. Yuen, G. Berger, et al. 2007. Declining Transition Rate in Ultra High Risk (Prodromal) Services: Dilution or Reduction of Risk? *Schizophr. Bull.* **33**:673–681. [11]

Yung, A. R., H. P. Yuen, P. D. McGorry, et al. 2005. Mapping the Onset of Psychosis: The Comprehensive Assessment of At-Risk Mental States. *Aust. N. Z. J. Psychiatry* **39**:964–971. [11]

Zai, C. C., A. K. Tiwari, G. C. Zai, M. S. Maes, and J. L. Kennedy. 2018. New Findings in Pharmacogenetics of Schizophrenia. *Curr. Opin. Psychiatry* **31**:200–212. [8]

Zeevi, D., T. Korem, and E. Segal. 2016. Talking About Cross-Talk: The Immune System and the Microbiome. *Genome Biol.* **17**:50. [7]

Zhang, B., B. Suarez-Jimenez, A. Hathaway, et al. 2012. Developmental Changes of Rhesus Monkeys in Response to Separation from the Mother. *Dev. Psychobiol.* **54**:798–807. [5]

Zhang, C., C. W. Phang, X. Zeng, et al. 2015. Circadian Rhythms in Socializing Propensity. *PLoS ONE* **10**:e0136325. [6]

Zheng, Y. 2013. Comparative Studies on Survey Sampling Bias in Cross-Cultural Social Research, 59th ISI World Statistics Congress, Hong Kong. http://2013.isiproceedings.org/Files/CPS015-P3-S.pdf. (accessed Sept. 26, 2018). [5]

Ziermans, T. B., P. F. Schothorst, H. G. Schnack, et al. 2010. Progressive Structural Brain Changes During Development of Psychosis. *Schizophr. Bull.* **38**:519–530. [11]

Subject Index

Strüngmann Forum Report Series*

The Neocortex
Edited by Wolf Singer, Terrence J. Sejnowski and Pasko Rakic
ISBN: 9780262043243

Interactive Task Learning: Humans, Robots, and Agents Acquiring New Tasks through Natural Interactions
Edited by Kevin A. Gluck and John E. Laird, ISBN: 9780262038829

Agrobiodiversity: Integrating Knowledge for a Sustainable Future
Edited by Karl S. Zimmerer and Stef de Haan
ISBN: 9780262038683

Rethinking Environmentalism: Linking Justice, Sustainability, and Diversity
Edited by Sharachchandra Lele, Eduardo S. Brondizio, John Byrne, Georgina M. Mace and Joan Martinez-Alier
ISBN: 9780262038966

Emergent Brain Dynamics: Prebirth to Adolescence
Edited by April A. Benasich and Urs Ribary
ISBN: 9780262038638

The Cultural Nature of Attachment: Contextualizing Relationships and Development
Edited by Heidi Keller and Kim A. Bard
Hardcover: ISBN: 9780262036900, ebook: ISBN: 9780262342865
Winner of the Ursula Gielen Global Psychology Book Award

Investors and Exploiters in Ecology and Economics: Principles and Applications
edited by Luc-Alain Giraldeau, Philipp Heeb and Michael Kosfeld
Hardcover: ISBN: 9780262036122, eBook: ISBN: 9780262339797

Computational Psychiatry: New Perspectives on Mental Illness
edited by A. David Redish and Joshua A. Gordon, ISBN: 9780262035422

Complexity and Evolution: Toward a New Synthesis for Economics
edited by David S. Wilson and Alan Kirman, ISBN: 9780262035385

The Pragmatic Turn: Toward Action-Oriented Views in Cognitive Science
edited by Andreas K. Engel, Karl J. Friston and Danica Kragic
ISBN: 978-0-262-03432-6

Translational Neuroscience: Toward New Therapies
edited by Karoly Nikolich and Steven E. Hyman, ISBN: 9780262029865

Trace Metals and Infectious Diseases
edited by Jerome O. Nriagu and Eric P. Skaar, ISBN 978-0-262-02919-3

Rethinking Global Land Use in an Urban Era
edited by Karen C. Seto and Anette Reenberg, ISBN 978-0-262-02690-1

* Available at https://mitpress.mit.edu/books/series/strungmann-forum-reports

Schizophrenia: Evolution and Synthesis
edited by Steven M. Silverstein, Bita Moghaddam and Til Wykes, ISBN 978-0-262-01962-0

Cultural Evolution: Society, Technology, Language, and Religion
edited by Peter J. Richerson and Morten H. Christiansen, ISBN 978-0-262-01975-0

Language, Music, and the Brain: A Mysterious Relationship
edited by Michael A. Arbib, ISBN 978-0-262-01962-0

Evolution and the Mechanisms of Decision Making
edited by Peter Hammerstein and Jeffrey R. Stevens, ISBN 978-0-262-01808-1

Cognitive Search: Evolution, Algorithms, and the Brain
edited by Peter M. Todd, Thomas T. Hills and Trevor W. Robbins, ISBN 978-0-262-01809-8

Animal Thinking: Contemporary Issues in Comparative Cognition
edited by Randolf Menzel and Julia Fischer, ISBN 978-0-262-01663-6

Disease Eradication in the 21st Century: Implications for Global Health
edited by Stephen L. Cochi and Walter R. Dowdle, ISBN 978-0-262-01673-5

Dynamic Coordination in the Brain: From Neurons to Mind
edited by Christoph von der Malsburg, William A. Phillips and Wolf Singer, ISBN 978-0-262-01471-7

Linkages of Sustainability
edited by Thomas E. Graedel and Ester van der Voet, ISBN 978-0-262-01358-1

Biological Foundations and Origin of Syntax
edited by Derek Bickerton and Eörs Szathmáry, ISBN 978-0-262-01356-7

Clouds in the Perturbed Climate System: Their Relationship to Energy Balance, Atmospheric Dynamics, and Precipitation
edited by Jost Heintzenberg and Robert J. Charlson, ISBN 978-0-262-01287-4
Winner of the Atmospheric Science Librarians International Choice Award

Better Than Conscious? Decision Making, the Human Mind, and Implications For Institutions
edited by Christoph Engel and Wolf Singer, ISBN 978-0-262-19580-5